STRENGTH OF MATERIALS

AUTHOR (S)

Dr. Uday Shanker Dixit
Professor, Department of Mechanical Engineering, Indian Institute of Technology Guwahati, Guwahati-781039, Assam, India

Dr. Nelson Muthu
Assistant Professor, Department of Mechanical Engineering, Indian Institute of Technology Guwahati, Guwahati-781039, Assam, India

Dr. S.M. Kamal
Assistant Professor, Department of Mechanical Engineering, Tezpur University, Tezpur-784028, Assam, India

REVIEWER

Dr. S.P. Harsha
Professor, Department of Mechanical and Industrial Engineering, Indian Institute of Technology Roorkee, Roorkee-247667, Uttarakhand, India

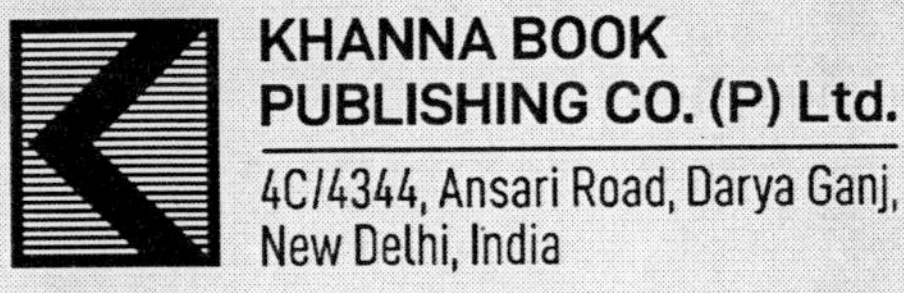

KHANNA BOOK PUBLISHING CO. (P) Ltd.
4C/4344, Ansari Road, Darya Ganj, New Delhi, India

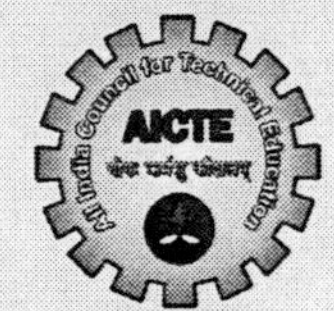

All India Council for Technical Education
Nelson Mandela Marg, Vasant Kunj, New Delhi, India

Dear Readers,

To prevent the piracy, this book is secured with HIGH SECURITY HOLOGRAM on the front title cover. In case you don't find the hologram on the front cover title, please write us to at contact@khannabooks.com or whatsapp us at +91-99109 09320 and avail special gift voucher for yourself.

Specimen of Hologram on front Cover title:

Moreover, there is a SPECIAL DISCOUNT COUPON for you with EVERY HOLOGRAM.

How to avail this SPECIAL DISCOUNT:

Step 1: Scratch the hologram

Step 2: Under the scratch area, your "coupon code" is available

Step 3: Logon to www.khannabooks.com

Step 4: Use your "coupon code" in the shopping cart and get your copy at a special discount

Step 5: Enjoy your reading!

ISBN: 978-93-5538-602-1

Book Code: UG423EN

Strength Of Materials

by Dr. Uday Shanker Dixit, Dr. Nelson Muthu and Dr. S.M. Kamal

First Edition: 2026

Originally Published by:
All India Council for Technical Education, Ministry of Education, GOI

Exclusively Published & Distributed by:
Khanna Book Publishing Co. (P) Ltd.
4C/4344, Ansari Road, Daryaganj,
New Delhi (INDIA)

Visit us at: **www.khannabooks.com**
Write us at: **contact@khannabooks.com**

To view complete list of books, Please scan the QR Code:

Printed in Bharat.

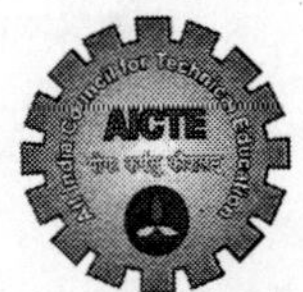

प्रो. टी. जी. सीताराम

अध्यक्ष

Prof. T. G. Sitharam

Chairman

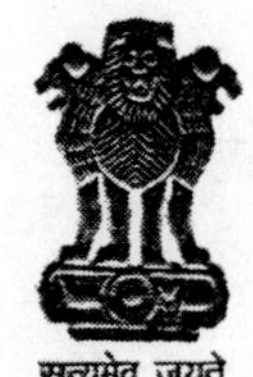

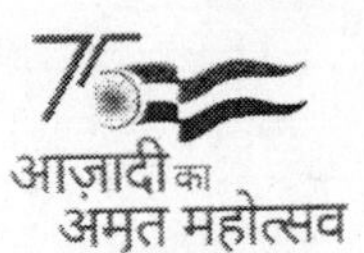

अखिल भारतीय तकनीकी शिक्षा परिषद्

(भारत सरकार का एक सांविधिक निकाय)

(शिक्षा मंत्रालय, भारत सरकार)

नेल्सन मंडेला मार्ग, वसंत कुंज, नई दिल्ली–110070

दूरभाष : 011–26131498

ई–मेल : chairman@aicte-india.org

ALL INDIA COUNCIL FOR TECHNICAL EDUCATION

(A STATUTORY BODY OF THE GOVT. OF INDIA)

(Ministry of Education, Govt. of India)

Nelson Mandela Marg, Vasant Kunj, New Delhi-110070

Phone : 011-26131498

E-mail : chairman@aicte-india.org

FOREWORD

Engineers are the backbone of any modern society. They are the ones responsible for the marvels as well as the improved quality of life across the world. Engineers have driven humanity towards greater heights in a more evolved and unprecedented manner.

The All India Council for Technical Education (AICTE), have spared no efforts towards the strengthening of the technical education in the country. AICTE is always committed towards promoting quality Technical Education to make India a modern developed nation emphasizing on the overall welfare of mankind.

An array of initiatives has been taken by AICTE in last decade which have been accelerated now by the National Education Policy (NEP) 2020. The implementation of NEP under the visionary leadership of Hon'ble Prime Minister of India envisages the provision for education in regional languages to all, thereby ensuring that every graduate becomes competent enough and is in a position to contribute towards the national growth and development through innovation & entrepreneurship.

One of the spheres where AICTE had been relentlessly working since past couple of years is providing high quality original technical contents at Under Graduate & Diploma level prepared and translated by eminent educators in various Indian languages to its aspirants. For students pursuing 2nd year of their Engineering education, AICTE has identified 87 books, which shall be translated into 12 Indian languages - Hindi, Tamil, Gujarati, Odia, Bengali, Kannada, Urdu, Punjabi, Telugu, Marathi, Assamese & Malayalam. In addition to the English medium, books in different Indian Languages are going to support the students to understand the concepts in their respective mother tongue.

On behalf of AICTE, I express sincere gratitude to all distinguished authors, reviewers and translators from the renowned institutions of high repute for their admirable contribution in a record span of time.

AICTE is confident that these outcomes based original contents shall help aspirants to master the subject with comprehension and greater ease.

T. G. Sitharam

(Prof. T. G. Sitharam)

ACKNOWLEDGEMENT

The authors are grateful to the authorities of AICTE, particularly Prof. M. Jagadesh Kumar, former Chairman; Prof. T.G. Sitharam, Chairman, Prof. M. P. Poonia, Vice-Chairman; Prof. Rajive Kumar, Member-Secretary and Dr Amit Kumar Srivastava, Director, Faculty Development Cell for their planning to publish the books on Strength of Materials. The authors sincerely acknowledge the valuable contributions of the reviewer of the book Prof. S.P. Harsha of Department of Mechanical and Industrial Engineering at IIT Roorkee for carefully going through the manuscript and offering valuable suggestions. We are overwhelmed by the encouragement and moral support provided by former Chairman of AICTE, Prof. Anil D. Sahasrabudhe.

This book is an outcome of various suggestions of AICTE members, experts and authors who shared their opinion and thought to further develop the engineering education in our country. Acknowledgements are due to the contributors and different workers in this field whose published books, review articles, papers, photographs, footnotes, references and other valuable information enriched us at the time of writing the book.

Dr. Uday Shanker Dixit,
Dr. Nelson Muthu,
Dr. S.M. Kamal

PREFACE

Strength of materials is an important course of civil and mechanical engineering. It has been taught to undergraduate students since decades and there are plenty of books on this subject. Hence, the natural question arises: Why this book?

The answer is that although the strength of material is an old course and hardly any significant change has taken place in its syllabus, yet there has been a substantial change in its pedagogy considering the students of 21st century. Engineering students of present time comprise a heterogeneous group with differing skills, interest and abilities. They are also having a lot of means of distraction. In fact, often the concerns are expressed over the declining interest of students for book reading. It has been observed that most of the students like very thin textbooks, rich in illustrative examples, at the cost of theoretical foundation. However, it may not be a wise idea on the part of the academicians to provide students a book that is devoid of sound fundamental concepts. An ideal book for modern age students should be concise, clear, rich in theoretical concepts and full of sufficient illustrative problems. It is a challenging problem of optimization. We have attempted to provide an optimal solution in the guise of this book.

While the book is on strength of material– so-called engineer's approach, basic concepts have been covered in a manner such that students can be prepared to study a course on theory of elasticity (so-called mathematician's approach) in later classes. Thus, the concept of stress at a point has been explained from a three-dimensional point of view, although the most of the examples in the book pertain to one- and two-dimensional situations only. We have provided a sufficient number of exercise problems too. Attempt has been made to keep exercise problems straightforward, so that students do not get distracted from grasping the subjects. Including a large number of problems in a book, in which several similar types of problems get repeated and many over-complex problems do not teach any new concept related to subject, demand more time from students, which is an inefficient way of learning. Considering a lot of load of other subjects on students, we cannot expect them to keep solving a large number of problems. Students have time to solve only a few problems. Students and teachers face difficulty in choosing sample problems from a book containing a huge number of problems. We hope that this book will not have such problem as it contains optimum number of problems, suitable for regular assignment sheets of the students.

This book can be used as a textbook for a one-semester course. There are already several books on strength of materials that can serve as reference books. In fact, after going through this book, students will find it easier to study higher level text and reference books. At the end of the book, we have recommended several books for further reading. Students can also take help of Massive Open Online Courses (MOOCs) available on internet. However, they should refrain from following any MOOC course or book blindly, but should use their intellect and wisdom. This book therefore puts more emphasis on science than empirical knowledge.

Enjoy reading the rest of the book...

Dr. Uday Shanker Dixit,
Dr. Nelson Muthu,
Dr. S.M. Kamal

OUTCOME BASED EDUCATION

For the implementation of an outcome based education the first requirement is to develop an outcome based curriculum and incorporate an outcome based assessment in the education system. By going through outcome based assessments evaluators will be able to evaluate whether the students have achieved the outlined standard, specific and measurable outcomes. With the proper incorporation of outcome based education there will be a definite commitment to achieve a minimum standard for all learners without giving up at any level. At the end of the programme running with the aid of outcome based education, a student will be able to arrive at the following outcomes:

PO1. **Engineering knowledge**: Apply the knowledge of mathematics, science, engineering fundamentals, and an engineering specialization to the solution of complex engineering problems.

PO2. **Problem analysis:** Identify, formulate, review research literature, and analyze complex engineering problems reaching substantiated conclusions using first principles of mathematics, natural sciences, and engineering sciences.

PO3. **Design / development of solutions:** Design solutions for complex engineering problems and design system components or processes that meet the specified needs with appropriate consideration for the public health and safety, and the cultural, societal, and environmental considerations.

PO4. **Conduct investigations of complex problems:** Use research-based knowledge and research methods including design of experiments, analysis and interpretation of data, and synthesis of the information to provide valid conclusions.

PO5 **Modern tool usage:** Create, select, and apply appropriate techniques, resources, and modern engineering and IT tools including prediction and modeling to complex engineering activities with an understanding of the limitations.

PO6. **The engineer and society:** Apply reasoning informed by the contextual knowledge to assess societal, health, safety, legal and cultural issues and the consequent responsibilities relevant to the professional engineering practice.

PO7. **Environment and sustainability:** Understand the impact of the professional engineering solutions in societal and environmental contexts, and demonstrate the knowledge of, and need for sustainable development.

PO8. **Ethics:** Apply ethical principles and commit to professional ethics and responsibilities and norms of the engineering practice.

PO9. **Individual and team work:** Function effectively as an individual, and as a member or leader in diverse teams, and in multidisciplinary settings.

PO10. **Communication:** Communicate effectively on complex engineering activities with the engineering community and with society at large, such as, being able to comprehend and write effective reports and design documentation, make effective presentations, and give and receive clear instructions.

PO11. Project management and finance: Demonstrate knowledge and understanding of the engineering and management principles and apply these to one's own work, as a member and leader in a team, to manage projects and in multidisciplinary environments.

PO12. Life-long learning: Recognize the need for, and have the preparation and ability to engage in independent and life-long learning in the broadest context of technological change.

COURSE OUTCOMES

CE: Course Outcomes

On completion of the course, the students will be able to:

CO-1: Describe the concepts and principles, understand the theory of elasticity including strain/displacement and Hooke's law relationship and perform calculations, relative to the strength and stability of structures and mechanical components

CO-2: Define the characteristics and calculate the magnitude of combined stresses in individual members and complete structures; analyze solid mechanics problems using classical methods and energy methods

CO-3: Analyse various situations involving structural members subjected to combined stresses by application of Mohr's circle of stress; locate the shear center of thin wall beams; and

CO-4: Calculate the deflection at any point on a beam subjected to a combination of loads; solve for stresses and deflections of beams under unsymmetrical loading; apply various failure criteria for general stress states at points; solve torsion problems in bars and thin walled members;

ME: Course Outcomes

CO-1: After completing this course, the students should be able to recognise various types loads applied on machine components of simple geometry and understand the nature of internal stresses that will develop within the components

CO-2: The students will be able to evaluate the strains and deformation that will result due to the elastic stresses developed within the materials for simple types of loading

Course Outcomes	Expected Mapping with Programme Outcomes: CE *(1- Weak Correlation: 2- Medium correlation; 3- Strong Correlation)*											
	PO-1	PO-2	PO-3	PO-4	PO-5	PO-6	PO-7	PO-8	PO-9	PO-10	PO-11	PO-12
CO-1	3	3	2	2	1	2	-	-	-	-	-	-
CO-2	3	3	2	2	-	-	-	-	-	-	-	-
CO-3	3	3	2	2	-	-	-	-	-	-	-	-
CO-4	3	3	3	2	1	-	-	-	-	-	-	-

Course Outcomes	Expected Mapping with Programme Outcomes: ME *(1- Weak Correlation; 2- Medium correlation: 3- Strong Correlation)*											
	PO-1	PO-2	PO-3	PO-4	PO-5	PO-6	PO-7	PO-8	PO-9	PO-10	PO-11	PO-12
CO-1	3	3	2	2	1	-	-	-	-	-	-	-
CO-2	3	3	2	2	1	-	-	-	-	-	-	-

GUIDELINES FOR TEACHERS

To implement Outcome Based Education (OBE) knowledge level and skill set of the students should be enhanced. Teachers should take a major responsibility for the proper implementation of OBE. Some of the responsibilities (not limited to) for the teachers in OBE system may be as follows:

- Within reasonable constraint, they should manoeuvre time to the best advantage of all students.
- They should assess the students only upon certain defined criterion without considering any other potential ineligibility to discriminate them.
- They should try to grow the learning abilities of the students to a certain level before they leave the institute.
- They should try to ensure that all the students are equipped with the quality knowledge as well as competence after they finish their education.
- They should always encourage the students to develop their ultimate performance capabilities.
- They should facilitate and encourage group work and team work to consolidate newer approach.
- They should follow Blooms taxonomy in every part of the assessment.

Bloom's Taxonomy

Level	Teacher should Check	Student should be able to	Possible Mode of Assessment
Create	Students ability to create	Design or Create	Mini project
Evaluate	Students ability to justify	Argue or Defend	Assignment
Analyse	Students ability to distinguish	Differentiate or Distinguish	Project/Lab Methodology
Apply	Students ability to use information	Operate or Demonstrate	Technical Presentation/ Demonstration
Understand	Students ability to explain the ideas	Explain or Classify	Presentation/Seminar
Remember	Students ability to recall (or remember)	Define or Recall	Quiz

GUIDELINES FOR STUDENTS

Students should take equal responsibility for implementing the OBE. Some of the responsibilities (not limited to) for the students in OBE system are as follows:

- Students should be well aware of each UO before the start of a unit in each and every course.
- Students should be well aware of each CO before the start of the course.
- Students should be well aware of each PO before the start of the programme.
- Students should think critically and reasonably with proper reflection and action.
- Learning of the students should be connected and integrated with practical and real life consequences.
- Students should be well aware of their competency at every level of OBE.

ABBREVIATIONS AND SYMBOLS

List of Abbreviations

General Terms			
Abbreviations	**Full form**	**Abbreviations**	**Full form**
BIS	Bureau of Indian Standards	SF	shear force
BM	bending moment	SFD	shear force diagram
BMD	bending moment diagram	UDL	uniformly distributed load
FBD	free body diagram		

List of Symbols

Symbols	Description	Symbols	Description
A	cross-sectional area of the bar	γ	change in the angle between two orthogonal lines
dF	force on infinitesimal area	δ	deformation or the extension
E	Young's modulus of elasticity	Δb	reduction in width
f	frequency of rotation	ΔL	change in length
F_{OS}	Factor of safety	ΔT	change in temperature
G	shear modulus or modulus of rigidity	Δt	reduction in thickness of the bar
I	moment of inertia	ε	true strain
K	bulk modulus of the material	ε_a	axial strain
k	stiffness	ε_t	lateral or transverse strain
L	length	ε_V	volumetric strain
M	moment	ε_x, ε_y *and* ε_z	strains in x, y and z directions, respectively
P	power	θ	angle
R	reaction force	v	Poisson's ratio
T	torque	σ	normal stress
U	Work done during deformation	τ	shear stress
U_r	resilience	ω	angular velocity
V	shear force	ΔA	area of the small circle
W	weight	$\hat{n}$	normal
y	distance from the neutral axis	$\Delta\vec{F}$	resultant of the distributed internal force
Z	section modulus	$\vec{t}_n$	traction
α	linear coefficient of expansion		

LIST OF FIGURES

Unit 1 Stresses and Strains

Unit 2 Compound Stresses and Strains

Unit 3 Shear Force and Bending Moment Diagrams

Unit 4 Bending Stresses

Unit 5 Shear Stresses in Beams

Unit 6 Deflection and Slope of Beams

Unit 7 Torsion of Circular Shafts

Unit 8 Thin and thick cylinders and spheres

CONTENTS

Unit 1

Stresses and Strains

UNIT SPECIFICS

The following topics are covered in this unit:

- Concept of stress and its different types;
- Stresses in axially loaded member;
- Concept of strain and its different types;
- Stress-strain diagram;
- Introduction to different elastic moduli and Poisson's ratio;
- Stresses and deformations in axially loaded member of varying cross-sections;
- Stresses and deformations in statically indeterminate axially loaded member;
- Analysis of stresses and strains in compound bars;
- Introduction to thermal stresses and strains;
- Strain energy in axial loading– gradually applied load, suddenly applied load and shock loading.

The topics are discussed providing real life applications for generating further curiosity and creativity. A moderate number of practice problems are also provided at the end including multiple choice questions, short and long answer type questions and numerical problems.

RATIONALE

Students have already learnt a course on engineering mechanics, where they primarily dealt with the rigid body mechanics. The rigid body is an abstraction and in reality, all bodies deform under the action of externally applied loads and due to change in temperature. In order to consider the deformation aspect of a solid under the action of forces, this course of strength of materials is introduced, which primarily deals with the deformable body mechanics. To begin the course, in this unit, the fundamental variables of deformable body mechanics, *viz*, stresses, strains and deformations are introduced. The evaluation of stresses, strains and deformations for the simplest one-dimensional loading, *i.e.*, axial loading is discussed in depth.

PRE-REQUISITIES

Engineering Mechanics

UNIT OUTCOMES

After completing this unit students will be able to

U1-O1: understand concept of stresses and strains in a solid and their different types.

U1-O2: compute stresses and deformations in an axially loaded bar of prismatic as well as varying cross-sections.

U1-O3: understand the stress-strain curve for a typical material and different salient points.

U1-O4: understand the concept of elastic moduli and Poisson's ratio.

U1-O5: understand the concept of strain due to change in temperature and compute thermal stresses.

U1-O6: Understand the concept of strain energy in gradually applied loading, suddenly applied loading and impact or shock loading.

Course Outcomes	Expected Mapping with Course Outcomes - CE (1- Weak Correlation; 2- Medium correlation; 3- Strong Correlation)			
	CO-1	CO-2	CO-3	CO-4
U1-O1	3	-	-	-
U1-O2	3	-	-	-
U1-O3	3	-	-	-
U1-O4	3	-	-	-
U1-O5	3	-	-	-
U1-O6	3	-	-	-

Course Outcomes	Expected Mapping with Course Outcomes - ME (1- Weak Correlation; 2- Medium correlation; 3- Strong Correlation)	
	CO-1	CO-2
U1-O1	2	2
U1-O2	3	3
U1-O3	2	2
U1-O4	2	2
U1-O5	3	3

1.1 Introduction

Strength of materials is a branch of physical science that studies the behaviour of solids, especially their strength and deformation, under the action of applied loading; loading can be in the form of force, change in temperature, phase change, etc. The strength of a deformable body is a measure of its capability to bear stresses and strain is a measure of deformation. Both stress and strain are internal effects produced in the material due to externally applied loads. In this unit, the concept of stresses and strains is introduced. Stresses and strains induced in simple structural members under simple loading conditions such as uniaxial loading are discussed. A thorough understanding of the several fundamental concepts arising from the concept of stress and strain, *e.g.*, Poisson's ratio, mechanical properties of materials and strain energy are provided in a systematic way.

1.2 Concept of Stress

In any engineering structures or systems, the individual components, which are in the form of solid bodies are subjected to external forces in service. These external forces arise either from the service conditions or from the environment in which the structure works. When we apply a force on a solid body, its particles are displaced. You can consider that even in a rigid body, the applied force produces displacement (although vanishingly small). The intensity of the internal force is called stress, which is the net internal force per unit area over which the internal forces are distributed.

In order to understand the concept of stress, let us consider an analogy of some students standing in a queue. As shown in Fig. 1.1, consider that Robert is standing with his back supported on a wall. In front of him is Shivam, then Narayan, then Umesh, and finally Joseph in a line. Now, if a wrestler pushes Joseph towards the wall, his motion is resisted by Umesh. After a few moments, Joseph will experience a force on his stomach applied by the wrestler and on his back, a force applied by Umesh. If Joseph is not moving, both these forces must be equal (net force zero, as per Newton's first law). As Umesh is applying a force on Joseph, he must also be getting the same amount of force by Joseph according to Newton's third law. As per Newton's second law, he gets some acceleration and moves toward Narayan, but gets stopped by Narayan, who then is able to apply the force equal to that of Joseph. This process continues. Ultimately, at steady state, each student is getting two equal and opposite forces, one at his stomach and the other at his back.

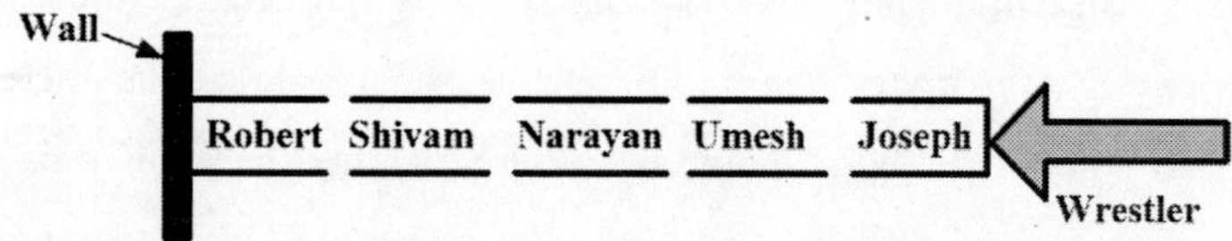

Fig. 1.1 Representation of push by a wrestler on Joseph against a wall on which Robert's back is resting

In order to know how much stress Narayan is facing, a free body diagram containing only Joseph, Umesh and Narayan is drawn in Fig. 1.2. In the free body diagram, the force of wrestler at one end and the force of Shivam (on Narayan) at the other end is shown. Note that we have broken the line of students hypothetically (In fact, we have not broken the line, but in our vision; we are only seeing Narayan, Umesh, Joseph and the two forces; we are not seeing two students and wall). Further, it is noted that in reality, the force of wrestler on Joseph and the force exerted by Shivam on Narayan are distributed in nature. However, for the purpose of analysis, we have shown them as concentrated forces by using the composition of forces and considered them to act through the centroidal axis of the line of students.

Now, if we are interested in finding out the intensity of the compressive force on the back of Narayan, it can be easily calculated. It is the force of Shivam divided by the area of the back of Narayan. We refer as the compressive stress on the back of Narayan. It is an average stress on the back of Narayan and in the standard international system (SI), its unit is N/m^2. However, the stress may differ from location to location. Can we find out stress at a point? How can we do it? A point does not have an area. How should we say stress is force divided by area here? This will be explained in Section 1.2.1.

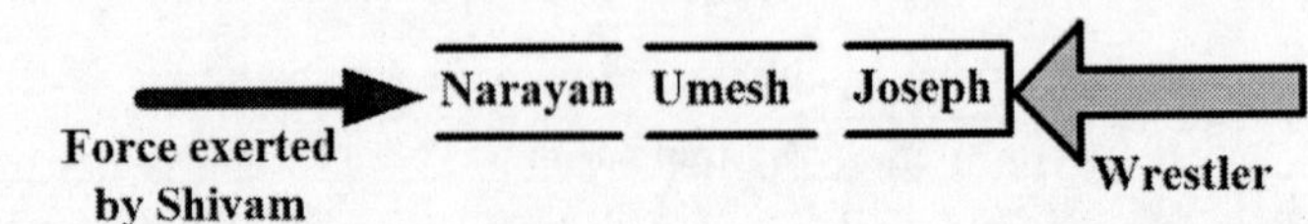

Fig. 1.2 Free body diagram of the system represented in Figure 1.1 considering Narayan, Umesh and Joseph in line.

1.2.1 Stress Vector or Traction at a Point

Stress is a measure of the intensity of internal forces generated in a body. In general, stresses in a body vary from point to point. In this section, we will define the traction or stress vector on a plane at point P of a body. Force is a vector quantity; hence, it is natural that force per unit area on the plane, i.e. stress, should also be a vector. However, from point P, an infinite number of planes can pass and one should be able to find out the stress vector at each plane. State of stress at a point means the information about the stress vector on each plane passing through that point. It can be shown that knowing the stress vector on three orthogonal planes is enough for finding out the stress vector on any plane. Hence, state of stress is specified by three stress vectors, which act on three orthogonal planes. This collection of three vectors acting on three orthogonal planes is called a tensor. Hence, state of stress is a tensor quantity. However, loosely people call stress at a point as a tensor quantity. In this section, however, we are very specific about calling stress as a vector, assuming that the plane on which it acts is specified along with the point P.

Let us consider an arbitrary body. The body is clamped at one part of the boundary and on some parts of the boundary, it is subjected to forces as shown in Fig. 1.3 (a). Under the action of the forces, the body gets deformed. The deformed configuration is shown in Fig. 1.3 (b). In the deformed configuration, the body is under the action of external forces. The external forces cause internal resistance to be developed at every point inside the body.

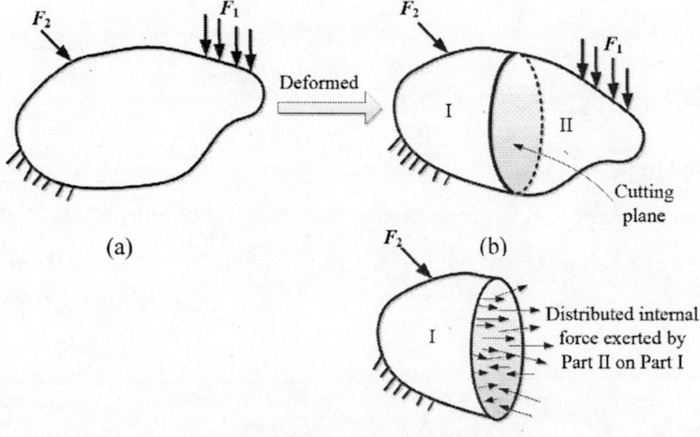

Fig. 1.3 An arbitrary solid body with an imaginary cut to reveal internal forces

In order to understand that internal effect, let us consider a plane that cuts the body into two parts– Part I and Part II. Now, if we isolate Part I from Part II, then on the entire internal cutting plane of the body, Part II will exert some force internally on Part I and that force will be distributed over the entire plane as depicted in Fig. 1.4. This distribution need not be uniform. Similarly, there are distributed internal forces on Part II exerted by Part I. Some portion may be subjected to pull and some portion may be subjected to push. Now, what is the intensity of the internal force with which Part II is exerting force on Part I?

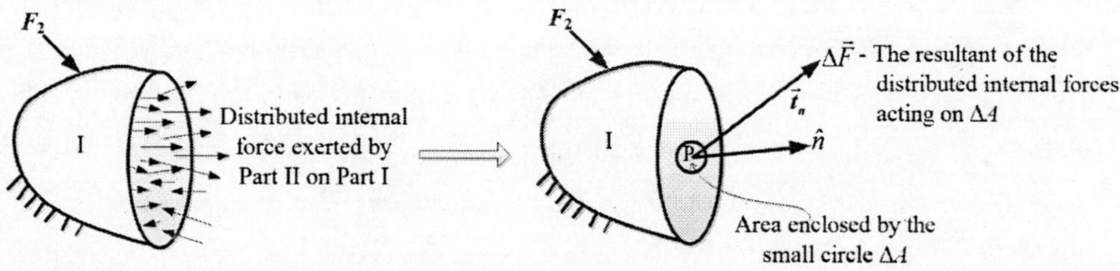

Fig. 1.4 Stress vector (traction) at a point

Let us come back to Part I again containing the cutting plane with the distributed internal forces. Suppose, we want to know the intensity of the internal force at some point on the cutting plane, say at point P. Let us now enclose point P by a small circle. The plane containing the point P enclosed by the small circle is represented by some normal $\hat{n}$. Let us say that the area of the small circle containing the point P is ΔA and the resultant of the distributed internal force on the area ΔA is $\Delta\vec{F}$. We need to quantify the intensity of the internal force at point P in the plane with normal $\hat{n}$.

Now, if we take the limit, that means when the area of the circle is shrunk to zero, the force applied by part II on that area is also going to decrease, but in the limit, it will attain a value and that value is called traction at that point. Thus, the traction at point P on the plane with normal $\hat{n}$ can be expressed mathematically as

$$\vec{t}_n(\vec{x},\hat{n}) = \lim_{\Delta A \to 0} \frac{\Delta\vec{F}}{\Delta A}, \tag{1.1}$$

where $\vec{x}$ is the position vector of point P.

Note that while shrinking the area of the circle, the circle must always contain the point P. The traction measures the intensity of the internal force at a point lying on a plane with normal $\hat{n}$. Thus, traction is basically telling us what is the intensity of the internal force at a given point, P on the plane with normal $\hat{n}$ with which one part of the body exerts a force on the other part of the body. Traction varies from point to point in a body. Even at a given point, traction on different planes is different. The magnitude of traction is expressed in terms of force per unit of area. Thus, it has the same unit as pressure, N/m^2. However, pressure is not the same as stress. Pressure is an externally applied load on a component during service, *e.g.*, pressure applied on the inner wall of a thick cylinder. On the other hand, stress is an internal effect, which gets developed due to the application of externally applied load, *e.g.*, stress induced across the wall thickness in a thick-walled cylinder due to the application of internal pressure at the inner wall. Moreover, when we apply pressure on a surface, it is always compressive in nature. However, stress can either be tensile or compressive in nature.

1.2.2 Types of Stresses

On a surface, stress vector, i.e. traction, can be resolved into normal to the plane and tangential to it. They are called normal stress and shear stress, respectively. The normal stress can be either tensile or compressive in nature. All other stresses are either combination of these basic stresses or similar to these. Let us now understand the normal and shear stress referring back to the traction on the cutting plane with normal $\hat{n}$ shown in Fig. 1.4.

On the cutting plane of the solid, the traction is not necessarily perpendicular to the plane, but is inclined in general (as in Fig. 1.4). Thus, traction $\vec{t}_n$ can be resolved perpendicular to the plane and along the plane. The component of $\vec{t}_n$ perpendicular to the plane is referred as the normal stress component, denoted by σ and the component of traction $\vec{t}_n$ along the plane is called the shear stress component and is denoted by τ. The normal and shear stress components on a plane are shown in Fig. 1.5.

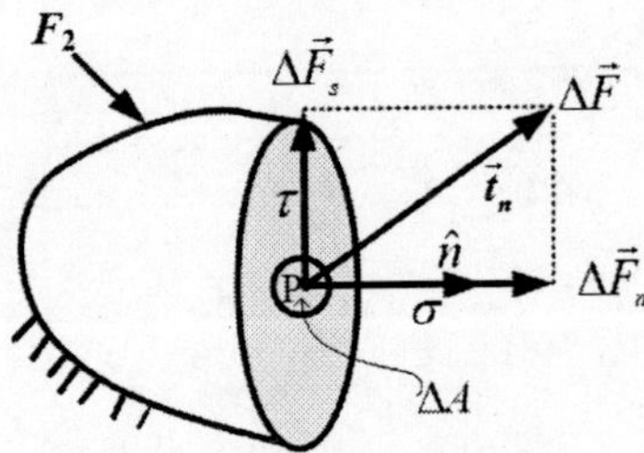

Fig. 1.5 The normal and shear stress components on a plane.

Taking the components of $\Delta\vec{F}$ perpendicular to the plane as $\Delta\vec{F}_n$ and that along the plane as $\Delta\vec{F}_s$, the component of traction $\vec{t}_n$ perpendicular to the plane, *i.e.*, the normal stress component is given by

$$\sigma = \lim_{\Delta A \to 0} \frac{\Delta\vec{F}_n}{\Delta A}. \tag{1.2}$$

If the normal stress component tends to pull on the area ΔA, as in Fig. 1.4, it is referred as tensile stress. On the other hand, if it tends to push on the area ΔA, then it is referred as compressive stress. The component of traction $\vec{t}_n$ along the plane, i.e., the shear stress component is given by

$$\tau = \lim_{\Delta A \to 0} \frac{\Delta\vec{F}_s}{\Delta A}. \tag{1.3}$$

The types of stresses are depicted in Fig. 1.6.

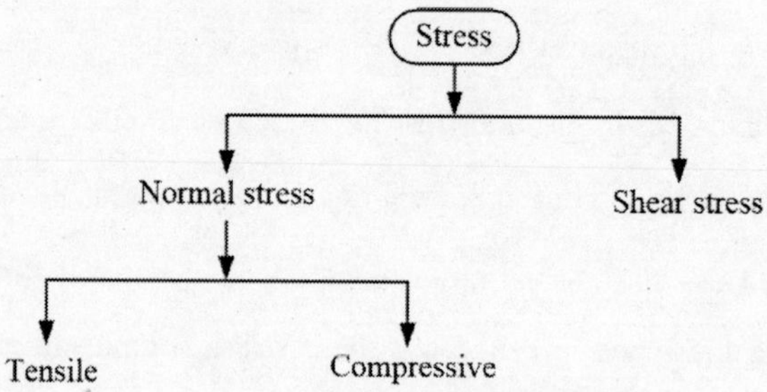

Fig. 1.6 Types of stresses

1.3 Stresses in Axially Loaded Bar

In this section, we will focus our attention on the determination of stresses on the vertical section of a prismatic bar loaded axially. It is assumed that the bar is a homogeneous continuum and isotropic i.e., it has the same physical and mechanical properties throughout its volume and in all directions. For the purpose of analysis, many engineering structures/components can suitably be approximated as homogeneous and isotropic materials.

Consider a prismatic rectangular bar with cross-sectional area A subjected to a uniform pull P as shown in Fig. 1.7 (a). It is assumed that P acts through the centroidal axis of the bar. Thus, it can be considered that at every point the same state of stress exists, which is not true in general. In order to evaluate the stress on a vertical plane, an imaginary vertical cutting plane is passed across the cross-section of the bar as shown in Fig. 1.7 (a), separating the bar into two parts. To maintain the equilibrium requirement of both the cut parts, the resultant internal normal force on the cut section must balance the externally applied load P. The distribution of the internal normal force on the cut section of the free body diagram of the left cut part of the bar is shown in Fig. 1.7 (b). As the same state of stress exists at every point on the cut section, the force on each infinitesimal area $\mathrm{d}A$ on the section is

$$\mathrm{d}F = \sigma \mathrm{d}A \tag{1.4}$$

Thus, the resultant normal force on the cut section can be obtained by integrating Eq. (1.4) over the area A as

$$\int \mathrm{d}F = \int_A \sigma \mathrm{d}A = \sigma \int_A \mathrm{d}A,$$

$$P = \sigma A,$$

$$\sigma = \frac{P}{A}, \tag{1.5}$$

where σ is the average tensile normal stress on any point on the vertical plane, P is the internal resultant normal force and A is the cross-sectional area of the bar. The resultant of the distributed internal normal force on the cut section of the left cut bar is shown in Fig. 1.7 (c). Nevertheless, a simplified free body diagram for this case is usually drawn as shown in Fig. 1.7 (d).

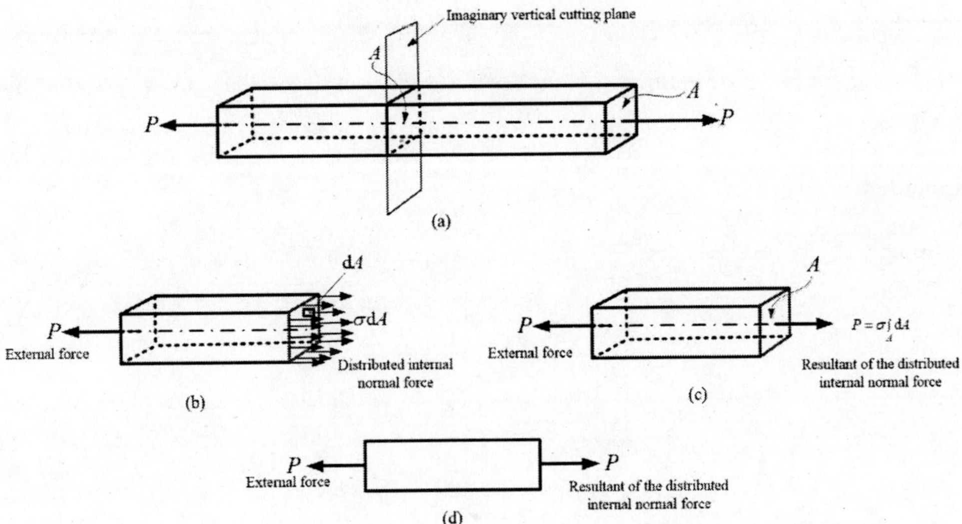

Fig. 1.7 A rectangular bar subjected to an axial pull: (a) cutting by an imaginary vertical plane, (b) the free body diagram of the left cut part of the bar showing the distributed internal normal force on the cut section, (c) the free body diagram of the left cut part of the bar showing the resultant of the distributed internal normal force on the cut section and (d) a simplified free body diagram of the left cut part of the bar.

Instead of pulling the rectangular bar, if one applies a push (the force is applied opposite to outward normal), uniform compressive normal stress is induced in the bar and is still given by Eq. (1.5). Only, a negative sign is associated with a compressive stress. The sign of tensile stresses is taken as positive. The state of stress in the present case is termed uniaxial stress as the stress acts only in one direction. The uniaxial stress state in the bar is usually represented by slicing out a thin rectangular element and showing the stresses on the left and right faces of the slice as shown in Fig. 1.8. In fact the thickness of the slice is very small, almost zero.

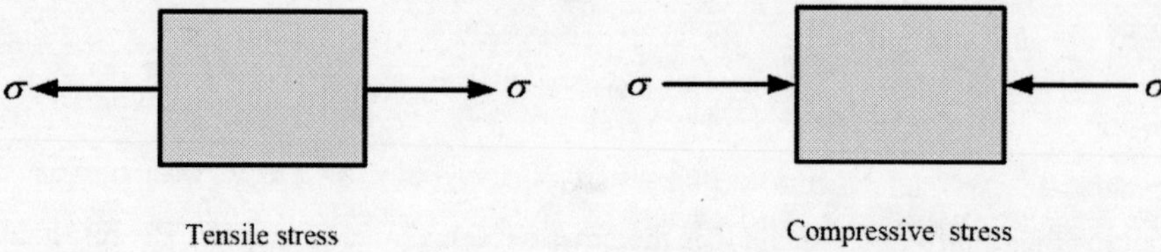

Fig. 1.8 Representative of a uniaxial state of stress in a rectangular element subjected to tension and compression.

Example 1.1 A steel bar AB of circular cross-section suspended from its top and supports a load of 50 kN at the bottom. If the diameter of the bar is 50 mm, then determine normal stress induced in the bar. If it is proposed to replace the steel bar with a wooden bar to withstand the same stress under the given loading, then what should be the dimeter of the wooden bar?

Solution

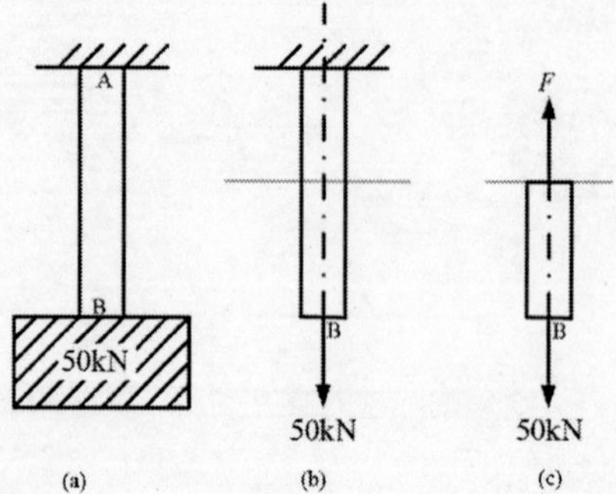

Assumptions: The weight of the bar is neglected. The only external force acting on the bar is W= 50 kN load that it is supporting at its bottom. This load is idealized as a concentrated force and supposed to act at the bottom face of the bar through the centroidal axis of the bar.

Now, we take an imaginary cut on the bar perpendicular to its axis and draw the free body diagram of the lower cut part of the bar. The use of static equilibrium equation provides the resultant internal force on the cut section as

$$F-W=0, \quad F=W=50 \text{ kN}.$$

Given the diameter of the steel rod, d=50 mm. Therefore, the cross-sectional area of the cut section where the internal force is acting is given by

$$A=\frac{\pi}{4}d^2=\frac{\pi}{4}(50)^2 \text{ mm}^2.$$

The normal stress induced in the member is computed as

$$\sigma = \frac{F}{A} = \frac{50 \times 10^3}{\frac{\pi}{4} \times 50^2} = 25.46\,\text{MPa}.$$

When the steel bar is replaced with a wooden bar to withstand the same stress under the same given loading, the diameter of the wooden bar must be same as that of the steel bar. It follows from the basic definition of stress that in order to withstand the same stress under the same given loading, the cross-sectional dimensions of all members must be same irrespective of the material of the bar.

1.4 Shear Stress

In Section 1.3, we considered that the bar is subjected to load, which is normal to the cross-section, that gives rise to a normal stress on a vertical cut section. Now, we will consider a situation, where the prismatic rectangular bar of cross-sectional area A is subjected to a set of equal and opposite forces parallel to its cross-section as shown in Fig. 1.9 (a). Passing an imaginary vertical plane of cut across the cross section of the bar, we obtain the free body diagram of the left half of the bar shown in Fig. 1.9 (b). The corresponding simplified free body diagram is shown in Fig. 1.9 (c). It is clear from the free body diagram that the resultant internal force V on the cut section of the left half of the bar is parallel to the cross-section and the equilibrium condition requires that this must be equal to P. This internal force V, which is distributed parallel to the cross-section concerned and tends to shear the material along the cut plane is referred as the shear force. The intensity of the shear force, *i.e.*, the shear force divided by the cross-sectional area resisting the shear is called as the average shear stress (τ). Mathematically, we can express it as

$$\tau = \frac{V}{A} = \frac{P}{A}. \tag{1.6}$$

1.4.1 Case of single shear

Let us take the case of a simple riveted butt joint of two plates as shown in Fig. 1.10 (a). If the plates are loaded in tension with a pair of equal and opposite force P, the rivet is subjected to shear forces tending to shear it off on one plane as indicated in Fig. 1.10 (b). This type of situation, where the shear forces tend to shear off the material only along one plane is termed as the case of single shear. Here, we have only one area A (the cross-sectional area of the rivet) that resists the shearing of the rivet due to the applied force P. Thus, the shear stress induced in the rivet is given by the applied force P divided by that one area A resisting shear as given in Eq. (1.6). Conversely, by drawing the free body diagram of the rivet half that lies above the shearing plane (Fig. 1.10 (c)), we see that a shear force V acts along the shear plane that equilibrates the external force P and the shear stress set up in the rivet is obtained same as in Eq. (1.6).

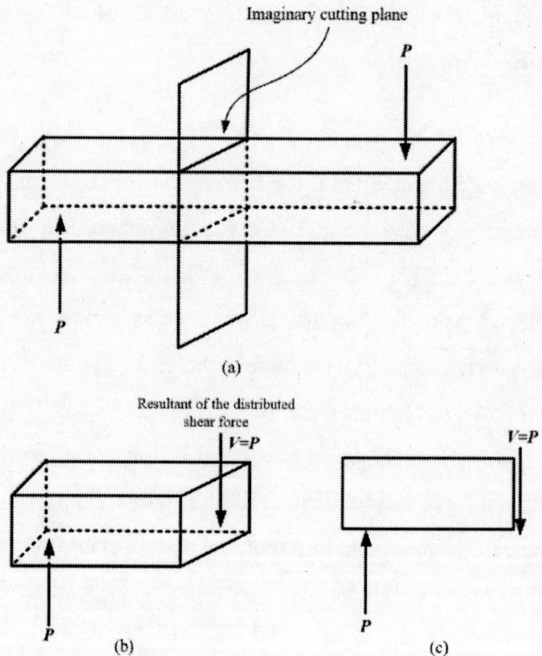

Fig. 1.9 A rectangular bar subjected to a set of equal and opposite forces parallel to its cross-section: (a) imaginary vertical cutting plane, (b) free body diagram of the left cut part of the bar revealing the resultant of the distributed shear force at the cut section, (c) a simplified free body diagram.

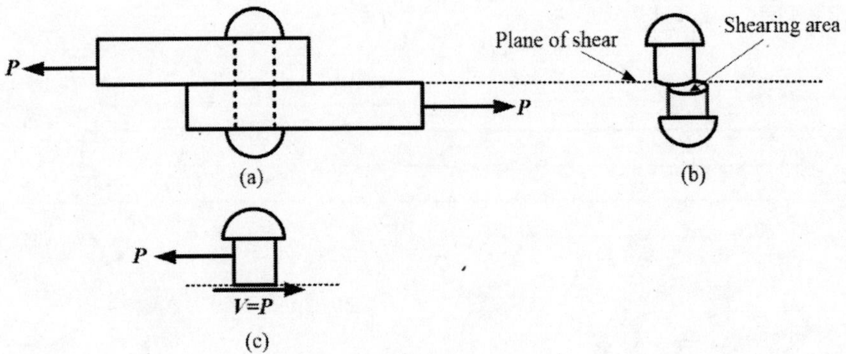

Fig. 1.10 A simple riveted butt joint: (a) joining two plates, (b) shearing of the rivet in single shear, (c) free body diagram of the rivet half above the shearing plane.

1.4.2 Case of Double Shear

Now, contrary to the riveted joint shown in Fig. 1.10, if we consider a riveted but joint with two cover plates as shown in Fig. 1.11 (a), the shearing of each rivet will take place on two faces of the rivets. Thus, we have two shear planes along which each rivet tends to shear as shown in Fig. 1.11 (b). This situation is referred as the double shear. Here, we have two shearing areas resisting the applied force. If we take each area resisting shear as A, the shear stress induced in each rivet is given by the applied force divided by the two shearing areas, *i.e.*,

$$\tau = \frac{P}{2A}. \tag{1.7}$$

Alternatively, from the free diagram of the rivet section containing the two shear planes as shown in Fig. 1.11 (c) we get

$$P = V + V = 2V,$$

where V is the shear force. Thus,

$$V = \frac{P}{2}.$$

Hence, the shear stress induced is given by

$$\tau = \frac{V}{A} = \frac{\frac{P}{2}}{A} = \frac{P}{2A}, \tag{1.8}$$

which is same as Eq. (1.7).

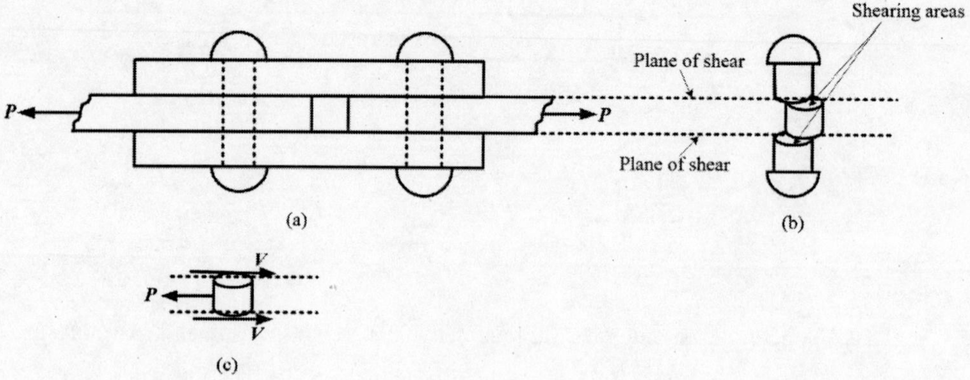

Fig. 1.11 Illustration of double shear: (a) a riveted butt joint joining two plates using two cover plates, (b) shearing of rivet in double shear, (c) free body diagram of the rivet section containing the two shear planes.

Example 1.2 A block of mass 10 kg is resting on a floor. The Coulomb's coefficient of friction is 0.1. If a horizontal (parallel to floor) force of 3 N is applied on the block and nominal area of the interface between block and floor is 0.1 m^2, then determine the average shear stress on the floor.

Solution

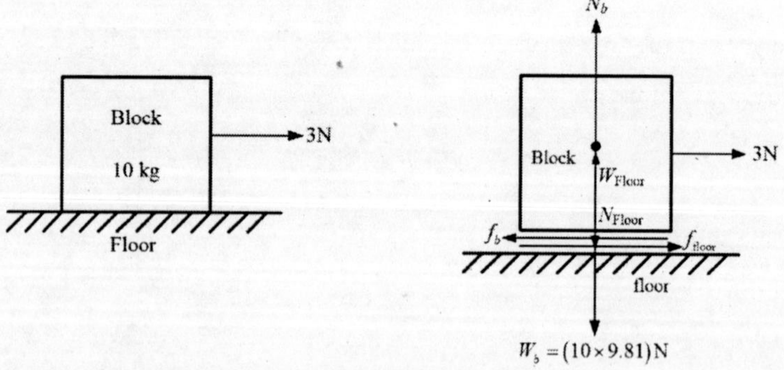

Drawing the free body diagram and using the equilibrium equation parallel to the floor, the average internal frictional force acting on the block tangential to its bottom face is obtained as

$$f = 3 \text{ N}.$$

The above force will act tangential to the floor in the opposite direction according to Newton's third law. The nominal area of the interface between the block and the floor is given as $A = 0.1\ \text{m}^2$. Thus, the average shear stress acting on the floor is given by

$$\tau_{av} = \frac{f}{A} = \frac{3}{0.1} = 30\ \text{N/m}^2.$$

Know More

1.5 Concept of Strain

So far in the preceding sections, we discussed stress induced in a solid body when it is subjected to external forces. In this section, we are going to introduce one more important concept called 'strain'. Strain is a relative measure of deformation. To understand the concept of strain, let us consider a bar of length L as shown in Fig. 1.12. Now, when the bar is subjected to either external forces or a change in temperature, it undergoes deformation and in the course of strength of materials, we are interested to define a quantity in terms of those deformations. For the time being, we will not consider the deformation due to temperature change, rather we consider that the bar is subjected to an axial tensile force. Due to this tensile force, the bar gets extended to a length $(L+\delta)$, where δ is the deformation or the extension of the bar. Now, if we define a quantity, which is the ratio of this deformation δ to the original undeformed length L, then we call that quantity as strain. We denote strain by ε. Thus, in this case, we can write

$$\varepsilon = \frac{\delta}{L}. \tag{1.9}$$

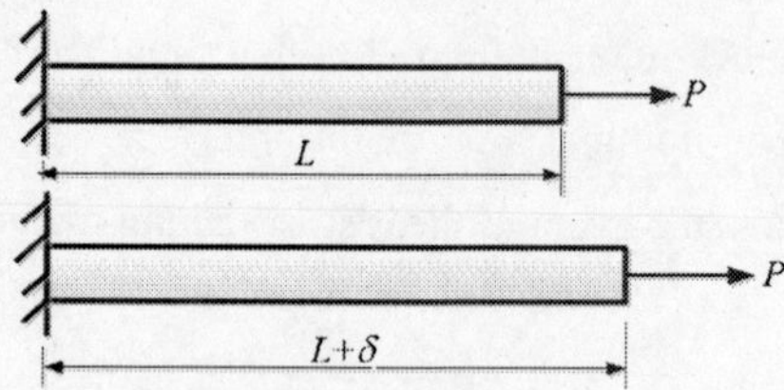

Fig. 1.12 A bar of length L getting elongated due to application of an axial tensile force P.

In the present case, we assume that the deformation is uniform at any point along the length of the bar and therefore, the same state of strain exists everywhere in the bar. We have already learnt that when the bar is loaded axially, then in the cross section of the bar we get a normal stress. Aligned with that the strain due to the axial loading given by Eq. (1.9) is called the normal strain. As the deformation is in the axial direction we also call it as axial or longitudinal strain. Strain is a dimensionless quantity.

The strain caused due to tensile force is termed as tensile strain and it is a positive quantity. On the other hand, instead of a tensile axial force, if the bar in Fig. 1.12 is subjected to an axial compressive force, the bar gets shortened and the resulting normal strain obtained is a negative quantity. The negative strain is termed as compressive strain.

1.6 Types of Strains

Just like stress, there are two basic types of strains that a solid body can experience— normal strain and shear strain. There are various other types of strains, such as thermal strain, which is a form of normal strain only and volumetric strain which arises due to changes in volume induced by normal strains. We have already discussed the concept of normal strain in Section 1.5. The other type of strain, *i.e.* shear strain, is discussed in the following section.

1.7 Shear strain

As we have the normal strain associated with the normal stress, likewise, we get shear strain associated with shear stress. Let us consider an infinitesimal rectangular element subjected to shear stress as shown in Fig. 1.13. There will be angular deformation in this case. The change in the angle between two orthogonal lines (ad and ab in the element) after deformation is called the shear strain. It is denoted by γ. The shear strain in this case can be expressed as

$$\gamma = \angle_{\text{undeformed}} - \angle_{\text{deformed}} = \frac{\pi}{2} - \frac{\pi}{2} + \phi = \phi. \tag{1.10}$$

It is measured in radians and is a non-dimensional quantity. By convention, a reduction in angle is positive shear. For measuring shear strain, the angle between any two lines is taken as 90° in the undeformed configuration.

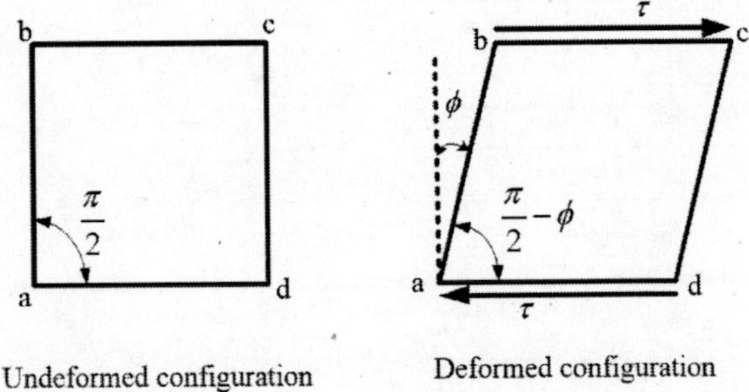

Fig. 1.13 Deformation of an infinitesimal rectangular element subjected to shear stress

1.8 Strain at a Point

Consider a bar and let A and B be any two points close to each other on the bar as shown in Fig. 1.14. Initially, these were at a distance of x_1 and x_3 from the assumed origin. After deformation due an axial tension, have moved to x_2 and x_4 distances, respectively. Now, if the travel of point A or (x_2-x_1) is the same as the travel of point B or (x_4-x_3), it is obvious that line element AB has simply travelled a distance without any change in length. Thus, there is no strain induced in the line element AB. However, if the distance travelled by points A and B are different, then the length of the line element will change. This provides strain developed in the bar. Thus, in the limit, when the length of the line $AB \rightarrow 0$, the strain experienced by the line element is given by

$$\varepsilon = \operatorname*{Lim}_{AB \rightarrow 0} \frac{A'B' - AB}{AB}. \tag{1.11}$$

Eq. (1.11) means the strain obtained at a point A or B, where A and B are coincident. It is to be noted that strains cannot occur without displacements; however, displacements are possible without strains.

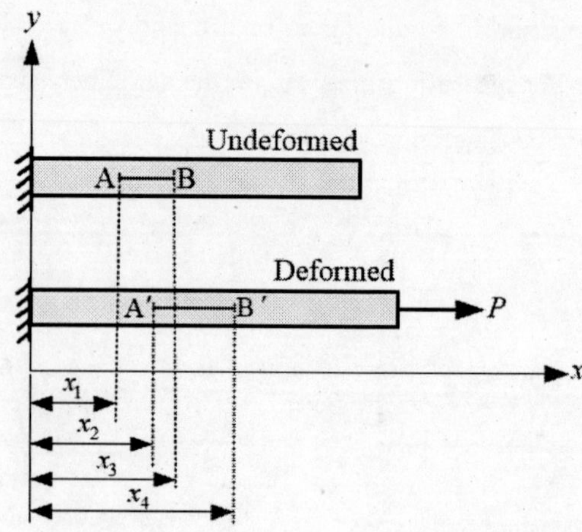

Fig. 1.14 Deformation of a line element AB on a bar subjected to tension.

Example 1.3 A member AB of length L is held in horizontal equilibrium position by means of a hinge at end A to a vertical wall AC and the other end B by means of a steel cable BC as shown in the figure. The vertical span AC is also equal to L. When there is no load acting on the member AB, then the angle θ=45°. Now a load W is hung from the end B of the member AB. This causes the cable to stretch and the angle θ becomes 46°. Determine the normal strain induced in the steel cable BC.

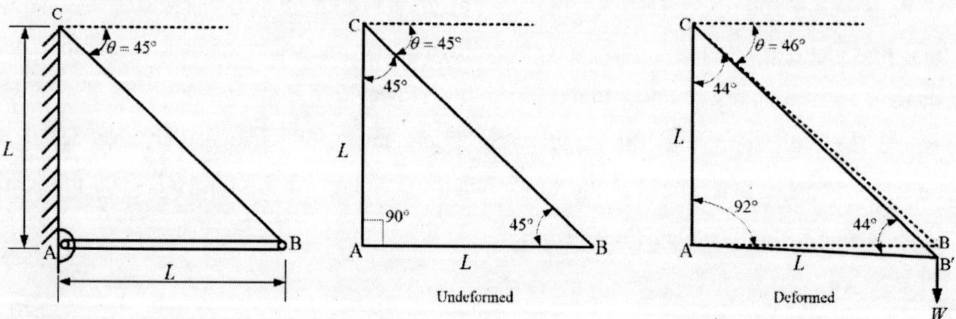

Solution

When there is no load applied to the member, the steel cable in its unstretched state and it makes and angle of 45° each to the member AB and the wall AC. In this case, the member AB, cable BC and the wall AC forms an isosceles right angle triangle. Thus, the unstretched length of the cable BC in terms of L is obtained as

$$BC = \sqrt{L^2 + L^2} = \sqrt{2}L$$

Now, when a weight W is hang from the end B of the member AB, the cable gets stretched making angle θ=46°. This makes the point B to move slightly downward, but the length of the member remains equal to L. The new position of the point B is taken as B′. Thus, the cable makes an angle 44° each with the member AB′ and the wall AC. The angle between the member AB′ and the wall AC then becomes 92°. At this stage, the triangle AB′C turns out to be isosceles. Now, using the cosine law, we can obtain the stretched length of the cable $B'C$ as

$$L^2 = L^2 + \left(B'C\right)^2 - 2L\left(B'C\right)\cos 44°,$$

$$B'C = 2L\cos 44°.$$

Now, the change in length of the cable, $\delta = B'C - BC = 2L\cos 44° - \sqrt{2}L.$

Thus, the normal strain induced in the cable is obtained as

$$\varepsilon = \frac{\delta}{L} = \frac{2L\cos 44° - \sqrt{2}L}{L} = 0.0245.$$

Example 1.4 A triangular plate ABC is deformed into the shape AB′C shown by the dotted line as a result of some loading. Determine the average shear strain developed at corner A relative to the edges AB and AC.

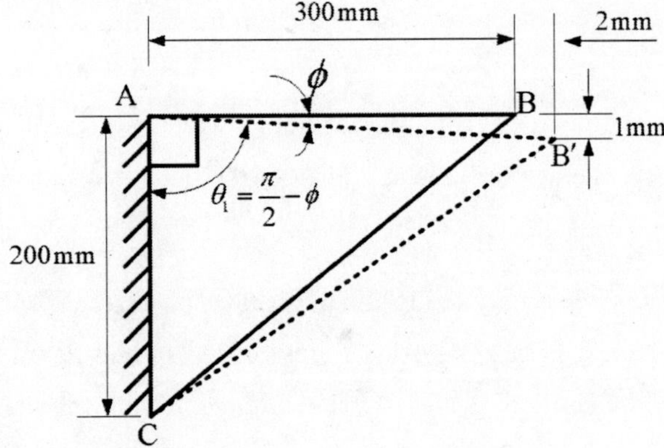

Solution

The 90° angle between the sides AB and AC *i.e.* angle BAC of the plate changes to θ_1 due to the displacement of point B to B′ in the deformed configuration. As the change in the angle between the undeformed and deformed configuration at corner A is the shear strain γ at A, thus,

$$\gamma = \frac{\pi}{2} - \theta_1 = \frac{\pi}{2} - \left(\frac{\pi}{2} - \phi\right) = \phi = \tan^{-1}\left(\frac{1}{300+2}\right) = 0.1897° = 0.0033 \text{ rad.}$$

1.9 Stress-Strain Diagram

To know the load-deformation characteristics of a material, the stress-strain diagrams are of interest to engineers. A uniaxial tensile test is usually performed in order to plot the incremental loads over the cross-sectional area on the ordinate and incremental deformations over the original length of the specimen concerned on the abscissa to obtain a stress-strain diagram. Instead of plotting the stress-strain in the uniaxial tensile test, one can also simply plot the load-deformation diagram. However, it is not plotted. In order to measure different strength parameters of a given material, a stress-strain diagram is always preferred over the load-deformation diagram. This aspect is discussed in Subsection 1.9.1.

1.9.1 Genesis of the Stress-Strain Curve

To measure the load-deformation characteristics of a particular material, one can simply take a solid cylindrical rod specimen of that material and then load it in tension at the ends. For each increment of the load, the corresponding deformations are recorded. Let us consider three different specimens of the same material with different lengths L_1, L_2, L_3 and cross-sectional areas A_1, A_2 and A_3 as shown in Fig. 1.15 (a). Now, suppose one loads these specimens gradually up to loads P_1, P_2 and P_3, respectively so that they undergo very small deformation. Plotting the deformation δ for each increment of the load for all three specimens, one will get three different load-deformation curves as shown in Fig. 1.15 (b). This poses difficulty in characterizing the load-deformation behaviour of a material as one has to perform a separate test for each specimen of the same material with different lengths and cross-sectional areas.

Instead of plotting simply the load-deformation, if one replots them by normalizing loads divided by the original cross-sectional areas of the specimens on the ordinate and by normalizing the deformations divided by the original lengths of the specimens on the abscissa, then one will arrive at a single curve as shown in Fig. 1.15 (b). This greatly simplifies the problem of determining the load-deformation characteristics of a material. Therefore, a single test plotting the stress on the ordinate and strain on the abscissa is sufficient to determine the load-deformation characteristics of a material and the curve thus obtained is called the stress-strain curve.

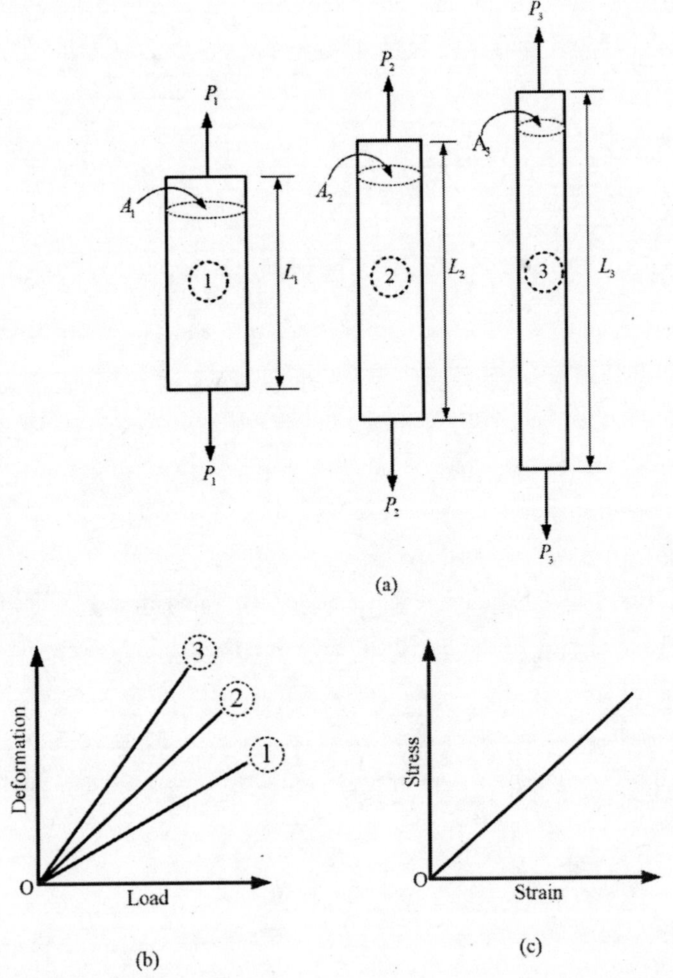

Fig. 1.15 (a) Three bars of same material with different lengths and cross-sectional areas subjected to loads to produce same maximum extension, (b) Load-deformation and (c) stress-strain diagram of three bars.

1.9.2 The uniaxial tensile test

To establish a relationship between stress and strain, a uniaxial tensile test is conducted. The test is usually performed on a solid cylindrical bar specimen of a given material with different cross-sectional forms as shown in Fig. 1.16. The grip portion of the specimen is inserted in a tensile testing machine and the whole bar is then pulled. Initially, a distance between two predefined points on the central uniform portion of the test specimen bar is fixed away from the grips, referred as the gauge length. This is done so that the length on which we focus our attention during the test is not affected by the distribution of the load in the grip portion but is only affected by the resultant longitudinal load.

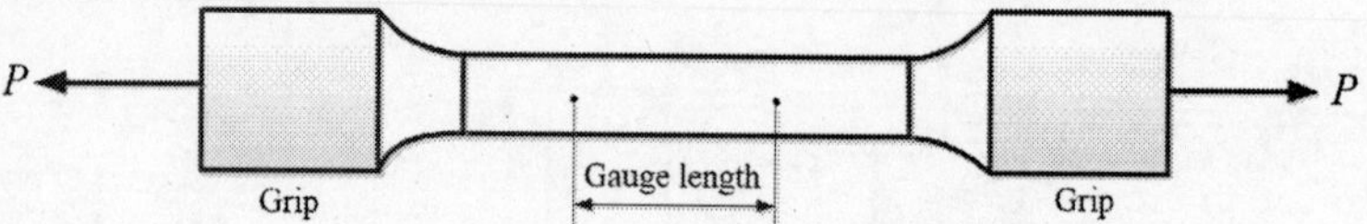

Fig. 1.16 The tensile test specimen.

Now, we apply a pull P on the bar gradually and the bar undergoes deformation causing the change in the gauge length. If we can measure the increment in gauge length (the deformation), then we can easily compute the strain. Similarly, for each increment of the load, we can compute the stress. Note that while evaluating the stress for each load increment, if the load at each increment is divided by the original cross-sectional area of the bar, then the stress is referred as the engineering stress or nominal stress. Also, in evaluating the strains, if the change in gauge length for each load increment is divided by the original undeformed gauge length of the bar, then the strain measured is referred as the engineering strain or nominal strain. If the original cross-sectional area of the central uniform portion of the specimen is A_0, the original undeformed gauge length of the specimen is L_0, and ΔL is the change in gauge length, the measure of engineering stress (σ_0) and engineering strain (e) are determined as

$$\sigma_0 = \frac{P}{A_0}, \quad e = \frac{\Delta L}{L_0}. \tag{1.12}$$

When the stress σ_0 is plotted against strain e, one obtains an engineering stress-strain curve. On the other hand, if the stress is evaluated by dividing the load by the current cross-sectional area (reduced area), then it is termed as the true stress. In a similar way, if the strain is measured with reference to the current extended length of the bar, it is termed as the true strain or natural strain, or logarithmic strain. Taking the current cross-sectional area as A and the current gauge length as L, the true stress (σ) and true strain (ε) for each load increment can be determined using the following equations:

$$\sigma = \frac{P}{A}, \quad \varepsilon = \ln\left(\frac{L}{L_0}\right). \tag{1.13}$$

If we plot stress σ against strain ε, we get a true stress-strain diagram. The stress-strain diagram of mild steel is discussed in Subsection 1.9.3 along with all the salient points.

1.9.3 The stress-strain curve of mild steel

A typical engineering stress-strain relationship for a mild steel bar is represented in Fig. 1.17 by plotting the engineering stress (σ) against engineering strain (e) during a uniaxial tensile test. The salient points of the stress-strain diagram shown in Fig. 1.18 are marked as A, B, C, D, E and F and they are discussed in the following paragraphs.

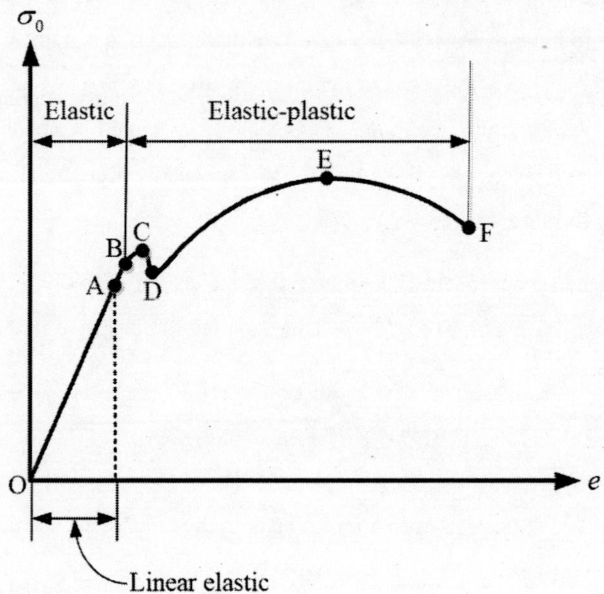

Fig. 1.17 The engineering stress-strain diagram for mild steel

Point A: It is observed from the stress-strain diagram that up to point A, the stress is directly proportional to the strain giving a straight line OA. Thus, the point A is termed as the proportional limit. The material remains elastic and linearity of stress-strain holds good up to this point.

Point B: For a short span beyond point A, the material still behaves elastically up to the point B. This point B is called the elastic limit. It is that point up to which the load is applied on the body and upon releasing the load the body springs back to its original state.

Point C and Point D: Beyond elastic limit, point C is reached where the deformation in the bar no longer remains elastic and plastic deformation initiates in the bar. This point is called the upper yield point and corresponds to the maximum stress required to initiate yielding. After that stress falls slightly to a point D, called the lower yield point. The lower yield point D signifies the minimum stress required to maintain the yielding of the material. If the bar is loaded beyond the yield point, the specimen does not come back to its original state upon releasing the load. Some amount of deformation is permanently set within the bar. The stress corresponding to the yield point is referred as the yield stress of the material.

Point E: If we keep on applying load beyond yield point, without much increase in the load we are going to have excessive deformation and we reach to a point E where the stress level is the maximum. This point is called the ultimate stress point. The stress corresponding to the ultimate stress point is the maximum stress that the specimen material can withstand without failure and is termed as the ultimate strength or tensile strength of the material. Just after point E, neck formation takes place.

Necking: As failure approaches, the material stretches very rapidly, causing the cross section to narrow down, as shown in Fig. 1.18. This is called as necking of the tensile test specimen.

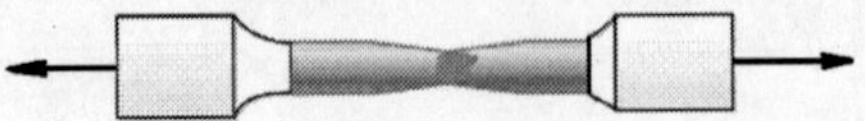

Fig. 1.18 Formation of neck in the tensile test specimen

Point F: Beyond the ultimate stress point E, the bar cannot take much load and there is a loading down on the bar. Also, due to necking, there is a larger reduction in the cross-sectional area. One will observe that at a certain point F the specimen fails with a cup and cone failure as shown in Fig. 1.19. This point F is called the fracture point. The value of the stress corresponding to point F in the stress-strain diagram is known as the fracture strength of the specimen material.

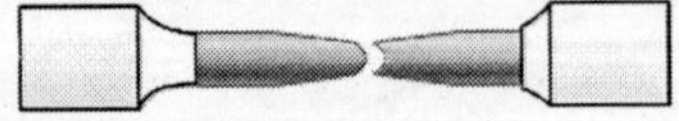

Fig. 1.19 Cup and cone failure of the tensile test specimen

Now, if one plots the true stress-strain curve for the same mild steel specimen, the stress-strain diagram as shown in Fig. 1.20 is obtained. The corresponding salient points with the same physical significance as depicted in Fig. 1.17 are also shown. For small strains such as elastic strains, the true strain values are essentially same as that of the engineering strains.

Also, true stresses in the elastic region are almost same as that of the engineering stress as there is little reduction in area during elastic deformation. Thus, the true stress-strain diagram and engineering stress-strain diagram seems to coincide for elastic deformation. Only when the specimen experiences plastic deformation, the deformations of the bar become comparatively larger causing a significant reduction in area. This makes the true stress-strain curve rise upward from lower yield point to the fracture point F as shown in Fig. 1.20. It is to be noted that beyond the initial yielding, the stress required to cause the continued plastic deformation increases with strain. This behaviour during plastic deformation of the material is called strain hardening.

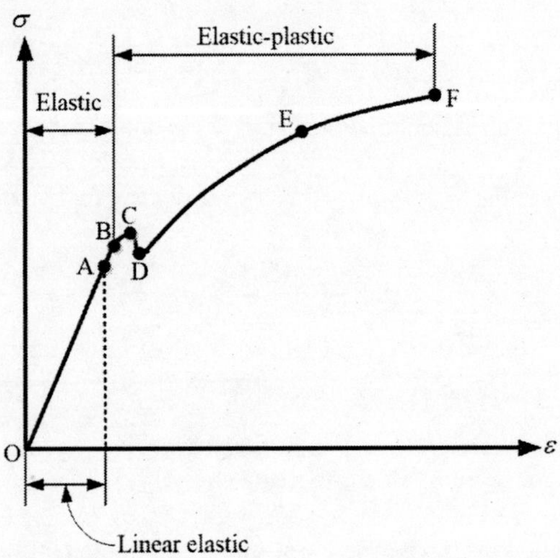

Fig. 1.20 The true stress-strain curve for mild steel

1.9.4 Relationship between engineering stress-strain and true stress-strain

The measure of engineering stress-strain and true stress-strain of a material subjected to uniaxial tension are given by Eqs. (1.12) and (1.13), respectively. As there is no volume change during plastic deformation, one can write

$$A_o L_o = AL,$$

$$A = \left(\frac{L_o}{L}\right) A_o \tag{1.14}$$

The current length L in terms of the change in length ΔL can be expressed as

$$L = L_0 + \Delta L. \tag{1.15}$$

Using the value of L from Eq. (1.15) in Eq. (1.14) and then substituting it in the expression of true stress σ in Eq. (1.13) we get

$$\sigma = \frac{P}{\left(\frac{L_o}{L_0 + \Delta L}\right) A_o} = \frac{P}{A_o}\left(\frac{L_0 + \Delta L}{L_o}\right),$$

$$\sigma = \sigma_0 \left(1 + \frac{\Delta L}{L_0}\right),$$

$$\sigma = \sigma_0 (1 + e). \tag{1.16}$$

Eq. (1.16) relates the true stress with engineering stress and engineering strain.

Substituting Eq. (1.15) in the expression of true strain in Eq. (1.13), one obtains

$$\varepsilon = \ln\left(\frac{L_0 + \Delta L}{L_0}\right) = \ln\left(1 + \frac{\Delta L}{L_0}\right),$$

$$\varepsilon = \ln(1 + e). \tag{1.17}$$

Eq. (1.17) relates the true strain with engineering strain.

1.9.5 Mechanical properties derivable from uniaxial tensile test

Following are the parameters that signify the mechanical properties of a material, which can be derived from the stress-strain diagram plotted during a uniaxial tensile test:

Ductility: It is observed from the strain-strain diagram in Fig. 1.17 that beyond the elastic limit B, plastic deformation initiates in the material at point C and the plastic deformation continues up the point of fracture at F with a relatively rapid increase in strain without much corresponding increase in the stress. This causes the stress-strain curve to cover a much larger portion of the strain axis as compared to the elastic range. This ability of the material to undergo a large range of plastic deformation before fracture is termed as the ductility of the material. The materials that possess the property of ductility are called *ductile materials.* Otherwise, they are termed as *brittle materials,* that means there is little plastic deformation before they fracture. The ductility of a material can be quantified either in terms of percentage elongation strain at fracture point or percentage reduction in area given by

$$\%\text{elongation strain at fracture point} = \frac{\text{Increase in gauge length to fracture point}}{\text{Original gauge length}} \times 100\%, \qquad (1.18)$$

$$\%\text{reduction in area} = \frac{\text{Reduction in cross sectional area of the necked portion}}{\text{Original cross sectional area}} \times 100\%. \qquad (1.19)$$

Strengths: The yield stress and ultimate stress are the important strength parameters dictated by the stress-strain curve of the material concern. In many design applications, we do not want a structural member or a machine element to deform plastically. If we allow to deform the member plastically, there might be a misalignment of the component concerned and the structure or machine as a whole become noisy during its service. In order to avoid such untoward situation, it is desirable to design such components based on the maximum stress that circumvents plastic deformation. The limiting stress that prevents the plastic deformation of a material is the yield stress corresponding to the yield point of the stress-strain diagram. Usually, for ductile materials, designers want to keep the stress in the material during its service without exceeding its yield stress.

In certain cases, a designer may be interested in the maximum stress that the component may withstand without failure. As we have learnt in the stress-strain diagram, we refer this stress as the ultimate stress or tensile strength of the material (Point E in Fig. 1.17). While designing for brittle materials, the optimum size of the components is decided based on the tensile strength.

Toughness: The energy absorbed per unit volume up to the point of fracture, *i.e.*, the area of stress-strain plot (the shaded area in Fig. 1.21) is known as the toughness of the material.

The above parameters are termed as the mechanical properties, because their values remain constant for a given homogeneous and isotropic material irrespective of its shape and size at a specified temperature.

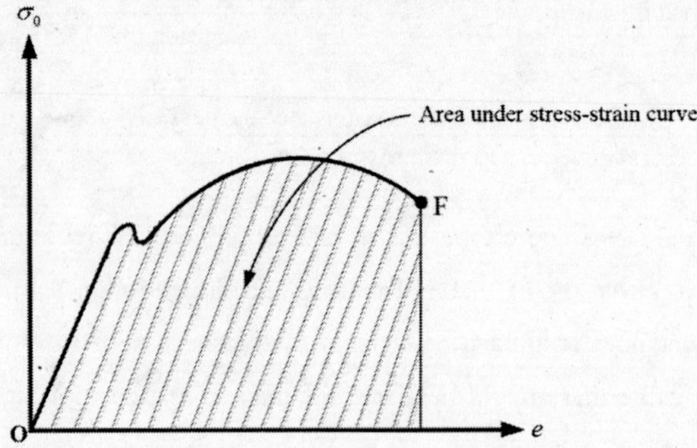

Fig. 1.21 The area under stress-strain curve signifying the toughness of a material

1.9.6 Stress-strain diagram for brittle material

A brittle material exhibits very small plastic deformation or little plastic deformation before fracture. It does not show any indication before fracture unlike necking in the case of ductile materials and suddenly gets separated into two pieces. A typical stress-strain diagram for a brittle material such as cast iron and steels with high carbon content is shown in Fig. 1.22.

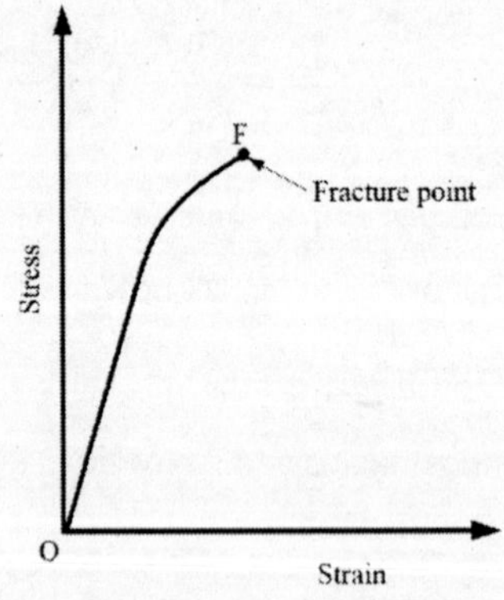

Fig. 1.22 A typical stress-strain curve for brittle materials

1.9.7 Proof stress

We have seen in the stress-strain diagram of mild steel bar that a well-defined yield point exists. Correspondingly we have a definite value of yield stress for that material, denoted by σ_Y. However, some materials such as aluminium, do not possess a definite yield point. In strength of materials, when we deal with the stresses within the elastic limit, it is of interest to know what is the value of the yield stress beyond which a material starts deforming plastically. When we do not observe any definite yield point on the stress-strain curve plotted during the uniaxial tensile test of the concerned material as shown in Fig. 1.23, it is difficult to know precisely what is the value of the yield stress. In such cases, to compute the yield stress an offset method is used. It is observed that the strain corresponding to the yield stress value is of the order of 0.2% or 0.002. Thus, in the offset method, a tangent is drawn to the stress-strain curve passing through the origin and a line offsetting at 0.2% strain value parallel to the tangent is drawn as shown in Fig. 1.23. Now, the point at which the line corresponding to 0.2% strain cuts the stress-strain curve is taken as the yield point and the corresponding stress is considered as the yield stress σ_Y. The yield stress evaluated using this offset method is termed as the proof stress.

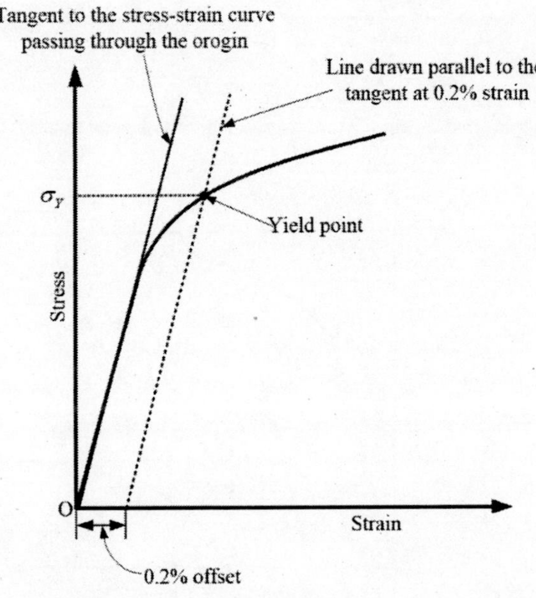

Fig. 1.23 Proof stress (yield stress at 0.2% offset)

1.9.8 Elasticity and Plasticity

The elasticity refers to the ability of a material to spring back to its original configuration (recovering both shape and size) after the removal of externally applied load. In the stress-strain diagram, the property of elasticity is valid up to the elastic limit (e.g., up to point B in Fig. 1.17). The range marked up to the point B in the stress-strain diagram is the elastic range of the material. If one loads the material to any point in this range and then unloads, the unloading follows the same path as in the loading. This situation is shown in Fig.

1.24 by plotting the stress-strain diagram up to any point in the elastic range for a typical material. Many materials behave elastically following a linear stress-strain relationship as shown in Fig. 1.24 (a) but some materials have nonlinear behavior in the elastic range as shown in Fig. 1.24 (b).

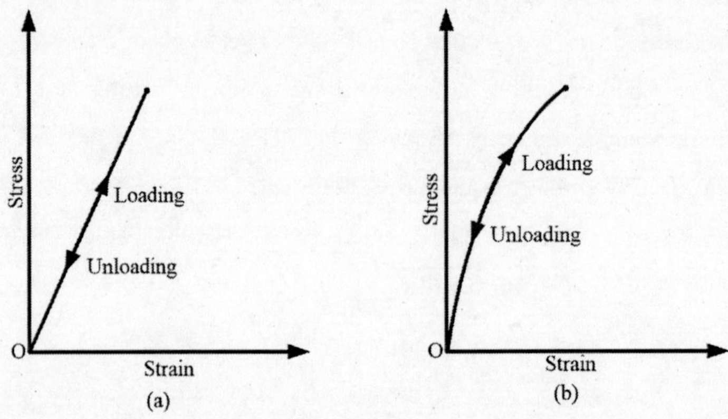

Fig. 1.24 The elastic behaviour of materials (a) linear elastic, (b) nonlinear elastic.

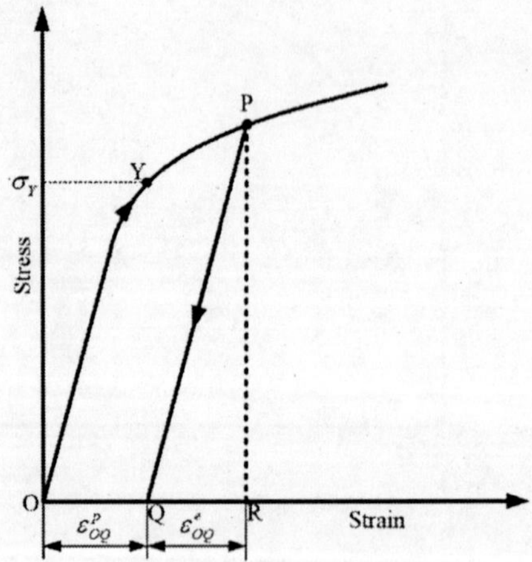

Fig. 1.25 The plastic behaviour of material when loaded beyond yield point

Plasticity is the behaviour of a material to undergo permanent (so-called plastic) deformation at a stress greater than the yield stress. When a load sufficient to cause plastic deformation is employed, deformation comprises elastic as well as a plastic portion. After the removal of the load, only the elastic part of the deformation or the strain is recovered. Some amount of permanent set is left in the material after unloading. The phenomenon of plasticity can be understood from the general stress-strain diagram shown in Fig. 1.25. As shown in Fig. 1.25, let's say the material is loaded beyond the yield point up to the point P. The loading path is shown by the arrowhead directed upward towards point P. Now, if unloading is carried out, it does not follow the same path as in the elastic case. For most of the practical purposes, it is reasonable to consider the unloading process to be purely elastic, it follows a path parallel to the initial straight portion of the stress-strain curve from point P to point Q on the strain axis. It is to be noted that when we load the material up to point P, it comprises both elastic (OY) as well as plastic (YP) portions. While unloading following the path PQ, the elastic deformation, *i.e.*, the elastic part of the strains equal to ε_{QR}^{e} is recovered leaving a permanent set (plastic strain) in the material equal to ε_{OQ}^{p}. Thus, the addition of the plastic and elastic parts of the strains will give the total strain at point P.

1.9.9 Hooke's law

For most of the structural materials, up to certain limit, the stress induced in the bar is proportional to the strain. This simple linear relationship between the stress and strain was first formulated by the English scientist Robert Hooke in 1678 and is named after him. It is popularly known as Hooke's law. Mathematically, Hooke's experimental law can be expressed as

$$\sigma \propto \varepsilon \quad \text{or} \quad \sigma = E\varepsilon, \tag{1.20}$$

where E is the constant of proportionality called the Young's modulus of elasticity.

If P is the tensile pull producing extension δ of the bar, L is the length and A is the cross-sectional area of the bar, then Eq. (1.21) can be expressed as

$$\frac{P}{A} = E\frac{\delta}{L}, \quad \delta = \frac{PL}{AE}. \tag{1.21}$$

In establishing the stress-strain relationship by tensile testing of a bar, we observed that the two points, proportional limit and elastic limit are in the very close vicinity to each other on the stress-strain curve and virtually it is difficult to distinguish these two points. Thus, the proportionality of stress-strain can be considered up to the elastic limit on the stress-strain curve. This extends the validity of Hooke's law approximately up to the elastic limit of the material.

1.9.10 Axial stiffness

For an axially loaded bar shown in Fig. 1.26 (a), if we know the axial pull P, cross-sectional area A, length of the bar L and the material with which the bar is made of (*i.e.*, the modulus of elasticity of the material E), then we can evaluate the amount of axial deformation of the bar using Eq. (1.21). Eq. (1.21) can be rewritten in the following form:

$$\delta = \frac{P}{\frac{AE}{L}}. \tag{1.22}$$

Consider a spring of stiffness k and subjected to a tensile force P as shown in Fig. 1.26 (b). If the material of the spring is linear and elastic, then the extension δ of the spring can be expressed as

$$\delta = \frac{P}{k}. \tag{1.23}$$

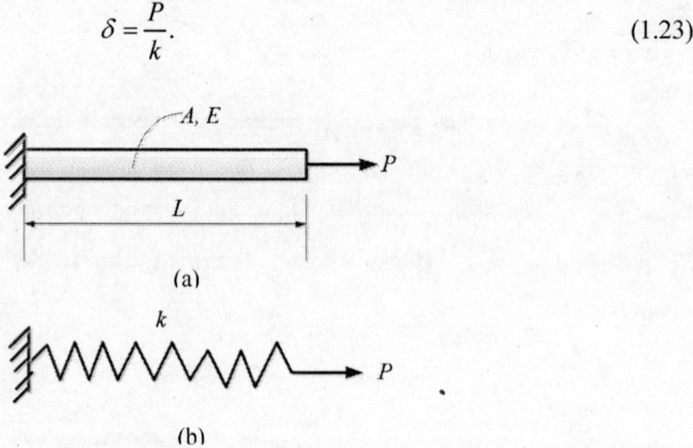

Fig. 1.26 (a) An axially loaded prismatic bar, (b) a linear spring pulled by a load P.

Now, by using the analogy between Eqs. (1.22) and (1.23), one can express the denominator of Eq. (1.22) as

$$k_a = \frac{AE}{L}, \tag{1.24}$$

which is termed as the axial stiffness of the bar. The SI unit of stiffness is N/m. The reciprocal of stiffness is called the flexibility of the bar. The unit of flexibility in SI is m/N.

Example 1.5 Consider the following information for the tensile test of a steel specimen of initial diameter 12 mm and gauge length 56 mm:

A typical load within the elastic range is 24 kN producing a corresponding elongation of 0.06 mm,

The load corresponding to the yield point=33 kN,

The maximum load= 40.5 kN,

Load at fracture = 28 kN,

Minimum diameter after fracture = 6.5 mm,

The gauge length measured at fracture =70.56 mm.

Using the above information, determine,

(a) the Young's modulus of elasticity of the material,

(b) the tensile strength of the material,

(c) the yield strength of the material,

(d) the percentage reduction of area,

(e) the percentage elongation,

(f) the nominal and true stress at fracture.

Solution

(a) It is given that a typical load within the elastic range is 24 kN producing a corresponding elongation of 0.06 mm. Now, for this given data, within the elastic range, we can calculate the stress and strain as

$$\sigma = \frac{24\times10^3}{\frac{\pi}{4}\times12^2} = 212.21\text{ MPa},$$

$$\varepsilon = \frac{0.06}{56} = 0.00107.$$

Thus, the Young's modulus of elasticity (E) is evaluated as

$$E = \frac{\sigma}{\varepsilon} = \frac{212.21}{0.00107} = 198.33\times10^3\text{ MPa} = 198.33\text{ GPa}.$$

(b) The tensile strength or the ultimate tensile stress (σ_u) of the material is

$$\sigma_u = \frac{\text{The maximum load}}{\text{Nominal cross-sectional area}} = \frac{40.5\times10^3}{\frac{\pi}{4}\times12^2} = 358.10\text{ MPa}.$$

(c) Yield strength (σ_Y) of the material is

$$\sigma_Y = \frac{\text{Load at yield point}}{\text{Nominal cross-sectional area}} = \frac{32\times10^3}{\frac{\pi}{4}\times12^2} = 291.78\text{ MPa}.$$

(d) Given original diameter of the specimen, D=12 mm and

Minimum diameter after fracture, d=6.5 mm

Now, the percentage reduction of area is calculated using Eq. (1.19) as

$$\text{Percentage reduction of area} = \frac{\frac{\pi}{4}D^2 - \frac{\pi}{4}d^2}{\frac{\pi}{4}D^2} \times 100$$

$$= \frac{\frac{\pi}{4}\times 12^2 - \frac{\pi}{4}\times 6.5^2}{\frac{\pi}{4}\times 12^2} \times 100 = 70.66\%.$$

(e) The original gauge length of the specimen, L=56 mm and

The gauge length at fracture L_1= 70.56 mm.

Now, the percentage elongation is determined by using Eq. (1.18) as

$$\text{Percentage elongation} = \frac{L_1 - L}{L} \times 100 = \frac{70.56 - 56}{56} \times 100 = 26\%.$$

(f) The nominal stress at fracture, $(\sigma_0)_f$ is

$$(\sigma_0)_f = \frac{\text{Load at fracture}}{\text{nominal cross-sectional area}} = \frac{28 \times 10^3}{\frac{\pi}{4}\times 12^2} = 247.57 \text{ MPa}.$$

The true stress at fracture, σ_f is

$$\sigma_f = \frac{\text{Load at fracture}}{\text{reduced cross-sectional area}} = \frac{28 \times 10^3}{\frac{\pi}{4}\times 6.5^2} = 843.80 \text{ MPa}.$$

Example 1.6 Yield strength of a steel rod is 200 MPa. If the Young's modulus of elasticity is 200 GPa. What is the maximum strain in a tensile test to keep the rod in elastic state?

Solution

As we know that, the maximum strain to keep the rod in elastic state, $(\varepsilon) = \frac{\sigma_y}{E}$,

where σ_y is the yield strength and E is the modulus of elasticity.

Hence, the maximum strain, $\varepsilon = \frac{200}{200 \times 10^3} = 0.001.$

Example 1.7 Determine the total deformation of an aluminium bar with circular cross-section of diameter 6 mm and length 20 m, subjected to an axial load of 250 N. Take the Young's modulus of elasticity of aluminium as E=70 GPa. Also, determine the axial stiffness of the bar.

Solution

Given: diameter of the bar, d=6 mm, length, L=20 m, axial load, P=250 N, E=70 GPa.

The total deformation of the bar, $\delta = \frac{PL}{AE} = \frac{250 \times 20}{\frac{\pi}{4} \times (0.006)^2 \times 70 \times 10^9} = 2.53 \times 10^{-3}\ \text{m} = 2.53\,\text{mm}.$

Axial stiffness of the bar, $k_a = \frac{P}{\delta} = \frac{250}{2.53 \times 10^{-3}} = 98.81$ kN/m.

Example 1.8 Refer to the true stress-strain diagram for an aluminum alloy as shown obtained from an uniaxial tensile test of a specimen of circular cross-section. Note in the stress-strain diagram that the specimen of this material is stressed to 560 MPa (point B), determine the plastic strain in the material when it is unloaded to point C following a path BC parallel to the initial elastic portion OA.

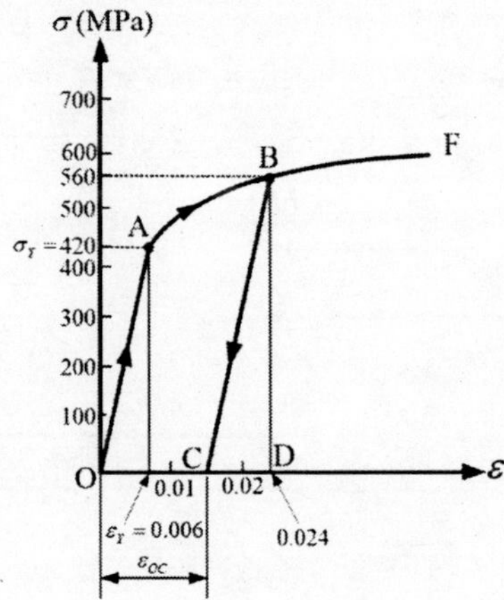

Solution

From the given stress-strain diagram of the aluminium alloy, the material remains elastic up to point A, where the stress level is σ_Y = 420 MPa. The corresponding strain at point A is 0.006. The slope of the lone OA will provide the Young's modulus of elasticity of the material (E). Thus,

$$E = \text{Slope of line OA} = \frac{\sigma_Y}{\varepsilon_Y} = \frac{420}{0.006} = 70 \text{ GPa}.$$

When the material is loaded to point B, it strain hardens initiating from point A. The stress corresponding to point B is 560 MPa and the corresponding total strain is 0.024 (point D). The unloading is taking place along the path BC parallel to OA. Thus, the line BC has the same slope as OA. The recovered elastic strain after unloading (*CD*) is then obtained from the slope of line BC as

$$\text{Slope of line BC} = \frac{BD}{CD} = E,$$

$$\frac{560}{CD} = 70 \times 10^3, \; CD = 0.008.$$

The total strain at point D is the additive decomposition of both the elastic part (CD) and plastic part (OC) of strains. Thus, the plastic part of the strain OC is obtained as

$$OC = 0.024 - CD = 0.024 - 0.008 = 0.016.$$

Example 1.9 Consider a bar of length L subjected to a uniaxial pull to elongate it to a final length of $2L$ (Case I). Now, the same elongated bar is subjected to a uniaxial push to bring it back to its original length L (Case II). During this entire procedure, what is the net engineering strain and net true strain induced in the bar? From the obtained solutions, comment which strain is a real measure of strain, engineering strain or true strain?

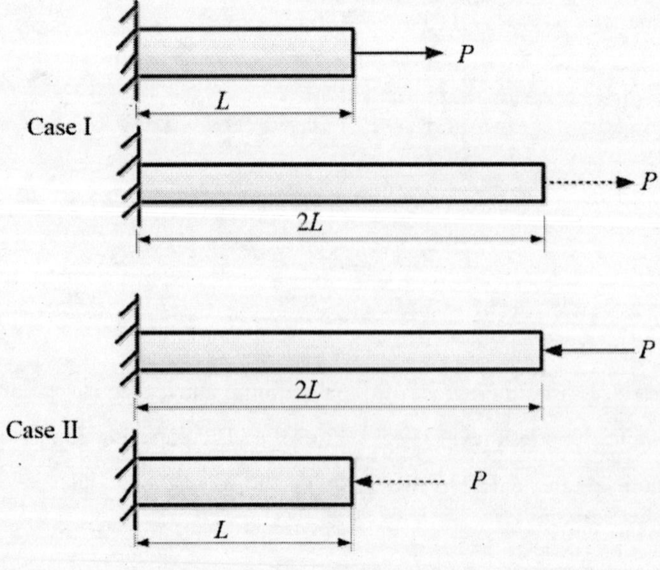

Solution

Case I (intermediate elongation):

Engineering strain, $e = \frac{2L - L}{L} = 1.$

True strain, $\varepsilon = \ln\left(\frac{2L}{L}\right) = \ln 2.$

Case II (Final compression):

Engineering strain, $e = \frac{L - 2L}{2L} = -0.5.$

True strain, $\varepsilon = \ln\left(\frac{L}{2L}\right) = -\ln 2.$

Now, the net engineering strain in the bar, $e_{net} = 1 - 0.5 = 0.5.$

The net true strain in the bar, $\varepsilon_{net} = \ln 2 - \ln 2 = 0.$

Thus, it can be seen that when the deformations are large, the engineering strain provides an erroneous measurement of strain; however, the true strain provides the actual measure of strain.

1.10 St. Venant's principle

In considering the stresses in an axially loaded bar, we assumed that the normal stresses are uniformly distributed in any section perpendicular to the axis of the bar. This kind of assumption is not true in the immediate vicinity of the point of application of load. If we consider a bar subjected to tension as shown in Fig. 1.7 (a), then in the immediate vicinity of the point of application of load the stress is highly localized and not uniform as shown in Fig. 1.27. very near to the load application point, the actual stress is much larger than P/A. However, it is observed that at a certain distance away from the point of application of load, the stress induced in the bar is uniform everywhere equal to P/A. This indicates that the assumption of uniform stress is true anywhere in the bar away from the point of application of load and the stress state is unaffected by the precise manner in which the load is applied at the ends (*e.g.*, one may grip the ends of the bar and pull the bar as in the case of tensile test, one may make a hole at the end and insert a hook to pull the bar, etc.) so long as the resultant load P is unchanged. This observation was first made by St. Venant in 1855 and is known as St. Venant's principle. The principle of St. Venant can be stated as follows: "*Stress distribution can be assumed to be independent of the mode of load application except in the immediate vicinity of load application points so long as the resultant load remains the same*".

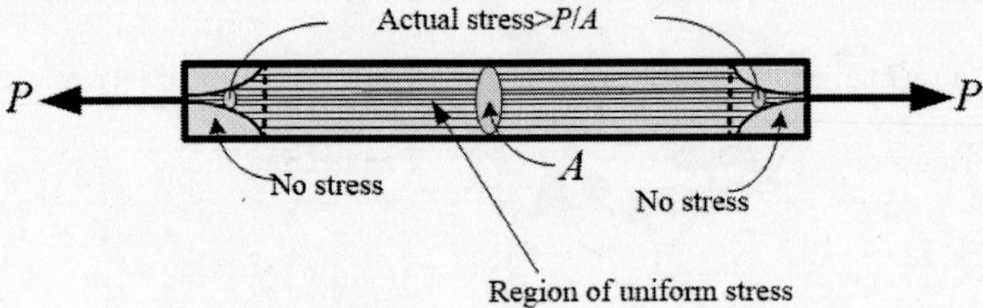

Fig. 1.27 Highly localized stress distribution in a bar in the immediate vicinity of the load application point due to St. Venant.

1.11 Working Stress and Factor of Safety

In designing a structural or machine component, it is important to safeguard the component against the maximum stress that it can withstand without failure. It is desirable to restrict the stress level in the component in its service within a certain limit corresponding to the suitable strength criterion (the maximum stress at failure such as yield stress or ultimate stress) of the component material. This is crucial to the design of the component such that it can perform its intended design function during its service. The value of stress in the component, which is set to work at a stress less than the specified maximum stress at failure is usually termed as the working stress or allowable stress.

It is now understood that no structural or machine component is designed to bear the maximum stress that it can withstand. Every designer follows a more conservative approach and wants to keep the stress level in the component well below its maximum strength. This is to take into account for the uncertainties in loading conditions on the component in the actual working environment, manufacturing faults, material deficiency and assembly stresses that may affect the actual performance of the component. In order the safeguard the component against all such untoward situations, designers usually incorporate a safety factor in their design called as factor of safety (Fos) and is given by

$$F_{OS} = \frac{\text{Maximum stress limit at failure}}{\text{Working stress}}. \tag{1.22}$$

If one wants safeguard the component against yielding, that means the plastic deformation is not all desirable by design, Eq. (1.22) can be modified as

$$F_{OS} = \frac{\text{Yield stress}}{\text{Working stress}}. \tag{1.23}$$

If the design is based on the tensile strength of the material, the factor of safety can be modified accordingly by replacing maximum stress at failure in the numerator by the ultimate stress. The value of factor of safety must be greater than 1 in order to safeguard the component against potential failure.

Example 1.10 Referring back to Example Problem 1.1, find out the required diameter of the bar in order withstand a load of 50 kN. The yield stress of steel =205 MPa. Use a factor of safety =1.5 against yielding.

Solution

Given, Yield stress, σ_Y=205 MPa, factor of safety, Fos=1.5.

Now, allowable working stress, $\sigma_{allowable} = \frac{\sigma_Y}{F_{OS}} = \frac{205}{1.5} = 136.67\,\text{MPa}$.

Let us assume that the required diameter of the bar to withstand a load P=50 N is d. Then we can write

$$\sigma_{allowable} = \frac{P}{A} = \frac{P}{\frac{\pi}{4}d^2},$$

$$136.67 = \frac{50\times10^3}{\frac{\pi}{4}d^2}, \quad d = 21.58 \text{ mm}.$$

Thus, the required minimum diameter of the steel bar to withstand a load of 50 kN is obtained as d=21.58 mm.

1.12 Lateral Strain

If a bar is stretched by an axial force, there is contraction in the transverse or lateral dimensions. For example, if we consider a rectangular bar fixed at one end and the other is pulled by applying a tensile load P, it gets extended by an amount δ as shown in Fig. 1.28. While stretching, the bar also experiences an effective uniform contraction in all lateral directions as depicted in Fig. 1.28, *i.e.*, there is reduction in the width and thickness of the bar. If we now define a quantity by taking either the ratio of change in width to the original width or the change in thickness to the original thickness, we call that quantity as the lateral strain. For a uniform tension of an isotropic material, the lateral or transverse strain (ε_l) in the width and thickness directions of the bar is the same. Thus,

$$\varepsilon_t = -\frac{\Delta b}{b} = -\frac{\Delta t}{t}, \tag{1.24}$$

where Δb is the reduction in width and Δt is the reduction in thickness of the bar when stretched. The negative sign in Eq. (1.24) indicates the contractions in the respective lateral dimensions. Instead of a rectangular bar, if we consider a bar of circular cross-section with diameter d and pull it, then the bar is subjected to diametral contraction in the transverse direction. If the diametral contraction is taken as Δd, the lateral strain, in that case, is given by

$$\varepsilon_t = -\frac{\Delta d}{d}. \tag{1.25}$$

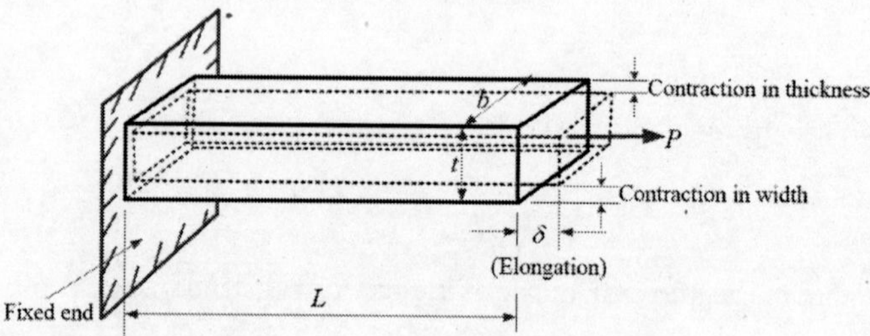

Fig. 1.28 A rectangular bar subjected to lateral contractions in its width and thickness while pulling by a load P.

1.13 Poisson's Ratio

For stress within proportional limit, Poisson demonstrated that the ratio of the transverse strain (ε_t) to the axial strain (ε_a) is constant. This constant is called Poisson's ratio. It is denoted by ν and can be expressed as follows:

$$\nu = -\frac{\varepsilon_t}{\varepsilon_a}. \tag{1.26}$$

The Poisson's ratio is usually positive for engineering materials. As the lateral strain experienced by material is negative, the expression of Poisson's ratio (ν) is accompanied by a negative sign so that one arrives at a positive value of ν. There are some materials that expand in the lateral direction when stretched, *e.g.*, polymer foams. As both the axial and lateral strains are positive, it follows from Eq. (1.26) that the Poisson's ratio of such materials is negative. There are also certain materials that do not deform in the transverse direction upon stretching. Thus, those materials possess zero Poisson's ratio. One such material is cork.

Referring back to Fig. 1.28, the bar of length L undergoes a deformation δ in the axial direction while pulling by a load P. Thus the axial strain in this case is given by,

$$\varepsilon_a = \frac{\delta}{L}. \tag{1.27}$$

The lateral strain in the bar is given by Eq. (1.24). Thus, the Poisson's ratio for the present case can be given by either

$$\nu = -\frac{-\frac{\Delta b}{b}}{\frac{\delta}{L}} = \frac{\frac{\Delta b}{b}}{\frac{\delta}{L}}, \text{ or } \nu = -\frac{-\frac{\Delta t}{t}}{\frac{\delta}{L}} = \frac{\frac{\Delta t}{t}}{\frac{\delta}{L}}. \tag{1.28}$$

Example 1.11 Consider an aluminium rod of diameter 8 mm is subjected to a uniaxial tension of 2000 N within the elastic range. As a result, the diameter of the rod is decreased by a value of 0.0013 mm. If the Young's modulus of elasticity of the aluminium rod is 70 GPa, determine the lateral strain and Poisson's ratio of the material.

Solution

Given, diameter of the rod, d=8 mm.

Axial tension, P=2000 N.

Young's modulus of elasticity, E=70 GPa.

Change in diameter of the rod, Δd=0.0013 mm.

Stress induced by a load of 2000 N in the rod is $\sigma = \frac{P}{A} = \frac{2000}{\frac{\pi}{4}\times 8^2} = 39.79\,\text{MPa}.$

From Hooke's law, axial or longitudinal strain, $\varepsilon_a = \frac{\sigma}{E} = \frac{39.79}{70\times 10^3} = 0.00057.$

The lateral or transverse strain induced in the rod, $\varepsilon_t = -\frac{\Delta d}{d} = -\frac{0.0013}{8} = -0.000162.$

Therefore, Poisson's ratio, $\nu = -\frac{\varepsilon_t}{\varepsilon_a} = -\frac{-0.000162}{0.00057} = 0.284.$

1.14 Modulus of Rigidity

In the case of an axial pull applied to a bar, we observed that up to the proportional limit, stress is directly proportional to strain. In a similar way, when a body is under the action of shear force, within the proportional limit, shear stress (τ) is directly proportional to the shear strain (γ). Mathematically,

$$\tau \propto \gamma,$$

$$\tau = G\gamma, \tag{1.29}$$

where G is the constant of proportionality known as the modulus of rigidity or shear modulus. It has the unit of stress.

1.15 Biaxial and triaxial state of stress

So far we are familiar with the uniaxial stress, wherein the stress acts in a body only in one direction. For example, the stress induced in any section of a bar due to an axial tension. In this section, we will introduce some more types of stress states that may exist in a body such as bi-axial and tri-axial states of stress.

If two mutually perpendicular normal stresses act on a body, it is termed as the state of biaxial stress. The state of biaxial stress can be easily represented using a two-dimensional rectangular element sliced out from a loaded body in Cartesian x-y coordinate system as shown in Fig. 1.29 (a). The stress on the face normal to the x-axis is represented as σ_x and the stress on the face normal to the y-axis is represented as σ_y. Similarly, if three normal stresses act on the three mutually perpendicular faces of a body, it is referred as the triaxial state of stress. The triaxial state of stress is shown in Fig. 1.29 (b) on a cube element sliced out from a loaded body. The normal stresses σ_x, σ_y and σ_z acts on the three faces of the cube, which are perpendicular to the x, y and z-axis, respectively.

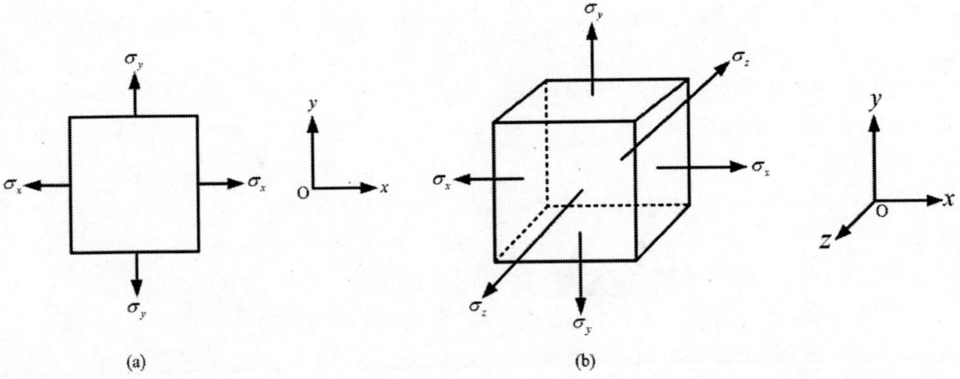

Fig. 1.29 State of stress with no shear stresses: (a) Biaxial stress state, (b) Triaxial stress state

1.16 Hydrostatic stress

The state of hydrostatic stress in a body is the state of uniform tensile or compressive stress acting on all directions. The state of hydrostatic stress is shown in Fig. 1.30 acting on a rectangular cube element. The effect of hydrostatic stress is to change the volume of the body. This gives rise to the concept of another strain, called volumetric strain. The hydrostatic stress can also be called as the volumetric stress as it tends to change the volume of a body and is given by the average of the normal stresses acting in *x*, *y* and *z*- directions in a Cartesian coordinate frame. Next, we will discuss the volumetric strain.

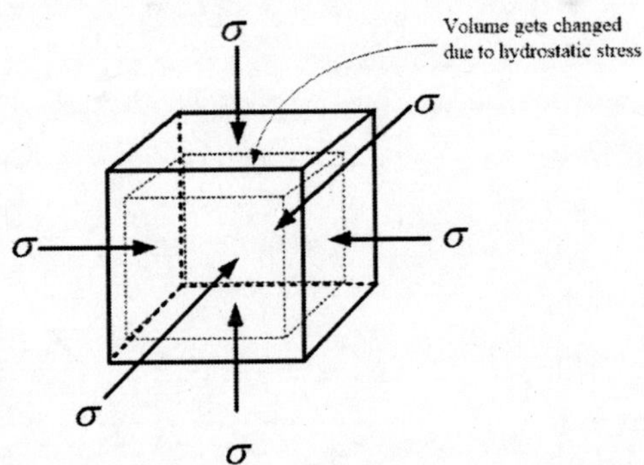

Fig. 1.30 State of compressive hydrostatic stress

1.16.1 Volumetric strain

Normal stresses acting on the body tend to change its volume. If this change in volume is expressed per unit of the original volume of the body, then it is called as the volumetric strain. It is denoted by ε_V and given by

$$\varepsilon_V = \frac{\text{Change in volume}}{\text{Original volume}} = \frac{\Delta V}{V}. \tag{1.30}$$

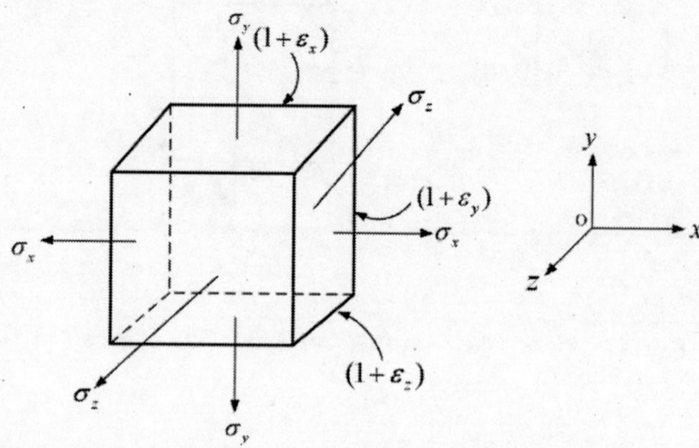

Fig. 1.31 A rectangular cube element of unit initial volume subjected to normal stresses in all directions.

Now, to obtain an expression for volumetric strain, let us consider a cube element of a homogeneous isotropic material as shown in Fig. 1.31. let us say the in its unstressed state, the volume of this cube element is unity, i.e. V_0=1 and its each side is of unit length. The cube element gets deformed into a rectangular parallelepiped under the action of normal stresses σ_x, σ_y and σ_z. The volume of the deformed shape becomes

$$V = (1+\varepsilon_x)(1+\varepsilon_y)(1+\varepsilon_z), \tag{1.31}$$

where ε_x, ε_y and ε_z are the strains in *x*, *y* and *z* directions respectively, which also indicate the change in length in the respective directions for the present case. Since ε_x, ε_y and ε_z are much smaller than unity, Eq. (1.31) reduces to

$$V = 1+\varepsilon_x+\varepsilon_y+\varepsilon_z. \tag{1.32}$$

Now, change in volume is given by

$$\Delta V = V - V_o = 1+\varepsilon_x+\varepsilon_y+\varepsilon_z - 1 = \varepsilon_x+\varepsilon_y+\varepsilon_z. \tag{1.33}$$

Using Eq. (1.30), the volumetric strain is obtained as

$$\varepsilon_V = \varepsilon_x+\varepsilon_y+\varepsilon_z. \tag{1.34}$$

The value given by Eq. (1.34) is called the dilatation of the material.

1.16.2 Bulk modulus

As a special case of interest, let us say the cube element of Fig. 1.31 is subjected to uniform hydrostatic pressure p. Now, the element is under the action of a triaxial compressive stress (state of hydrostatic stress) given by

$$\sigma_x = \sigma_y = \sigma_z = \sigma = -p. \tag{1.35}$$

The stress given by Eq. (1.35) is the volumetric stress that causes a volumetric strain ε_V. Within the proportional limit, the volumetric strain is directly proportional to the volumetric stress. Thus,

$$\varepsilon_V \propto (-p),$$

$$p = -K\varepsilon_V, \tag{1.36}$$

where K is the constant of proportionality known as the bulk modulus of the material. The reciprocal of bulk modulus of elasticity is called compressibility. The unit of bulk modulus is expressed in the unit of stress.

1.17 Elastic Moduli

In studying the elastic behaviour of homogeneous isotropic materials under normal, shear and hydrostatic loading we came across a total of four different elastic constants, *viz.*, Young's modulus of elasticity (E), Poisson's ratio (ν), modulus of rigidity (G) and bulk modulus (K). Rewriting Eqs. (1.20), (1.29) and (1.36), the different elastic moduli can be expressed as follows within the proportional limit:

$$E = \frac{\sigma}{\varepsilon}, \tag{1.37}$$

$$G = \frac{\tau}{\gamma}, \tag{1.38}$$

$$K = -\frac{p}{\varepsilon_V}. \tag{1.39}$$

The expression for Poisson's ratio (ν) is given by Eq. (1.26). It is to be noted that, not all of these four elastic constants are independent. Given any two of the elastic constants, the other two can be obtained using certain relations among them. Thus, there are only two independent elastic constants. We will establish a relationship among the elastic constants in Unit 2, as it requires an understanding of compound stresses and strains.

Example 1.12 A steel cube of side 60 mm has its bottom face fixed to the ground. Consider a tangential force of 100 kN is applied to the upper face of the cube, which causes it to displace by 0.02 mm. The block remains in the proportional range during deformation. Determine the modulus of rigidity of the cube.

Solution

Tangential force applied to the upper face, V= 100 kN=100×10^3 N.

Area on which the tangential force is distributed, A=60×60=3600 mm^2.

Thus, shear stress, $\tau = \frac{V}{A} = \frac{100\times10^3}{3600} = 27.78$ MPa.

The shear strain for the present case is given by

$$\gamma = \tan^{-1}\left(\frac{-0.02}{60}\right)\times\frac{\pi}{180} = 3.33\times10^{-4} \text{ rad.}$$

Now, the modulus of rigidity of the steel cube,

$$G = \frac{\tau}{\gamma} = \frac{27.78}{3.33\times10^{-4}} = 83.42\times10^3 \text{ MPa=83.42 GPa.}$$

Example 1.13 A rectangular block is subjected to compression from all directions as shown. Find the volumetric stress and change in volume of the block after deformation. Also, calculate the bulk modulus of the block material. Take the associated strains in the x, y and z-directions as ε_x= -0.378×10^{-6}, ε_y= 0.185×10^{-6}, ε_z= -0.226×10^{-6}.

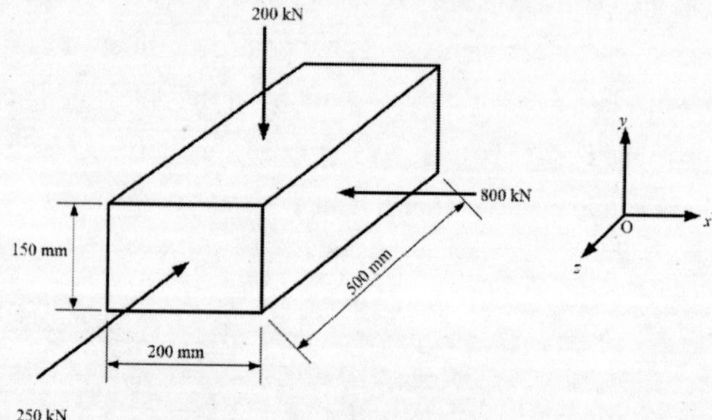

Solution

With reference to the given Cartesian coordinate frame of reference,

The compressive stress in the x, y and z- directions are calculated as,

$$\sigma_x = -\frac{800\times10^3}{500\times150} = -10.67\text{MPa,}$$

$$\sigma_y = -\frac{200\times10^3}{500\times200} = -2\text{MPa,}$$

$$\sigma_z = -\frac{250\times10^3}{200\times150} = -8.33\text{MPa.}$$

Therefore, the volumetric stress is given by the average of the above stresses. Thus, volumetric stress,

$$\sigma_V = \frac{\sigma_x + \sigma_y + \sigma_z}{3} = \frac{-10.67 - 2 - 8.33}{3} = -7\,\text{MPa}.$$

Given, the associated strains in the x, y and z-directions as $\varepsilon_x = -0.378\times10^{-6}$, $\varepsilon_y = 0.185\times10^{-6}$ and

$\varepsilon_z = -0.226\times10^{-6}$. Thus, volumetric strain is

$$\varepsilon_V = \varepsilon_x + \varepsilon_y + \varepsilon_z = (-0.378 + 0.185 - 0.226)\times10^{-6} = -0.419\times10^{-6}.$$

Now, using Eq. (1.30), the change in volume is obtained as

$$\Delta V = \varepsilon_V \times V = (-0.419\times10^{-6})\times(500\times200\times150) = -6.285\ \text{mm}^3,$$

where negative sign indicates the change in volume due to the volumetric stress.

The bulk modulus of the material, $K = \frac{\sigma_V}{\varepsilon_V} = \frac{-7}{-0.419\times10^{-6}} = 1.67\times10^4\ \text{GPa}.$

1.18 Bars of Varying Section

Till now we obtained the stresses and strains in a prismatic bar subjected to simple loading. In this section, we will consider bars of varying cross-section subjected to uniaxial loading and determine the stresses and deformations. First, we will consider the case of stepped bars and then bars of gradually varying cross section under axial loading and analyse the stresses and strains induced in such bars.

1.18.1 Stresses and deformations in stepped bars

Let us consider a bar with variable cross sections (stepped bar) as shown in Fig. 1.32 (a). It consists of three different segments- AB, BC and CD with different cross-sectional areas, A_1, A_2 and A_3, and lengths L_1, L_2, L_3, respectively. The entire bar is made up of the same material with Young's modulus of elasticity E. The bar is subjected to axial forces of P_1, P_2, P_3 and P_4 at points A, B, C and D respectively.

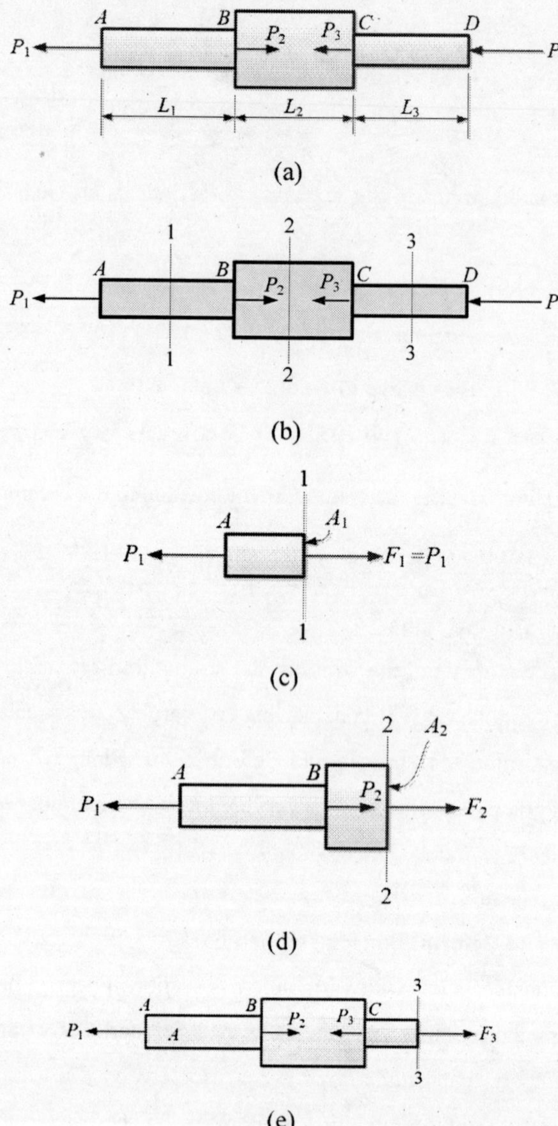

Fig. 1.32 An example of stresses and deformation in stepped bar: (a)A stepped bar with different cross-sectional areas subjected to axial load, (b) the stepped bar showing the different cutting planes, (c) FBD of the left cut section of the bar when a cut is taken on the segment AB, (c) FBD of the left cut section of the segment of the bar when a cut is taken on the segment BC and (d) FBD of the left cut section of the segment of the bar when a cut is taken on the segment CD.

Let us draw the free body diagram (FBD) of each of the segments taking an imaginary internal cut as shown in Fig. 1.32 (b) to find out the internal forces in each segment. Considering a cutting plane 1-1 in the segment AB, the FBD of the left side of the cut section is shown in Fig. 1.32 (c). The equilibrium requirement of this cut section provides that this section is subjected to an internal force of $F_1 = P_1$. Thus, the strain in the segment AB is given by

$$\varepsilon_{AB} = \frac{P_1}{A_1 E},$$

$$\frac{\delta_{AB}}{L_1} = \frac{P_1}{A_1 E}, \tag{1.40}$$

where δ_{AB} is the axial deformation of the segment AB. From Eq. (1.40),

$$\delta_{AB} = \frac{P_1 L_1}{A_1 E}. \tag{1.41}$$

Next, we consider a cutting plane 2-2 in the segment BC and the FBD of the left side of the cut section of the bar is shown in Fig. 1.32 (d). The equilibrium requirement provides that the segment BC is subjected to an internal force,

$$F_2 = P_1 - P_2. \tag{1.42}$$

If δ_{BC} is the extension of the bar segment BC due to load F_2, then

$$\delta_{BC} = \frac{(P_1 - P_2) L_2}{A_2 E}. \tag{1.43}$$

Similarly, by taking an internal cut 3-3 in the segment CD and considering the FBD of the left side of the cut section of the bar (Fig. 1.32(e)), we get the internal force in Section CD as

$$F_3 = P_1 + P_3 - P_2. \tag{1.44}$$

Thus, the extension of the bar segment CD due to load F_3 is given by

$$\delta_{CD} = \frac{(P_1 + P_3 - P_2) L_3}{A_3 E}. \tag{1.45}$$

Now, the total extension of the bar can be computed as

$$\delta_{Net} = \delta_{AB} + \delta_{BC} + \delta_{CD},$$

$$\delta_{Net} = \frac{P_1 L_1}{A_1 E} + \frac{(P_1 - P_2) L_2}{A_2 E} + \frac{(P_1 + P_3 - P_2) L_3}{A_3 E}. \tag{1.46}$$

If the bar is composed of n number of segments of different materials with different lengths and uniform cross-sections, then Eq. (1.46) can be recast into the following general form to obtain the net axial deformation of the bar:

$$\delta_{Net} = \sum_{i=1}^{n} \frac{P_i L_i}{A_i E_i}. \tag{1.47}$$

The stress induced in the different segment of the bar is different as different uniform stepped segment has a different cross-sectional area and are subjected to different internal load. The stresses in different segments (AB, BC and CD) of the stepped bar can be obtained as follows:

$$\sigma_{AB} = \frac{F_1}{A_1} = \frac{P_1}{A_1}, \tag{1.48}$$

$$\sigma_{BC} = \frac{F_2}{A_2} = \frac{P_1 - P_2}{A_1}, \tag{1.49}$$

$$\sigma_{CD} = \frac{F_3}{A_3} = \frac{P_1 + P_3 - P_2}{A_1}. \tag{1.50}$$

It is to be noted that the expressions for stresses in the prismatic segments AB, BC and CD given by Eqs. (1.48)–(1.50) are not valid in the vicinity of the load application points as well as in the vicinity of abrupt change in cross-sectional areas of the bar. At other places, they provide a fairly good estimate thanks Saint-Venant's principle.

1.18.2 Stresses and deformations in axially loaded bars of gradually varying cross-section

Contrary to the axially loaded prismatic bar discussed in Section 1.3, let us consider a bar with a gradually varying cross section subjected to an axial pull as shown in Fig. 1.33. We assume that the area of the cross section of the bar is varying linearly between A_1 and A_2 over the length of the bar L. The cross section of the bar can be circular, where diameter could be varying over the length or it can be rectangular section with uniform thickness, where the cross-sectional area is varying due to gradual changes in its width over the length of the bar.

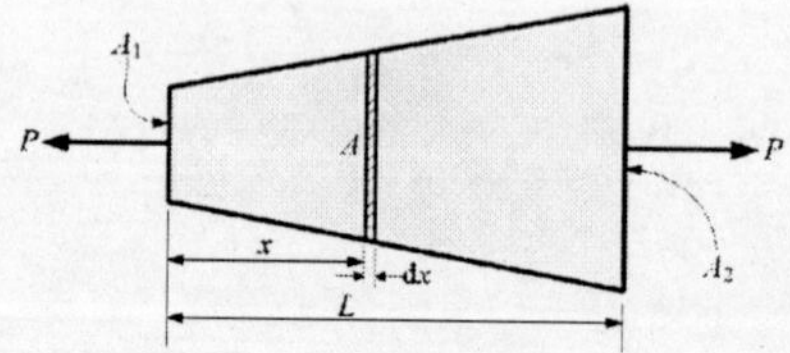

Fig. 1.33 An axially loaded bar of gradually varying cross-section

Let us take an infinitesimal element of length dx in the bar that undergoes an axial deformation dδ due to load P. The strain in the element is then obtained as

$$\varepsilon = \frac{\mathrm{d}\delta}{\mathrm{d}x},$$

$$\mathrm{d}\delta = \varepsilon \mathrm{d}x. \tag{1.51}$$

Using the basic definition of axial strain ε, one can recast Eq. (1.51) in the following form

$$\mathrm{d}\delta = \frac{P}{AE}\mathrm{d}x, \tag{1.52}$$

where E is the material constant, the Young's modulus of elasticity and A is the cross-sectional area which is varying over the length and thus, is a function of x. The net axial deformation experienced by the bar over the entire length L can be obtained by integrating Eq. (1.52) as

$$\delta = \int_0^L \frac{P}{A(x)E}\mathrm{d}x. \tag{1.53}$$

An example: Gradually varying bar of circular cross-section

As a simple case, if we consider the cross-section of the bar to be circular with diameters varying from d_1 to d_2 over the length L as shown in Fig. 1.34, then the diameter d of the bar at a distance x from the left end is given by

$$d = d_1 + \left(\frac{d_2 - d_1}{2}\right)\left(\frac{x}{L}\right) \times 2,$$

$$d = d_1 + (d_2 - d_1)\left(\frac{x}{L}\right), \tag{1.54}$$

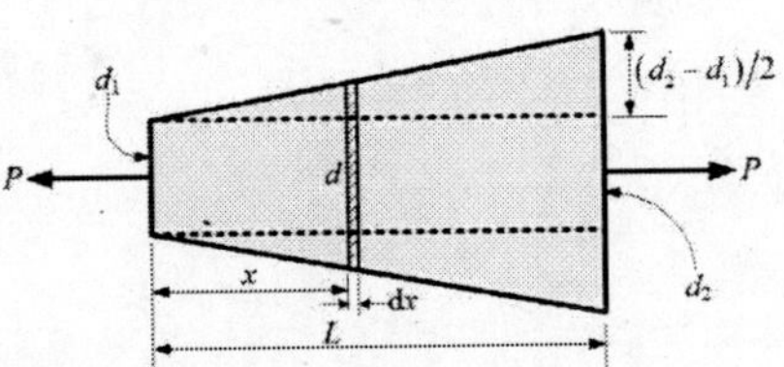

Fig. 1.34 Axially loaded bar with varying circular cross-section

The cross-sectional area of the bar segment of length dx is given by

$$A(x) = \frac{\pi}{4}d^2 = \frac{\pi}{4}\left\{d_1 + (d_2 - d_1)\left(\frac{x}{L}\right)\right\}^2. \tag{1.55}$$

Now, substituting Eq. (1.55) in Eq. (1.53), the deformation in the bar can be computed as follows:

$$\delta = \int_0^L \frac{P}{A(x)E} \mathrm{d}x$$

$$\delta = \frac{P}{E} \int_0^L \frac{\mathrm{d}x}{\frac{\pi}{4}\left\{d_1 + (d_2 - d_1)\left(\frac{x}{L}\right)\right\}^2},$$

$$\delta = \frac{4P}{\pi E} \int_0^L \frac{\mathrm{d}x}{\left\{d_1 + (d_2 - d_1)\left(\frac{x}{L}\right)\right\}^2}. \tag{1.56}$$

Let

$$d_1 + (d_2 - d_1)\left(\frac{x}{L}\right) = c. \tag{1.57}$$

Taking the derivative of Eq. (1.57) with respect to x,

$$\frac{\mathrm{d}c}{\mathrm{d}x} = \frac{d_2 - d_1}{L},$$

$$\mathrm{d}x = \left(\frac{L}{d_2 - d_1}\right)\mathrm{d}c. \tag{1.58}$$

The limit of the integral Eq. (1.56) with the change of the variable is changed as follows: when $x = 0,\ c = d_1$ and when $x = L,\ c = d_2$. Now, the integral Eq. (1.56) in terms of the changed variable can be expressed and evaluated as

$$\delta = \frac{4P}{\pi E} \int_{d_1}^{d_2} \left(\frac{L}{d_2 - d_1}\right)\frac{\mathrm{d}c}{c^2},$$

$$= \frac{4P}{\pi E}\left(\frac{L}{d_2 - d_1}\right)\left[\frac{c^{-2+1}}{-2+1}\right]_{d_1}^{d_2},$$

$$= \frac{4P}{\pi E}\left(\frac{L}{d_1 - d_2}\right)\left[\frac{1}{c}\right]_{d_1}^{d_2},$$

$$= \frac{4P}{\pi E}\left(\frac{L}{d_1 - d_2}\right)\left(\frac{1}{d_2} - \frac{1}{d_1}\right),$$

$$\delta = \frac{4PL}{\pi E d_1 d_2}. \tag{1.59}$$

As a special case, if we take $d_1 = d_2 = d$ in Eq. (1.59), it turns out to be the case of deformation in an axially loaded prismatic bar of circular cross-section given by

$$\delta = \frac{4PL}{\pi E d^2}. \tag{1.60}$$

In the present case, the stress induced in the bar is not constant and it is a function of x as the cross-sectional area of the bar is gradually varying along the length. Thus, stress induced at any section as a function of x can be given by

$$\sigma(x) = \frac{P}{A(x)}. \quad (1.61)$$

Example 1.14 A stepped steel bar with two uniform segments of different cross sectional areas subjected to axial loads at different points (B, C and D). Calculate the net deformation in the bar. What is the stress induced in each segment? Take the Young's modulus of elasticity of steel as E=200 GPa.

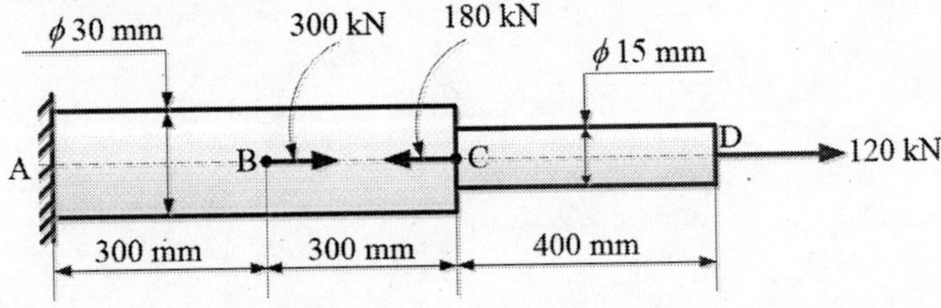

Solution

Considering the axial loading condition, the given bar is divided into three segments–CD, BC and AB. Let us name these segments as 1, 2 and 3 as shown in the figure. The cross-sectional areas of segments 1, 2 and 3 are taken as A_1, A_2 and A_3, respectively. The lengths of the corresponding segments are L_1=400 mm, L_2=300 mm and L_3=300 mm.

Now, in order to determine the internal force in each segment, we take imaginary cuts in each segment and then draw the free body diagram (FBD) of one half of the cut section for each segment. First taking a cut 1-1 in the segment 1 (CD) and then drawing the FBD of the right cut section of the segment, we get the internal force F_1 in the segment from the axial force equilibrium Eq. as F_1=120 kN.

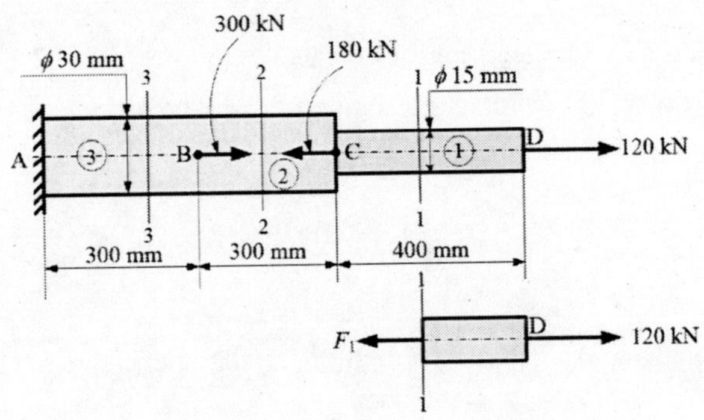

Next, we take an imaginary cut 2-2 in the segment 2 (BC) and we draw the FBD of the right cut half of the segment as

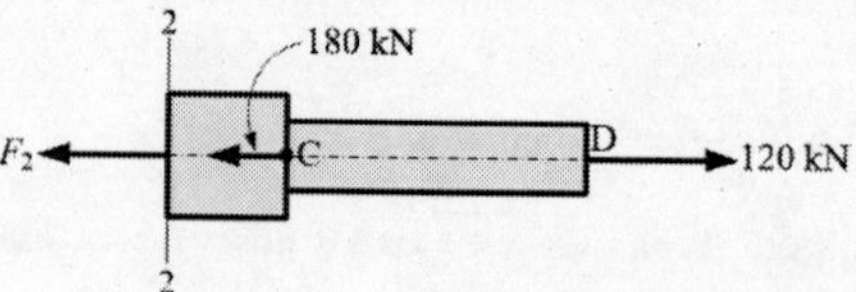

Now, the axial force equilibrium provides the internal force F_2 in the segment as

$$120-180-F_2=0,\quad F_2=-60\text{ kN}.$$

Similarly, by taking a cut 3-3 in the segment 3 (AB) the FBD of the right half of the cut section is shown below:

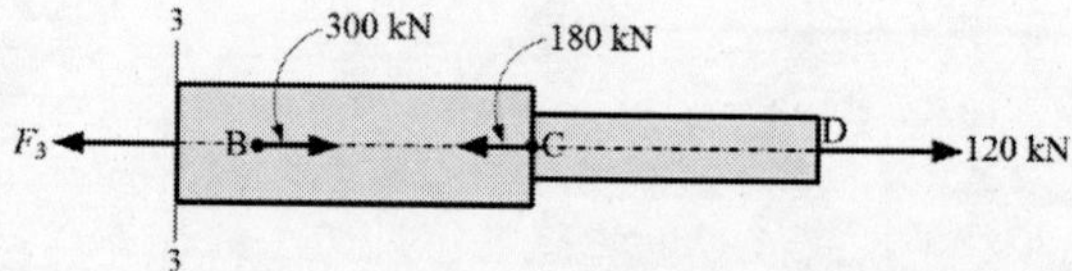

The axial force equilibrium equation provides the internal force F_3 in the segment 3 as

$$120-180+300-F_3=0,\quad F_3=240\text{ kN}.$$

Now, the axial deformation of the bar can be obtained by using Eq. (1.47) as

$$\delta_{Net}=\frac{F_1L_1}{A_1E_1}+\frac{F_2L_2}{A_2E_2}+\frac{F_3L_3}{A_3E_3}.$$

Here, $E_1=E_2=E_3=200$ GPa, as all the segments are composed of the same material. Also, as F_2 is negative (compressive), this will cause the shortening of the corresponding segment. Thus, we get

$$\delta_{Net}=\frac{120\times10^3\times400}{\frac{\pi}{4}\times15^2\times200\times10^3}+\frac{(-60)\times10^3\times300}{\frac{\pi}{4}\times30^2\times200\times10^3}+\frac{240\times10^3\times300}{\frac{\pi}{4}\times30^2\times200\times10^3}=1.74\text{ mm.}$$

The stress induced in each segment is calculated as follows:

$$\sigma_1=\frac{F_1}{A_1}=\frac{120\times10^3}{\frac{\pi}{4}\times15^2}=679.06\,\text{MPa},$$

$$\sigma_2=\frac{F_2}{A_2}=\frac{(-60)\times10^3}{\frac{\pi}{4}\times30^2}=-84.88\,\text{MPa},$$

$$\sigma_3=\frac{F_3}{A_3}=\frac{240\times10^3}{\frac{\pi}{4}\times30^2}=339.53\,\text{MPa}.$$

Example 1.15 The cross-section of a circular rod AB varying gradually from diameter 30 mm to 20 mm is connected to another uniform circular segment BC of diameter 20 mm. The entire rod with segments AB and BC is made of the same material with Young's modulus of elasticity E=200 GPa. The length of the segment AB is 1.5 m and that of the segment BC is 0.5 m. When the rod is subjected to an axial tension of 100 kN, determine the net axial deflection of the rod.

Solution

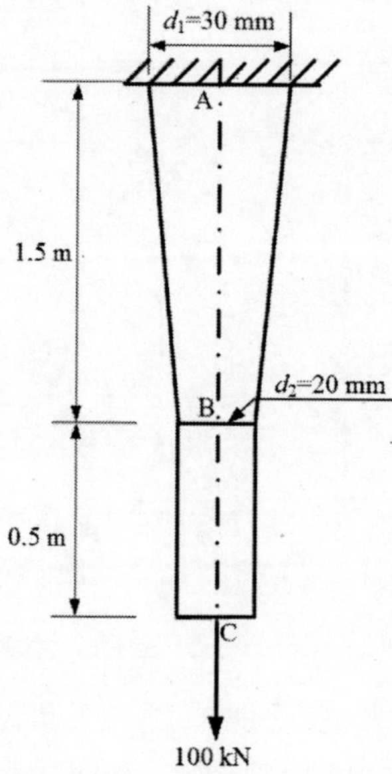

The axial elongation of the gradually varying circular segment AB is given by

$$\delta_{AB} = \frac{4PL_{AB}}{\pi E d_1 d_2}.$$

Here, d_1=30 mm, d_2=20 mm, E=200 GPa, L=1.5 m=1500 mm. Taking a cut in the segment and then using equilibrium of any half of the cut section, the internal force in any of the segments (both AB and BC) is obtained as P=100 kN. Thus,

$$\delta_{AB} = \frac{4\times 100\times 10^3 \times 1500}{\pi \times 200\times 10^3 \times 30\times 20} = 1.59\,\text{mm}.$$

In the uniform segment, BC, the axial elongation is obtained as

$$\delta_{BC} = \frac{PL_{BC}}{AE} = \frac{100\times 10^3 \times 500}{\frac{\pi}{4}\times 20^2 \times 200\times 10^3} = 0.796\,\text{mm}.$$

Thus, the net elongation of the bar is

$$\delta_{Net} = \delta_{AB} + \delta_{BC} = 1.59 + 0.796 = 2.386\,\text{mm}.$$

Know More

1.19 Stresses and Deformation Produced in a Bar Due to its Own Weight

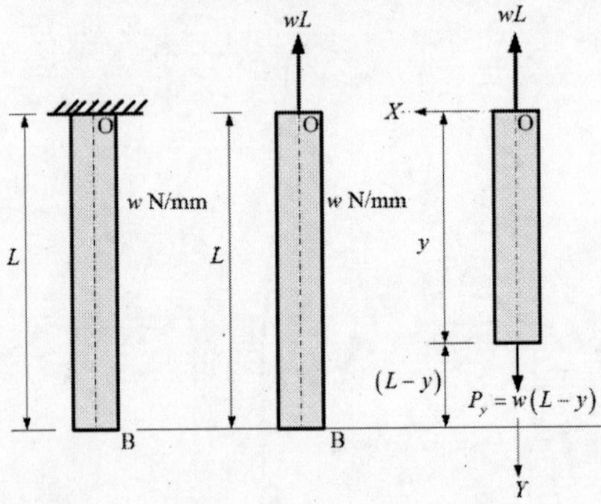

Fig. 1.35 A bar suspended from its top bearing its own weight

Let us consider a bar of length L and cross sectional area of A suspended from its top as shown in Fig. 1.35. The own weight of the bar is taken as w N/mm. The Young's modulus of elasticity of the bar is E. As the entire weight of the bar is supported at its top, the force acting at the built-in upper cross-section is wL. Now, let us take a section at a distance y from the top. At that section, the axial force on the bar as a function of position due to its own weight will be

$$P(y) = w(L - y). \tag{1.62}$$

Now, the stress induced in the bar as a function of position at any section along its length can be computed as

$$\sigma(y) = \frac{P(y)}{A} = \frac{w(L-y)}{A}. \tag{1.63}$$

Let us now proceed to evaluate the deformation produced in the bar. The change in length of the bar at a generic position y can be estimated as,

$$\delta(y) = \int_0^y \frac{P(y)\mathrm{d}y}{AE} = \frac{1}{AE}\int_0^y w(L-y)\mathrm{d}y,$$

$$\delta(y) = \frac{w}{AE}\left(Ly - \frac{y^2}{2}\right). \tag{1.64}$$

The axial deflection of the bar at point B can be obtained by substituting y=L in Eq. (1.64) as

$$\delta(L) = \frac{w}{AE}\left(L^2 - \frac{L^2}{2}\right) = \frac{wL^2}{2AE} = \frac{WL}{2AE}, \tag{1.65}$$

where W=wL is the total weight of the bar.

In addition to the own weight of the bar, if a concentrated axial force P is also acting at point B, then it contributes to an additional deflection of the bar equal to PL/AE. The total deflection δ of the bar at point B is then can be obtained by superposing the deflection due to its own weight and the deflection due to the axial load P under the assumption that the bar is subjected to small elastic deformations. Thus,

$$\delta = \frac{PL}{AE} + \frac{WL}{2AE} = \frac{L}{AE}\left(P + \frac{W}{2}\right). \tag{1.66}$$

This has been done using the principle of superposition.

1.20 The Principle of Superposition

"If the response of a structure is linear, then effects of different loadings can be superposed."

In arriving at the total axial deflection of point B due to the self-weight of the bar and an axial load P acting at point B in Section 1.19 (Eq. (1.66)), we simply added the individual deformations caused by each individual force at point B algebraically. This approach of obtaining the net effect caused by several forces at a point in a solid elastic body is termed as the principle of superposition. A formal statement of principle of superposition can be given as follows: "*If response of materials/structures are linear (elastic materials) and undergo small linear deformations, then effects of different loadings can be superposed.*"

The principle of superposition is a very useful principle of strength of materials, which can be used to obtain the net response at a material point due to several forces acting on a linear elastic body. Although it is a very useful principle, it has certain limitations. The principle of superposition is applicable only when

(i) the material is elastic,

(ii) the material follows a linear stress-strain relationship and

(ii) deformations experienced by the body are small (infinitesimal strain).

The principle of superposition is not valid for non-linear elastic materials.

Example 1.16 Consider an aluminium alloy rod of diameter 40 mm is suspended from its top bearing its own weight. In order to withstand the maximum stress of 450 MPa under its own weight, determine the required length of the rod. Take the density of aluminium alloy rod is 2700 kg/m^3. Also, find out the axial deformation of the rod under its own weight.

Solution

Diameter of the rod d=40 mm.

Therefore, cross-sectional area $A = \frac{\pi}{4} d^2 = \frac{\pi}{4}^2 (40)^2$ mm^2.

Total weight of the rod can be calculated as

$$W = \rho g A L,$$

where ρ is the density of the material, g is the acceleration due to gravity (9.81 m/s^2) and L is the suspended length of the rod. The rod bears its entire weight at the top and thus bears the maximum stress σ_{max}=450 MPa at the top. Thus,

$$\sigma_{max} = \frac{W}{A} = \frac{\rho g A L}{A} = \rho g L,$$

$$450 \times 10^6 = 2700 \times 9.81 \times L,$$

$$L = \frac{450 \times 10^6}{2700 \times 9.81} = 16.99 \approx 17\,\text{m},$$

which is the required length of the rod to bear its own weight.

Now, the axial elongation of the rod of length 17 m under its own weight is estimated using Eq. (1.65) as

$$\delta = \frac{WL}{2AE} = \frac{\rho g A L L}{2AE} = \frac{\rho g L^2}{2E} = \frac{2700 \times 9.81 \times 17^2}{2 \times 200 \times 10^9} = 1.91 \times 10^{-5}\,\text{m} = 0.0191\,\text{mm}.$$

1.21 Axially Loaded Bars: Statically Indeterminate Problems

In all our preceding sections, we obtained the reactive forces and internal forces by employing the equations of equilibrium. Now, if the equilibrium equations are not sufficient to evaluate the reactive/internal forces in a given problem, such types of problems are categorized as the statically indeterminate problems.

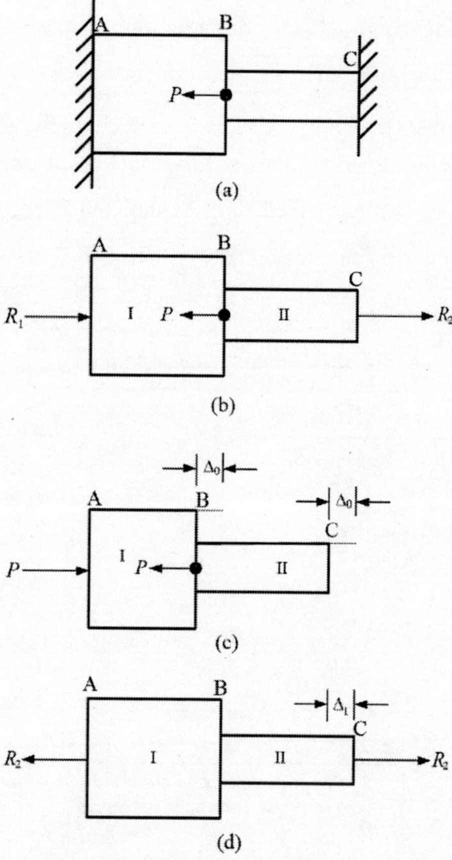

Fig. 1.36 An example of a statically indeterminate structure: (a) A statically indeterminate axially loaded stepped bar, (b) FBD of the stepped bar, (c) Contraction of the bar when reaction R_2 is removed temporarily, (d) extension of the unloaded bar.

As an example, let us consider a problem of an axially loaded stepped bar consisting of two uniform segments of different materials AB and BC fixed between two walls as shown in Fig. 1.36 (a). The axial load P is applied at the junction between the two segments *i.e.* at point B. By drawing the free body diagram as shown in Fig. 1.36 (b), one will find that there are two unknown reactions R_1 and R_2 to be obtained. However, for this problem, one can write only one equation of equilibrium *i.e.*, the force equilibrium equation in the x-direction. This single equilibrium equation is not sufficient to determine the two unknown reactions and the problem turns out to be a statically indeterminate problem. Here, we need one more equation to completely evaluate the unknown reactive forces. Now, the question is from where does this additional equation come? A statically indeterminate problem always has some geometric restrictions imposed on its deformation. When one expresses those geometric restrictions mathematically, one arrives at an equation which is termed as compatibility equation. The compatibility equations will help in determining the unknown reactive forces along with the equilibrium equations. In the procedure of obtaining the unknown reactive forces, the geometric compatibility equations are expressed in terms of forces using Hooke's law. The solution procedure for unknown reactive forces in case of a statically indeterminate problem is represented in terms of a flow chart as shown in Fig. 1.37.

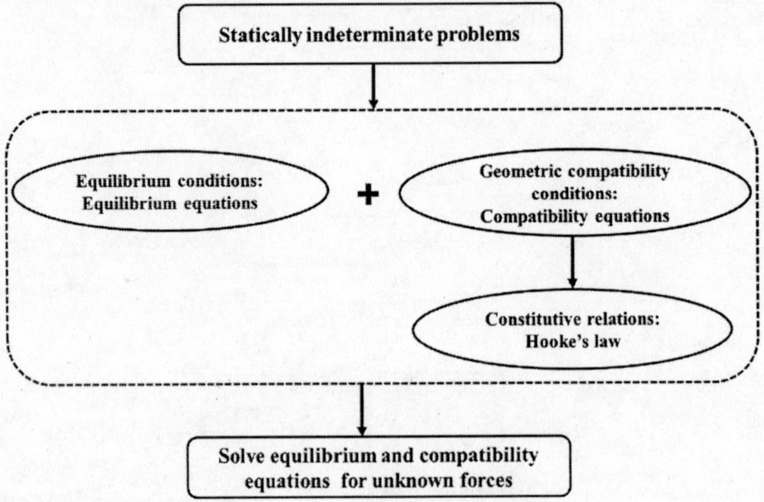

Fig. 1.37 Solution procedure to solve for unknown forces in a statically indeterminate problem

Let us now go back to the problem stated in Fig. 1.36. In order to solve this problem, one of the unknown reactive force (arbitrarily chosen) is temporarily removed making the problem statically determinate. Let's say the reaction R_2 is removed temporarily allowing both the bar segments to deform as shown in Fig. 1.36 (c). The static equilibrium requirement provides that the reaction R_1 becomes equal to P. In this case, only the segment AB is subjected to stress (compressive). Thus, the same axial contraction Δ_0 will produce at point C as that at point B. If A_1 and L_1 are the cross-sectional area and length of the segment AB and E_1 is the Young's modulus of elasticity of the material of the segment AB, then the axial contraction Δ_0 is given by

$$\Delta_0 = -\frac{PL_1}{A_1E_1}, \tag{1.67}$$

where negative sign indicates the contraction. This result violates the geometric boundary condition at C. To offset this, the axial deformation Δ_1 is obtained next caused by the reaction R_2 acting on the unloaded bar as shown in Fig. 1.36 (d). This is caused by stretching of both the bar segments. Thus, the net axial extension of the bar due to R_1 is given by

$$\Delta_1 = \left(\frac{L_1}{A_1 E_1} + \frac{L_2}{A_2 E_2} \right) R_2, \tag{1.68}$$

where A_2 and L_2 are the cross-sectional area and length of the segment BC and E_2 is the Young's modulus of elasticity of the material of the segment BC.

The compatibility requirement of deformation at point C dictates that

$$\Delta_0 + \Delta_1 = 0. \tag{1.69}$$

Substituting Eqs. (1.67) and (1.68) in Eq. (1.69), one obtains

$$-\frac{PL_1}{A_1 E_1} + \left(\frac{L_1}{A_1 E_1} + \frac{L_2}{A_2 E_2} \right) R_2 = 0,$$

$$R_2 = \left(\frac{f_1}{f_1 + f_2} \right) P, \tag{1.70}$$

where f_1 and f_2 are the flexibilities of the segments AB and BC, respectively, given by

$$f_1 = \frac{L_1}{A_1 E_1}, \quad f_2 = \frac{L_2}{A_2 E_2} \tag{1.71}$$

Writing the force equilibrium equation in the x-direction, we get

$$R_1 = P - R_2. \tag{1.72}$$

Substituting the expression for R_2 from Eq. (1.70) in Eq. (1.72), the reaction R_1 is obtained as

$$R_1 = \left(\frac{f_2}{f_1 + f_2} \right) P. \tag{1.73}$$

Example 1.17 A rigid bar AB is supported by a pin at B and by two rods as shown in the figure. Find the stress in each rod. Cross-sectional area of steel rod is 500 mm^2 and that of aluminium rod is 400 mm^2. Neglect the weight of the bar. Take the Young's modulus of elasticity of steel and aluminium as 200 GPa and 70 GPa, respectively.

Solution

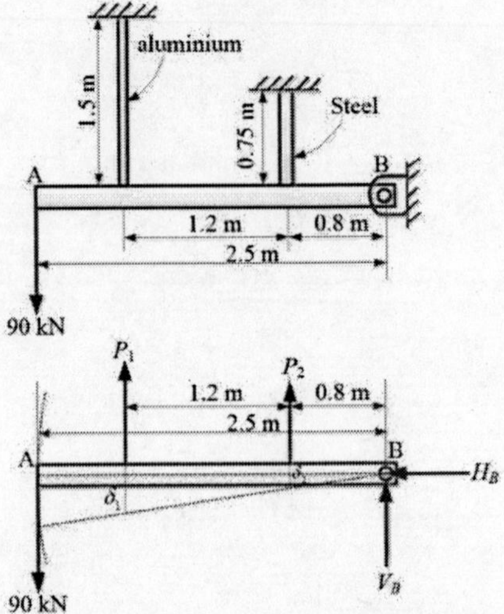

The free body diagram of the system is drawn revealing all the internal forces and support reactions. Now, using the moment equilibrium equation (taking moment about point B):

$$2P_1 + 0.8P_2 = 90\times 10^3 \times 2.5 = 225\times 10^3, \qquad \text{(i)}$$

where P_1 and P_2 are the internal reactive forces acting on the bar provided by the aluminium and the steel rods, respectively.

The geometric compatibility provides,

$$\frac{\delta_1}{2} = \frac{\delta_2}{0.8}, \ \delta_1 = \frac{2}{0.8}\delta_2,$$

$$\frac{P_1L_1}{A_1E_1} = \frac{2}{0.8}\left(\frac{P_2L_2}{A_2E_2}\right), \qquad \text{(ii)}$$

where A_1, A_2 are the cross-sectional areas and L_1, L_2 are the lengths of the aluminium and steel rods respectively; E_1 and E_2 denote the Young's modulus of elasticity of the aluminium and steel rods, respectively. Substituting the values of L_1, L_2, A_1, A_2, E_1 and E_2 in Eq. (ii), we get

$$5.357P_1 = 1.875P_2, \ P_2 = 2.857P_1.$$

Substituting the above value of P_2 in terms of P_1 in Eq. (i), the value of P_1 as $P_1 = 46.32\text{kN}$.

Thus, P_2 is obtained as $P_2 = 132.34\,\text{kN}$.

Now, the stress in the aluminium rod:

$$\sigma_{\text{Aluminium}} = \frac{P_1}{A_1} = \frac{46.32\times10^3}{400\times10^{-6}} = 115.80\,\text{MPa}.$$

The stress in the steel rod:

$$\sigma_{\text{Steel}} = \frac{P_2}{A_2} = \frac{132.34\times10^3}{500\times10^{-6}} = 264.68\,\text{MPa}.$$

1.22 Compound Bars

Certain engineering design applications demand the use of a combination of elements such as bars made of different materials in order to perform certain individual intended design functions. Such structures constructed from elements of different materials are usually termed as compound bars. For example, the overhead electric transmission cables are made of a set of copper wires for carrying current surrounded by steel wires as shown in Fig. 1.38. Here, the purpose of steel wires is to support the current carrying copper wires over a large span.

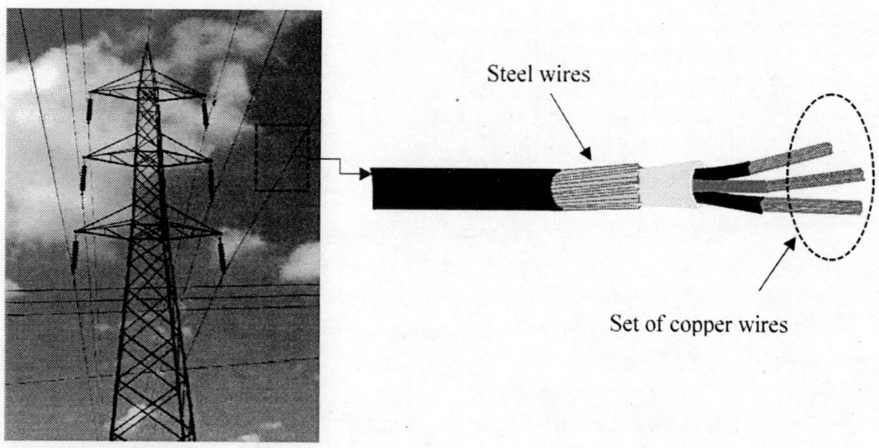

Fig. 1.38 The power transmission cable with different constituent materials.

1.22.1 Stresses and deformations in compound bars

In this section, we shall discuss stresses and deformations in compound bars which are symmetrically proportioned such that no bending results. Let us consider a compound bar consisting of n members of different materials as shown in Fig. 1.39. Each constituent member has the different length and cross-sectional area. It is assumed that the resultant axial load acts through the centre of gravity of the composite bar to produce the same extension in each member. If the common extension experienced by all members is y, then for the nth member, one can write

$$\frac{\sigma_n}{\varepsilon_n} = E_n = \frac{\frac{F_n}{A_n} L_n}{\frac{y}{L_n}},$$

$$F_n = \frac{E_n A_n y}{L_n}, \tag{1.74}$$

where F_n is the force in the nth member and A_n, L_n and E_n are the cross-sectional area, length and Young's modulus of elasticity of the nth member, respectively. The total load F carried by the compound bar can be obtained by superposing all such loads contributed by all members. Thus,

$$F = \sum \frac{E_n A_n y}{L_n} = y \sum \frac{E_n A_n}{L_n}. \tag{1.75}$$

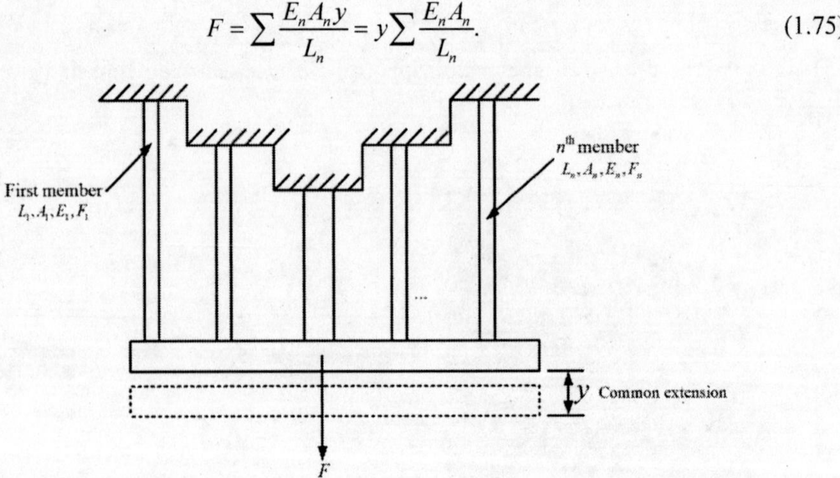

Fig. 1.39 A compound bar with n elements

From Eq. (1.74), the force in the first member F_1 can be expressed as

$$F_1 = \frac{E_1 A_1 y}{L_1}, \tag{1.76}$$

where A_1, L_1 and E_1 represents the cross-sectional area, length and Young's modulus of elasticity of the first member, respectively. From Eq. (1.75), the common extension y is given by

$$y = \frac{F}{\sum \frac{E_n A_n}{L_n}}. \tag{1.77}$$

Substituting y from Eq. (1.77) in Eq. (1.76), one obtains

$$F_1 = \frac{E_1 A_1}{L_1} \frac{F}{\sum \frac{E_n A_n}{L_n}} = \frac{\frac{E_1 A_1}{L_1}}{\sum \frac{EA}{L}} F. \tag{1.78}$$

Thus, each member contributes to a portion of the total load F proportional to its corresponding $(EA)/L$ value.

If the length of each individual member is the same then from Eq. (1.78), one can write

$$F_1 = \frac{E_1 A_1}{\sum EA} F. \tag{1.79}$$

The stress induced in the first member is then determined as

$$\sigma_1 = \frac{F_1}{A_1}. \tag{1.80}$$

Similarly, the stresses in the other individual members can be evaluated.

1.22.2 Equivalent or combined modulus

In order to conceive the idea of equivalent or combined modulus, we imagine the compound bar as an equivalent single bar made of a single material with an equivalent modulus E_c. To achieve the same strains in all members of the compound bar, it is necessary to assume that both the extension and the original lengths of the individual members are the same.

The total load on the compound bar is given by the summation of the forces in each individual member constituting the compound bar. This,

$$\text{Total load} = F_1 + F_2 + F_3 + ... + F_n,$$

$$\sigma\left(A_1 + A_2 + A_3 + ... + A_n\right) = \sigma_1 A_1 + \sigma_2 A_2 + \sigma_3 A_3 + \; ... \; + \sigma_n A_n, \tag{1.81}$$

where σ is the stress in the equivalent single bar, σ_1, σ_2, ...σ_n are the stresses in the individual members of the compound bar and A_1, A_2, ... A_n are the individual cross-sectional areas. Dividing Eq. (1.81) by the common strain ε on both sides,

$$\frac{\sigma}{\varepsilon}\left(A_1 + A_2 + A_3 + ... + A_n\right) = \frac{\sigma_1}{\varepsilon} A_1 + \frac{\sigma_2}{\varepsilon} A_2 + \frac{\sigma_3}{\varepsilon} A_3 + \; ... \; + \frac{\sigma_n}{\varepsilon} A_n,$$

$$E_c\left(A_1 + A_2 + A_3 + ... + A_n\right) = E_1 A_1 + E_2 A_2 + E_3 A_3 + ... E_n A_n,$$

$$E_c = \frac{E_1 A_1 + E_2 A_2 + E_3 A_3 + ... E_n A_n}{A_1 + A_2 + A_3 + ... + A_n} = \frac{\sum EA}{\sum A}. \tag{1.82}$$

Equation (1.82) provides the equivalent or combined modulus of the single bar. If an external load F is applied to the single equivalent bar, then stress and strains in the bar can be expressed as

$$\sigma = \frac{F}{\sum A}, \qquad \varepsilon = \frac{F}{E_c \sum A} = \frac{y}{L},$$

$$y = \frac{FL}{E_c \sum A}. \tag{1.83}$$

Equation (1.83) provides the extension of an equivalent single bar.

Example 1.18 A power transmission cable consists of twelve copper wires each of 1.5 mm diameter surrounding five steel wires each of 2.5 mm diameter. For this compound transmission cable determine the following:

a) The stresses in each of the wires when the cable supports a tension of 2 kN assuming all of the wires are of equal lengths

b) The combined Young's modulus of elasticity for the compound cable and hence determine the extension of a 30 m length of the cable.

Take the Young's modulus of elasticity of copper as E_1=100 GPa and that of steel as E_2=200 GPa.

Solution

a) From Eq. (1.79) the force in the copper wire is given by

$$F_{cu} = \frac{E_{cu} \times A_{cu}}{\Sigma EA} \times F$$

$$F_{cu} = \frac{100 \times 10^3 \times 12 \times \frac{\pi}{4} \times 1.5^2}{12(100 \times 10^3 . \times \frac{\pi}{4} \times 1.5^2) + 5(200 \times 10^3 \times \frac{\pi}{4} \times 2.5^2)} \times 2 \times 10^3 = 603.35\,\text{N}.$$

Therefore, the total force in the steel wire is

$$F_s = F - F_{cu} = 2000 - 603.35 = 1396.65 \text{ N}.$$

Now, the stresses in the copper and steel wires are calculated as

$$\sigma_{cu} = \frac{F_{cu}}{A_{cu}} = \frac{603.35}{12 \times \frac{\pi}{4} \times 1.5^2} = 28.45\,\text{MPa},$$

$$\sigma_s = \frac{F_s}{A_s} = \frac{1396.65}{5 \times \frac{\pi}{4} \times 2.5^2} = 56.90\,\text{MPa}.$$

b) The combined Young's modulus of elasticity (E_c) of the compound cable is obtained using Eq. (1.82) as

$$E_c = \frac{\Sigma EA}{\Sigma A} = \frac{\left(100 \times 10^3 \times 12 \times \frac{\pi}{4} \times 1.5^2\right) + \left(200 \times 10^3 \times 5 \times \frac{\pi}{4} \times 2.5^2\right)}{\frac{\pi}{4} \times \left(12 \times 1.5^2 + 5 \times 2.5^2\right)} = 153.65\,\text{GPa}.$$

The stress in the equivalent cable,

$$\sigma = \frac{2 \times 10^3}{\Sigma A} = \frac{2 \times 10^3}{\frac{\pi}{4}(12 \times 1.5^2 + 5 \times 2.5^2)} = 43.72\text{MPa}.$$

Now,

$E_c = \frac{\sigma}{\varepsilon}$, where ε is the strain in the equivalent cable

$$\Rightarrow \varepsilon = \frac{\sigma}{E_c} = \frac{43.72}{153.65 \times 10^3} = 2.845 \times 10^{-4}.$$

Therefore, the extension of a 30 m length cable is obtained as

$$\delta = \varepsilon \times L = 2.845 \times 10^{-4} \times 30 = 8.53 \times 10^{-3}\,\text{m} = 8.53\,\text{mm}.$$

1.23 Introduction to Thermal Stresses and Strains

When the temperature of a component is increased or decreased the material expands or contracts, respectively. If this expansion or contraction is not resisted in anyway, then they take place free of stress. However, if the expansion and contraction due to temperature change are restricted, then the component is subjected to stress. Now, in the following subsections, the strains and stresses caused by the temperature change are discussed.

1.23.1 Thermal strain

Consider a bar of material with a linear coefficient of expansion α. Let the original length of the bar be L and lying initially at a temperature T as shown in Fig. 1.40 (a). If the bar is free to expand or contract for a change in temperature ΔT as shown in Figs. 1.40 (b) and (c), then the change in length of the bar ΔL is given by

$$\Delta L = \alpha L \Delta T. \tag{1.84}$$

If this change in length of the bar due to a change in temperature ΔT of the bar is measured per unit original length of the bar, it is termed as the thermal strain. It is denoted by ε_T and is given by

$$\varepsilon_T = \frac{\alpha L \Delta T}{L} = \alpha \Delta T. \tag{1.85}$$

The value of ΔT is positive for expansion and negative for contraction. The uniform change in temperature throughout the body causes uniform thermal strain. The thermal strain is a dimensionless quantity.

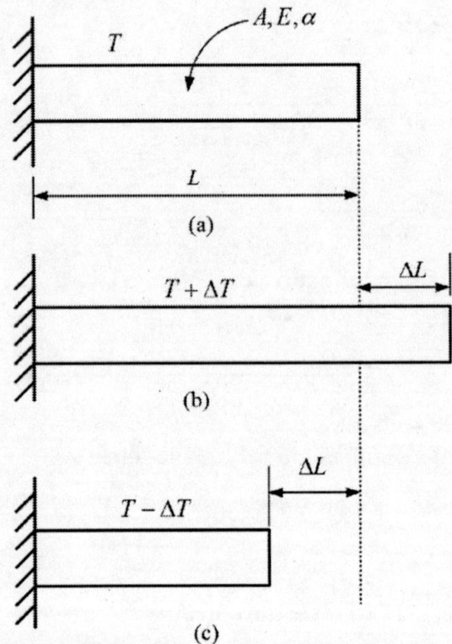

Fig. 1.40 Illustration of thermal strain: (a) a bar at temperature T, (b) Expansion of a bar due to an increase of temperature, (c) contraction of a bar due to a decrease of temperature

1.23.2 Thermal stress

No internal forces are induced in the body if the deformation due to temperature change is allowed to occur freely. Thus, no stress will be developed due to temperature change, but there will be thermal strain induced in the body. If the change in dimensions due to temperature change is restricted, internal forces are induced in the body, which resists forces due to thermal expansion or contraction. The stresses caused by these internal forces are termed as thermal stresses. If the expansion due to an increase in temperature is restricted, compressive thermal stress will be induced and if the contraction due to decrease in temperature is restricted, tensile thermal stress will be induced in the body.

In many engineering applications, designer has to carefully take into account the consequences of thermal stresses. For example, in the construction of railway tracks, instead of making them continuous, gaps are provided at certain distance intervals in order to accommodate the expansions due to temperature change. The temperature change is caused by hot weather as well as the passage of train over the rail. If the gaps between the rails were not provided or the designed gaps are not sufficient enough to accommodate the thermal expansion, there would have been excessive thermal stresses generated caused by constrained thermal expansion. Under this situation, the rails are susceptible to buckling leading to failure. A typical gap provided between railway tracks is shown in Fig. 1.41.

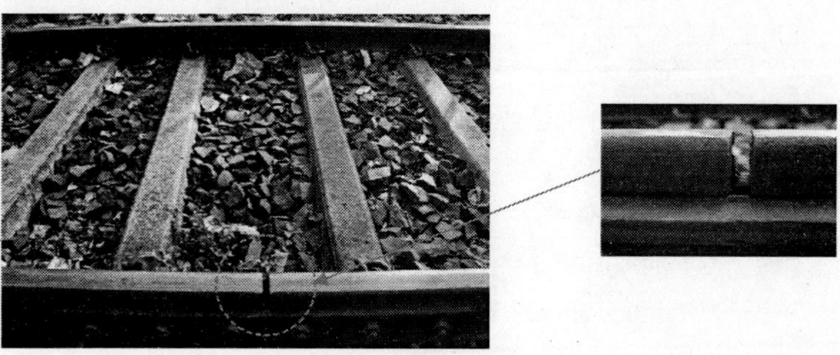

Fig. 1.41 A typical gap between rails to accommodate thermal expansion

Forces developed due to temperature change cannot be determined from equilibrium equations alone. Thus, the problem becomes statically indeterminate and we need the equation of compatibility. As an example, consider that a bar of length L, cross-sectional area A with a coefficient of thermal expansion α and Young's modulus of elasticity E is rigidly secured between two walls as shown in Fig. 1.42 (a). Now, let us say that the temperature of the bar is increased by ΔT. Due to this increase of temperature, the bar will try to expand, but the rigid supports at the ends will not allow it to expand freely. If any one of the supports would have not been there, it would have expanded freely. The moment we restrict the movement due to temperature change by putting the supports at the ends, it will induce an internal force in the bar. In order to obtain this internal force, one has to use both the equation of equilibrium and compatibility equation and solve them together as it becomes a statically indeterminate problem.

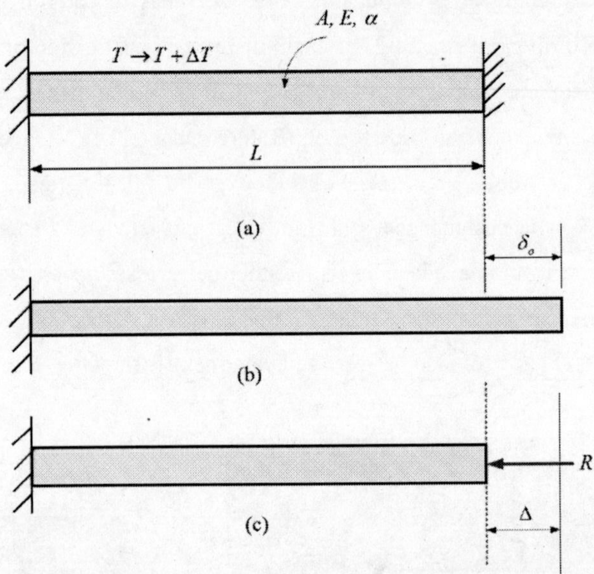

Fig. 1.42 A bar rigidly secured between two walls subjected to a temperature change: (a) actual scenario, (b) expansion if right support were not there, (c) support reaction counteracting the expansion

Now, to solve this problem, let us temporarily remove one of the support. In this case, we arbitrarily consider to remove the right support as shown in Fig. 1.42 (b) to allow the bar to expand freely due to change of temperature. Let's say if that right support would have not been there, the bar would have expanded freely by an amount δ_0, when the temperature is increased by ΔT. This free expansion is then given by

$$\delta_0 = \alpha L \Delta T. \tag{1.86}$$

The above result violates the geometric boundary condition at the right end. In order to comply with this, we now apply a compressive force R to the expanded bar to bring back the bar to its original position to hold it against the right support and in doing so we evaluate the deformation (contraction) produced in the bar. The situation is shown in Fig. 1.42 (c). Assuming that the axial contraction produced by the force R in the bar to be Δ, it is given by

$$\Delta = -\frac{RL}{AE}, \tag{1.87}$$

where the negative sign is used to indicate the contraction. Now, the geometric compatibility of deformation requires that the net deformation at the right support is zero. This provides,

$$\delta_0 + \Delta = 0. \tag{1.88}$$

Substituting Eqs. (1.86) and (1.87) in Eq. (1.88), one obtains

$$\alpha L\Delta T - \frac{RL}{AE} = 0,$$

$$R = \alpha \Delta TAE. \tag{1.89}$$

Once the value of R is obtained, taking any cut section in the bar, the internal force in the bar due to restriction in thermal expansion can be obtained by using the equation of equilibrium. In the present case, the internal force becomes equal to R. Thus, the thermal stress induced in the bar can be evaluated as

$$\sigma_T = \frac{R}{A} = \frac{\alpha \Delta TAE}{A} = \alpha \Delta TE. \tag{1.90}$$

Using Eq. (1.85), Eq. (1.90) can be expressed in terms of thermal strain as

$$\sigma_T = \varepsilon_T E. \tag{1.91}$$

1.23.3 Stresses in compound bars subjected to temperature change

Consider a compound bar of length L consists of two different materials say a steel bar and a brass bar are rigidly joined together as shown in Fig. 1.43 (a). As the coefficients of thermal expansion of the two materials forming the compound bar are not the same, on increasing the temperature each material will attempt to expand by different amounts. If the individual materials were allowed to expand freely (as if they are not rigidly joined), the steel bar would have expanded to its free length position B and the brass bar would have expanded to its free length position C as shown in Fig. 1.43 (b). The expansion of any length L due to an increase in temperature ΔT is given by Eq. (1.85).

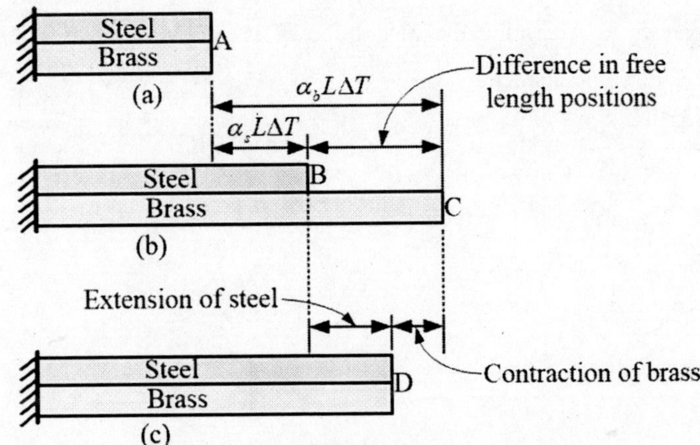

Fig. 1.43 Thermal expansion in compound bars

Let us take the coefficients of thermal expansion of steel and brass to be α_s and α_b, respectively. As α_b is greater than α_s, the difference of free expansion lengths is given by

$$\alpha_b L\Delta T - \alpha_s L\Delta T = (\alpha_b - \alpha_s) L\Delta T. \tag{1.92}$$

Now, if we consider that the bars are rigidly fixed to each other to form the compound bar, due to same temperature rise, each bar will try to expand to its free length position, but each bar will offer resistance to the movement of the other. Therefore, the bar with a higher coefficient of thermal expansion *i.e.*, the brass bar will seek to pull the steel bar which has a lower coefficient of thermal expansion up to its free length position. Similarly, the lower coefficient of thermal expansion steel bar will try to hold the higher coefficient of thermal expansion brass bar back to the free length position of steel. This counteraction causes the bars to reach a common position D as shown in Fig. 1.43 (c) by an effective compression of the brass from its free length position and an effective extension of the steel from its free length position. Now, from Fig. 1.43, the following observations can be made:

Extension of steel bar + compression of brass bar = difference in free length,

$$\frac{\sigma_s L}{E_s} + \frac{\sigma_b L}{E_b} = (\alpha_b - \alpha_s) L\Delta T, \tag{1.93}$$

where σ_s and σ_b are the thermal stress induced in steel and brass bars and E_s and E_b are their Young's modulus of elasticity. Further, using Newton's third law (equality of action and reaction pair), one can also write

Tensile force in steel = compressive force in brass,

$$\sigma_s A_s = \sigma_b A_b, \tag{1.94}$$

where A_s and A_b are the cross-sectional area of steel and brass bars. Eq. (1.93) and (1.94) are solved together to determine the magnitude of the thermal stresses induced in the bars constituting the compound bar.

Example 1.19 A bronze bar AB of length 3 m with a cross-sectional area of 320 mm^2 is placed between two rigid walls. At a temperature of –20 °C, there is a gap of 2 mm between the bar end B and the rigid wall on the right. Find the temperature at which the compressive stress in the bar will be 40 MPa.

Solution

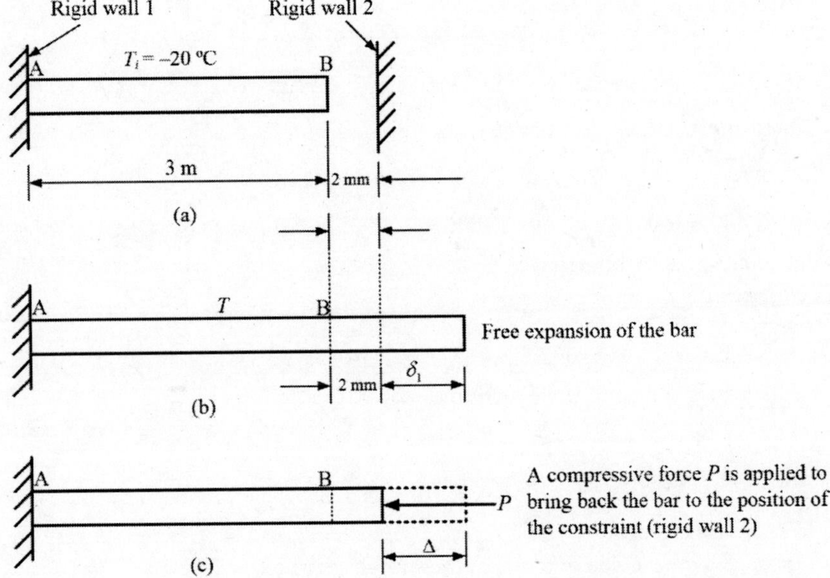

The bronze bar is at the initial temperature, T_i= – 20 °C. Let's say the temperature of the bar is increased to a final temperature T to induce a compressive thermal stress σ_T=40 MPa. Thus, the temperature of the bar is increased by an amount

$$\Delta T = T - T_i = T - (-20) = (T + 20).$$

When the temperature of the bar is increased to T, initially the bar expands freely in the gap (as shown in Fig. (a)) up to a distance of 2 mm just touching the rigid wall 2. Thereafter, any expansion will be resisted by the wall and induce a compressive internal force that gives rise to the thermal stress in the bar. In order to obtain this compressive force, we need to use the geometric compatibility of deformation at the rigid wall 2 due to temperature rise. Let us temporarily remove the wall in order to have an unconstrained expansion of the bar when the temperature increases to T. We assume that the bar can expand freely up to a length δ_1 from the rigid wall 2, if it is removed as shown in Fig. (b). Thus, the total free expansion of the bar is given by

$$\delta = 2 + \delta_1.$$

The free expansion (the change in length of the bar due to temperature change) is given by Eq. (1.84). Thus, using Eq. (1.84), the free expansion length in the present case can be expressed as

$$\delta = \alpha L \Delta T = 2 + \delta_1,$$

$$18 \times 10^{-6}(T+20) \times 3000 = 2 + \delta_1,$$

$$\delta_1 = 54 \times 10^{-3}(T+20) - 2,$$

where δ_1 is the free expansion from the rigid wall 2 if it is removed. This result violates the geometric boundary condition at the rigid wall 2. In order to comply with this, we apply a compressive force P to bring back the bar to the position of rigid wall 2 as shown in Fig. (c) such that it provides an equal amount of corresponding contraction. The contraction due to the application of compressive force P is given by

$$\Delta = -\frac{PL}{AE}.$$

Now, the geometric compatibility equation can be written as

$$\delta_1 + \Delta = 0,$$

$$54 \times 10^{-3}(T+20) - 2 - \frac{PL}{AE} = 0.$$

Recasting the above equation in terms of thermal stress σ_T ($\sigma_T = P/A$) as

$$54 \times 10^{-3}(T+20) - 2 - \frac{\sigma_T L}{E} = 0.$$

Substituting the values of L and E in the above equation, the temperature T at which compressive stress $\sigma_T = 40$ MPa can be estimated as

$$54 \times 10^{-3}(T+20) - 2 - \frac{40 \times 3000}{80 \times 10^3} = 0,$$

$$T = 44.81°\text{C}.$$

Example 1.20 A compound bar consists of three bars of width 30 mm and thickness 6 mm joined together rigidly to form an equivalent bar of width 30 mm and thickness 18 mm. Consider that the middle bar is of aluminium alloy with Young's modulus of elasticity E_{Al}= 70 GPa and the two steel bars are rigidly fixed to the aluminium alloy bar on its either side with Young's modulus of elasticity E_s = 200 GPa. If the bars are initially joined at 20 °C and the temperature of the whole assembly is then raised to 50 °C, determine the stresses set up in the steel and the aluminium alloy bars. Take the coefficient of thermal expansion of steel and aluminium alloy as α_s=12×10^{-6}/°C and α_{Al}=22×10^{-6}/°C, respectively.

Solution

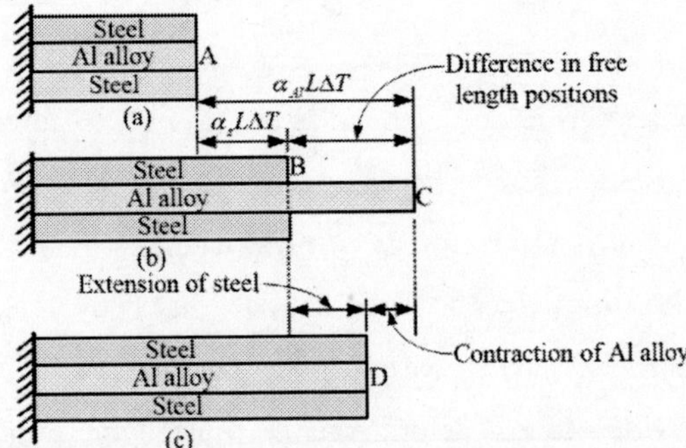

The compound bar of length L is shown in Fig. (a). As the coefficient of thermal expansion of aluminium alloy is more than that of steel, the free length expansion of aluminium alloy bar due to temperature rise will be more than steel if the bars are thought of as individual bars without any joint. This situation is shown in Fig. (b) above. Now if we consider the rigid connection among the bars, upon increasing the temperature, the aluminium alloy bar will attempt to pull the steel bar to its free length position and on the other hand, the steel par will attempt to hold the aluminium alloy bar back to its free length position. This counteraction causes all the three bars to expand to a common position D as shown in Fig. (c) inducing a tensile thermal stress in steel bars and compressive thermal stress in the aluminium alloy bar.

Let us assume that the stress in the aluminium alloy bar is x. As the tensile force in the two steel bars is equal to the compressive force in the aluminium alloy bar, we can write

$$2\sigma_s A_s = xA_{Al}.$$

Since the cross-sectional areas of steel bar A_s and aluminium alloy bar A_{Al} are the same, the above equation reduces to

$$\sigma_s = \frac{x}{2}.$$

Now, using Eq. (1.94), we get

$$\frac{\left(\frac{x}{2}\right)L}{E_s} + \frac{xL}{E_{Al}} = (\alpha_{Al} - \alpha_s)L\Delta T,$$

$$\frac{\left(\frac{x}{2}\right)}{200\times10^3} + \frac{x}{70\times10^3} = (22-12)\times10^{-6}\times(50-20),$$

$$x = 17.87\,\text{MPa}.$$

Thus, the compressive stress in the aluminium alloy bar is σ_{Al}=17.87 MPa.

The tensile stress in the steel bar is $\sigma_s = \frac{x}{2} = \frac{17.87}{2} = 8.93\,\text{MPa}$.

1.24 Strain Energy

In mechanics, energy is usually defined as the capacity to do work and it may exist in any of the many forms such as mechanical, thermal, chemical and nuclear energy. The potential energy of a body is a form of mechanical energy which is stored in a body as a result of the work which has previously been done on that body. *e.g.*, a drawn bow about a datum stores potential energy. When a solid body is subjected to deformation, it induces strain in the body. By virtue of this deformation or strain, some form of potential energy is stored within the material. This stored energy is referred as the strain energy.

Due to this strain energy, the material is then capable of doing an equivalent amount of work, when it returns to its original undeformed state. Thus, strain energy can be defined as the energy which is stored within a material when work has been done on the material during deformation. It is denoted by U and is given by

$$U = \text{Work done during deformation} = \text{Force} \times \text{deformation caused in the direction of force.} \tag{1.95}$$

It is assumed that when work is done on the material, it remains in the elastic state so that all of the stored energy can be fully recovered when load is removed. As there is no permanent set in the material, this strain energy associated with pure elastic deformation is called as the elastic strain energy. In this section, we will discuss the elastic strain energy in a bar subjected to uniaxial loading.

1.24.1 Strain energy in gradually applied uniaxial loading

Let us consider a bar of cross-sectional area A and Young's modulus of elasticity E, subjected to an axial pull P as shown in Fig. 1.44 (a). It is assumed that the axial pull to the bar is gradually applied from zero to reach a final value equal to P. The bar remains in the elastic state when it deforms under gradual application of load P. Consider a small element of length dx sliced out from the bar as shown in Fig. 1.44 (b). If one plots the load against an extension for this case, a load-extension diagram as shown in Fig. 1.44 (c) is obtained. Thus, for a gradually applied loading, the work done during deformation will provide the strain energy in the infinitesimal bar element, which is given by the shaded area under the load-extension curve, *i.e.*,

$$\mathrm{d}U = \frac{1}{2} P\delta, \tag{1.96}$$

where δ is the extension caused by the gradually applied load P.

Under the axial load P, the normal stress (σ) induced in the bar at any section slightly away from the load application point and support is equal to P/A. If δ is the extension of the element, the normal strain (ε) produced in the bar is $\delta/\mathrm{d}x$. The Young's modulus of elasticity from Hooke's law and using the expressions for stress and strain induced in the bar can be expressed as

$$E = \frac{\sigma}{\varepsilon} = \frac{\frac{P}{A}}{\frac{\delta}{\mathrm{d}x}} = \frac{P\mathrm{d}x}{A\delta}. \tag{1.97}$$

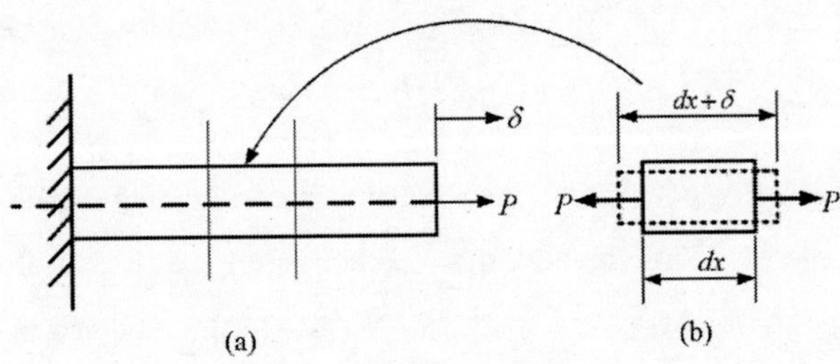

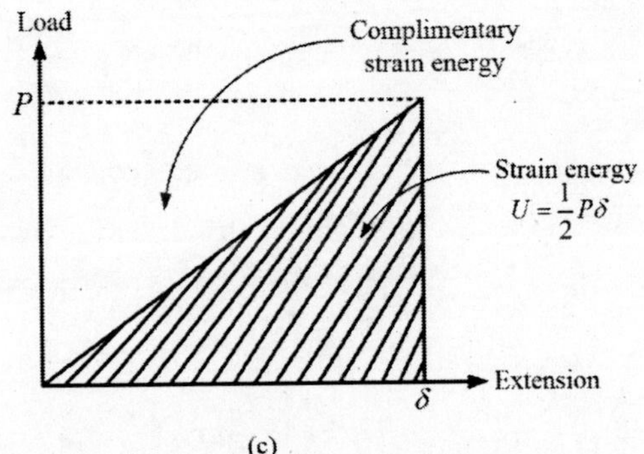

Fig. 1.44 (a) A bar subjected to gradual axial pull, (b) elemental bar of length subjected to deformation δ, (c) Load-extension curve for gradual axial loading.

From Eq. (1.97), the axial extension δ is given by

$$\delta = \frac{P\mathrm{d}x}{EA}. \tag{1.98}$$

Substituting the value of δ from Eq. (1.98) in Eq. (1.96), the strain energy in the elemental bar is given by

$$\mathrm{d}U = \frac{1}{2}\frac{P^2\mathrm{d}x}{EA}. \tag{1.99}$$

Now, the total strain energy in the bar of length L can be obtained by integrating Eq. (1.99) as

$$U = \int_0^L \frac{P^2 \mathrm{d}x}{2EA} = \frac{P^2 L}{2EA}. \tag{1.100}$$

Using Eq. (1.100) one can recast the expression of strain energy in terms of stress as

$$U = \frac{\left(\frac{P}{A}\right)^2 AL}{2E} = \frac{\sigma^2}{2E} V, \tag{1.101}$$

where V=AL is the volume of the bar. Using Hooke's law, Eq. (1.101) can be expressed in terms of stress and strain as

$$U = \frac{1}{2}\sigma\left(\frac{\sigma}{E}\right)V = \frac{1}{2}\sigma\varepsilon V. \tag{1.102}$$

It has already been mentioned that the area under the load-extension curve is the elastic strain energy. Consequently, the area above the load-extension curve is called as the complementary strain energy as depicted in Fig. 1.44 (c). For linear elastic material, the areas below and above the load-extension curve are equal. Thus, the strain energy and complementary strain energy are equal for a linear elastic solid. However, for nonlinear elastic material, this equality does not hold good.

1.24.2 Resilience

If the strain energy is expressed per unit volume of the material, it is termed as resilience. This is also called as strain-energy density. Rearranging Eq. (1.102), one can express the strain energy stored in an elastic solid per unit volume of material *i.e.*, resilience (U_r) as

$$U_r = \frac{U}{V} = \frac{1}{2}\sigma\varepsilon. \tag{1.103}$$

Eq. (1.103) signifies the area under the stress strain curve up to the proportional limit. From Eq. (1.101), resilience can also be expressed as

$$U_r = \frac{\sigma^2}{2E}. \tag{1.104}$$

Substitution of the value of stress at proportional limit in Eq. (1.104) for a given material provides a measure of material's ability to store or absorb energy without yielding. The quantity thus obtained is the measure of resilience or modulus of resilience for that particular material.

1.24.3 Strain energy in suddenly applied axial loading

Contrary to the situation considered in Subsection 1.24.1, now consider that a load P_1 is applied suddenly to the bar to produce the same amount of extension δ as in the case of gradual application of load P. This means that P_1 is applied with an instantaneous value, not gradually increasing from zero to P_1. In this case, if the load-extension curve is drawn, one will obtain it as a straight line parallel to the extension axis as shown in Fig. 1.45. The area under the load-extension curve of Fig. 1.45 will provide the strain energy for the present case. Thus, the strain energy due to suddenly applied axial loading is given by

$$U = P_1\delta. \tag{1.105}$$

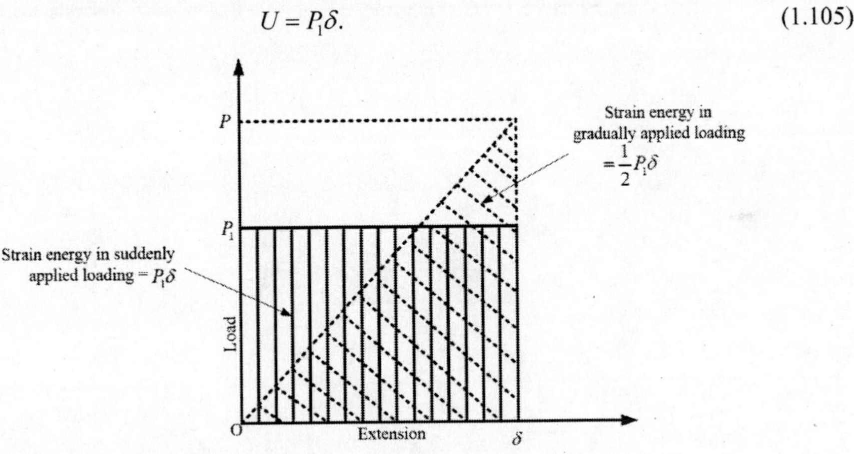

Fig. 1.45 Strain energy in suddenly applied loading

As the bar produces the same amount of extension δ as produced by the gradual loading P, the area under the load extension curves in both the cases must be same, *i.e.*, they provide the same strain energy. Thus,

$$P_1\delta = \frac{1}{2}P\delta,$$

$$P_1 = \frac{1}{2}P. \tag{1.106}$$

Eq. (1.106) shows that the suddenly applied load is equal to half the equivalent amount of static load in order to produce an equal amount of deformation or strain. Thus, it is clear that a suddenly applied load will produce twice the effect of the same load when gradually applied.

1.24.4 Impact or shock loading

The impact loading refers to the load or force delivered when a freely falling weight or a moving solid strikes a structure or machine element. When one encounters a problem involving such impact loading situations, for the purpose of analysis, it is necessary to idealize the system as elastic without any dissipation of energy at the point of impact. Further, the inertia of the system resisting an impact is usually neglected.

Let us Consider a bar of original length L and cross-sectional area A, suspended vertically from its top with a rigid collar firmly attached to its bottom as shown in Fig. 1.46. The load W is suspended by some means at a position y from the top of the collar and is free to slide vertically. When the load W is allowed to fall freely from the suspended position, it will strike the collar. Here, the weight of the bar along with the collar is neglected.

The work done during axial deformation of the bar resulting from impact will be stored as strain energy and is given by Eq. (1.101). Thus,

$$U = \frac{\sigma^2 AL}{2E}. \tag{1.107}$$

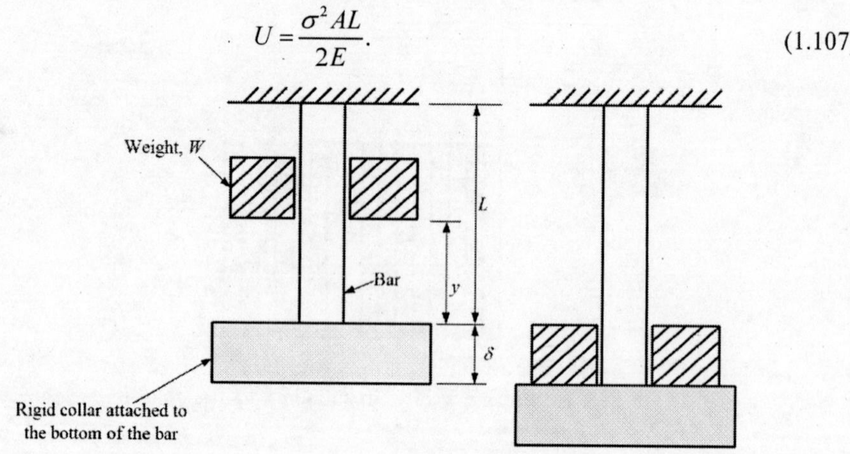

Fig. 1.46 Application of impact axial loading

In Eq. (1.107), σ is the instantaneous stress induced in the bar during impact. As the weight W travels through a distance $(y+\delta)$ after impact, the work done is also given by $W(y+\delta)$. Thus, one can write

$$\frac{\sigma^2 AL}{2E} = W\left(y+\delta\right). \tag{1.108}$$

From Eq. (1.108), the instantaneous stress σ is given by

$$\sigma = \sqrt{\frac{2WE\left(y+\delta\right)}{AL}}. \tag{1.109}$$

If δ is very small compared to y, it can be neglected and Eq. (1.109) becomes

$$\sigma = \sqrt{\frac{2WEy}{AL}}. \tag{1.110}$$

If δ is not negligible as compared to y, then it is expressed in terms of σ using Hooke's law as

$$\frac{\sigma}{\varepsilon}=E,\ \frac{\sigma}{\frac{\delta}{L}}=E,$$

$$\delta=\frac{\sigma L}{E}. \tag{1.111}$$

Substituting Eq. (1.111) in Eq. (1.108) one obtains

$$\frac{\sigma^2 AL}{2E}-\frac{WL}{E}\sigma-Wy=0,$$

$$\sigma^2-\frac{2W}{A}\sigma-\frac{2WEy}{AL}=0, \tag{1.112}$$

which is a quadratic equation in σ. Solving Eq. (1.112), the stress σ is obtained as

$$\sigma=\frac{W}{A}+\sqrt{\left(\frac{W}{A}\right)^2+\frac{2WEy}{AL}}. \tag{1.113}$$

The above equation provides the value of the maximum stress induced in the bar subjected to impact loading.

If the impact is sudden that means the weight W is not dropped, but suddenly applied effectively from $y=0$, then Eq. (1.113) provides

$$\sigma=\frac{W}{A}+\frac{W}{A}=\frac{2W}{A}. \tag{1.114}$$

Thus, it can be concluded that stress induced by a suddenly applied loading is twice of that induced by a gradually applied load of equal magnitude. It is therefore careful attention must be paid by a designer to exclude the application of sudden loading while designing a structure or machine component.

Example 1.21 Two identical solid circular bars AB and CD are of same material and length L are subjected to gradually applied equal axial tensile load P. The cross-sectional dimensions of the bars are different. It is given that the diameter of the bar CD is 16 mm. If the strain energy stored in bar CD is two times that of the bar AB, determine the diameter of the bar AB.

Solution

Since the bars AB and CD are of same material, they have the same value of Young's modulus elasticity E. It is given that the diameter of the bar CD is d_{CD}=16 mm. As the strain energy stored in bar CD is two times that of the bar AB, therefore, using Eq. (1.100), one can write

$$U_{CD} = 2U_{AB}$$
$$\frac{P^2L}{2EA_{CD}} = 2\frac{P^2L}{2EA_{AB}},$$
$$\frac{1}{2A_{CD}} = \frac{1}{A_{AB}},$$

where A_{AB} and A_{CD} represent the cross-sectional area of bars AB and CD, respectively. Now, the above equation provides the diameter of the bar AB as

$$\frac{1}{2\times\frac{\pi}{4}d_{CD}^2} = \frac{1}{\frac{\pi}{4}d_{AB}^2},$$
$$\frac{1}{2d_{CD}^2} = \frac{1}{d_{AB}^2},$$
$$d_{AB}^2 = 2d_{CD}^2,\quad d_{AB}^2 = 2\times16^2,$$
$$d_{AB} = 22.63\,\text{mm}.$$

Example 1.22 Referring back to Example Problem 1.8, determine the modulus of resilience of the material during loading.

Solution

Using Eq. (1.104), the modulus of resilience of the material from the stress-strain diagram of Example Problem 1.8 can be calculated as

$$U_r = \frac{\sigma^2}{2E} = \frac{420^2}{2\times70\times10^3} = 1.26\,\text{MJ/m}^3.$$

1.25 Summary

In this unit, the concept of stress and strain are introduced in a simple way. The understanding of the stress at a point, the basic types of stresses and strains are provided in general and then we proceed to discuss stresses, strains, and deformations induced in axially loaded bars. Different cases are considered– bars of prismatic section, stepped bars with uniform sections, bars with gradually varying cross-section and compound bars. The concept of shear stress as well as shear strains are provided for simple loading cases. The stress-strain diagram for a typical engineering material such as mild steel is discussed along with the description of the salient points and the mechanical properties derivable from the stress-strain diagram. The Hooke's law, understanding of elasticity and plasticity, proof stress, Poisson's ratio, different types of elastic moduli and the concept of thermal stress and strain are discussed and emphasis is provided on building the fundamentals along with practical applications. The unit is concluded with the concept of strain energy for uniaxially loaded bars for gradual, sudden, impact, or shock loading. All the fundamental concepts discussed in this unit are of vital importance because these concepts will form the basis for the engineering design of many practical structural members or machine elements.

Know  *More* 

EXERCISES

Multiple Choice Questions

1.1 SI unit of traction vector is

(a) N/m^2 (b) N/m

(c) N (d) Nm

1.2 A stress component is in the direction of normal to the plane. This will produce

(a) Tension (b) Compression

(c) Shear (d) No deformation

1.3 Consider two bars of the same cross-sectional areas, one is made of steel and the other is made of wood. If the bars are subjected to same axial tensile force, then

(a) Stress induced in steel bar is more. (b) Stress induced in the wooden bar is more.

(c) Stress induced in both the bars is same. (d) Cannot draw any conclusion from the given information\

1.4 Which of the following material has zero Poisson's ratio?

(a) Rubber (b) Cork

(c) Diamond (d) Glass

1.5 Toughness of a ductile material is the

(a) area under stress-strain curve up to the proportional limit. (b) area under stress-strain curve up to the elastic limit.

(c) area under stress-strain curve up to the yield point. (d) area under stress-strain curve up to the fracture point.

1.6 The stress concentration near the immediate vicinity of the support or load application point in a bar is due to the principle of

(a) Newton (b) Timoshenko

(c) St. Venant (d) Euler

1.7 A steel bar of square cross-section with each side equal to 10 mm and length 1 m is subjected to an axial load of 120 kN. If the Young's modulus of elasticity of the bar is 200 GPa, the flexibility of the bar is

(a) 5×10^{-5} mm/N (b) 5×10^{-5} N/mm

(c) 20×10^{3} N/mm (d) 5×10^{-3} mm/N

1.8 The type of stress induced in bolt while tightening it by placing a washer below it is

(a) Shear stress (b) Compressive stress

(c) Tensile stress (d) Both tensile and shear stress

1.9 In a uniaxial tensile test, a load of 450 kN produces a deformation of 0.05 mm in a specimen of gauge length 50 mm. The true strain induced in the specimen at this instant is

(a) 1×10^{-3} (b) 1×10^{-4}

(c) 9.99×10^{-4} (d) 9.95×10^{-3}

1.10 Two bars A and B of the same material with gradually varying cross-sections of equal lengths are subjected to an axial tensile load P. The largest diameter of each of the bars is d. The diameter of the bar A at its smaller end is $d/3$ and that of the bar B is $d/2$. What is the ratio of axial elongation of the bar A to that of the bar B?

(a) $\frac{2}{3}$ (b) $\frac{3}{2}$

(c) $\frac{1}{3}$ (d) $\frac{1}{2}$

1.11 A steel rod 12 mm in diameter and 0.5 m long is heated from 25°C to 100°C. The Young's modulus of elasticity of steel is E = 200 GPa and the coefficient of thermal expansion is $\alpha = 12 \times 10^{-6}$ /°C. If the rod is free to expand, the thermal stress developed in the rod is

(a) 0 MPa (b) 180 MPa (compressive)

(c) 180 MPa (tensile) (d) 90 MPa (compressive)

1.12 In Q. 11, the thermal strain induced in the material is

(a) zero (b) 0.0009

(c) –0.0009 (d) 0.00045

1.13 In Q. 11, if the rod is not allowed to expand freely, then the thermal stress induced in the rod is

(a) 0 MPa (b) 90 MPa (compressive)

(c) 180 MPa (tensile) (d) 180 MPa (compressive)

1.14 If the stress induced by a gradually applied load P is σ, then the equal magnitude of suddenly applied loading induces a stress equal to

(a) σ (b) $\frac{\sigma}{2}$

(c) 2σ (d) 4σ

1.15 The strain energy stored in an elastic body due to gradually applied load compared to when the same load is applied suddenly is

(a) the same (b) twice

(c) four times (d) $\frac{1}{4}^{th}$

Answers of Multiple Choice Questions

1.1 (a), 1.2 (a), 1.3 (c), 1.4 (b), 1.5 (d), 1.6 (c), 1.7 (a), 1.8 (c), 1.9 (c), 1.10 (b), 1.11 (a), 1.12 (b), 1.13 (d), 1.14 (c), 1.15 (d)

Short and Long Answer Type Questions

Category I

1.1 What is stress? How is it different from pressure?

1.2 Explain the stress at a point with a neat sketch.

1.3 What are the different types of stresses? Give example of each.

1.4 What is strain? What are the different types of strain?

1.5 What do you mean by strain at a point?

1.6 What is normal strain? What is its unit?

1.7 Define shear strain. What is its unit in SI?

1.8 Why is the stress-strain diagram of a material important?

1.9 Define engineering stress, engineering strain, true stress and true strain. Establish relations among them.

1.10 What is proof stress?

1.11 How will you distinguish a ductile material from a brittle material?

1.12 Which one is more stiff- rubber or steel? Justify your answer.

1.13 What is the difference between proportional limit and elastic limit?

1.14 Why the engineering fracture strength is less than the ultimate strength of a material? Does the actual fracture strength also show the same behaviour?

1.15 Why does a ductile material fail in a cup and cone manner in a uniaxial tensile test? Why this mode of failure is not observed in brittle materials?

1.16 State Hooke's law. What are its limitations?

1.17 Differentiate between elasticity and plasticity.

1.18 State St. venant's principle.

1.19 What is factor of safety? Why is it important to consider a factor of safety in the design of certain structures or machine elements?

1.20 Define Poisson's ratio? If a material does not contract when it is stretched in the axial direction, then what can you say about the Poisson's ratio of that material?

1.21 What is principle of superposition? What are its limitations?

1.22 What is thermal stress? Why is it important to take into account the effect of thermal stress in the design of railway tracks?

1.23 'When there is temperature rise, there is always thermal strain developed in the material; however, thermal stress may not induce'. Comment in support of the above statement.

1.24 Consider two bars A and B of different materials attached together rigidly. Assume that the coefficient of thermal expansion of material of bar A is higher than the coefficient of thermal expansion of material of bar B. In this case, which bar is subjected to compressive stress and which bar is subjected to tensile stress?

1.25 What is elastic strain energy? What is its physical significance? Is there any difference between the strain energy and resilience?

Category II

1.26 Draw the typical stress-strain diagram for mild steel. Show all the salient points and describe the importance of each point.

1.27 What are the different elastic constants? Define each of them.

1.28 Derive the axial extension for a bar of gradually varying rectangular cross section.

1.29 Show that the shear deformation cannot change the volume, it induces the shape change.

1.30 Consider a weight suspended by some means above a linear elastic spring as shown in the figure. When the weight is allowed to fall freely from a height *h*, it impacts the spring and causes it to undergo a compression of *y* and both the weight and the spring comes to rest. Derive an expression for the deformation y of the spring due to this impact.

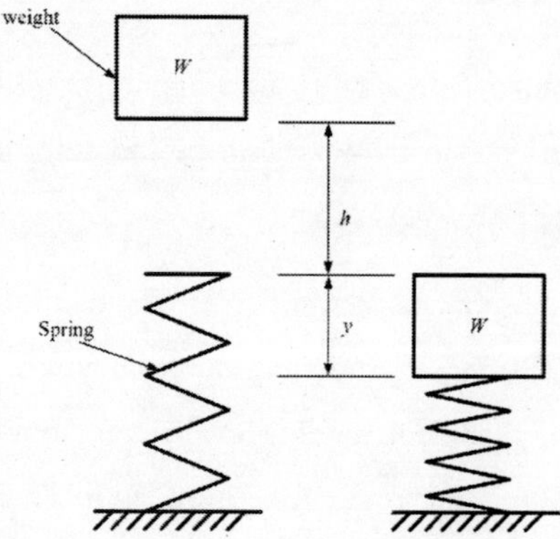

Numerical Problems

1.1 Determine stresses and strains in a circular bar of diameter 20 mm and length 1.5 m is subjected to an axial tensile force of 150 kN. Take the Young's modulus of elasticity of the bar is 210 GPa. (**Ans.** ε=0.0023, σ=460 MPa)

1.2 A hollow steel circular bar with outside diameter 20 mm and inside diameter 10 mm subjected to an axial tensile load of 50 kN. Determine the stress induced in the bar. If the stress in the bar is limited to 250 MPa, how much additional load that the bar will be able to withstand? (**Ans.** 212.21 MPa, 8.90 kN)

1.3 Consider a simple truss loaded as shown in the following figure. Find the stresses and their nature in each member of the truss if all the members constituting the truss are of circular cross-section with diameter 20 mm. (**Ans.** $\sigma_{AB} = \sigma_{AD}$ =220.52 MPa (Compressive), σ_{AC}=0 MPa $\sigma_{BC} = \sigma_{CD}$ 110.26 MPa (Tensile))

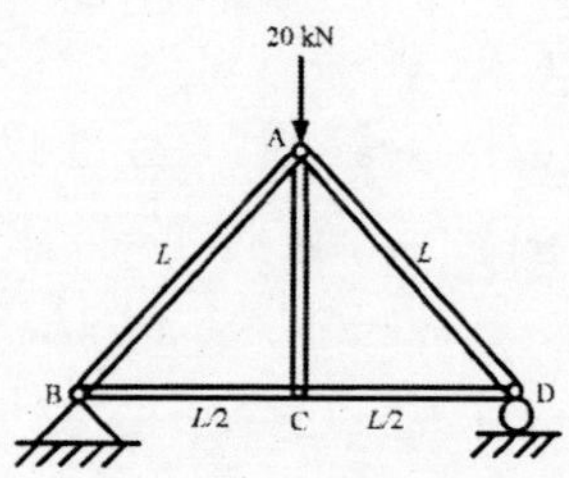

1.4 The top face of a rectangular block is subjected to a tangential force keeping its bottom face fixed. The height of the block is 40 mm and the cross-sectional dimension of the top and bottom face is 1 m ×1 m. The tangential force applied to the top faces causes the top face to displace by 0.025 mm. Determine shear strain, shear stress and the shear force in the rectangular block. Take the modulus of rigidity of the block as 80 GPa. (**Ans.** γ=0.00062 rad, τ=49.60 MPa, V=4.96×10^7 N)

1.5 In a tensile test, the gauge length of 10 mm diameter rod is 25 mm, which changes to 25.025 mm due to applied axial load. What will be the deformed diameter if the Poisson's ratio of the material is 0.28? (**Ans.** 9.9972 mm)

1.6 A bar is constructed by rigidly fastening two steel rods of diameter 15 mm each and one aluminium rod of diameter 30 mm as shown in the following figure. Determine the net axial deformation of the bar for the axial loading at different points as shown. Also, find the stresses in the steel and aluminium rods. Take the lengths of the steel bar segments as 800 mm and that of the aluminium bar segment as 400 mm. The Young's modulus of elasticity of steel and aluminium are 200 GPa and 70 GPa, respectively. (**Ans.** δ=0.986 mm, σ_{steel}=113.18 MPa, σ_{Al}=14.15 MPa)

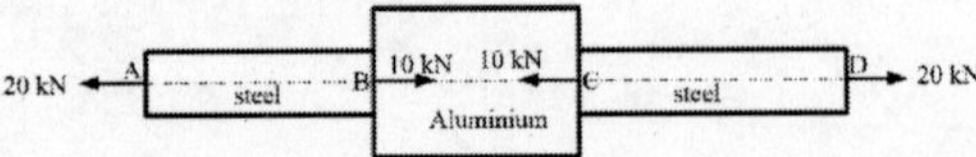

1.7 If the steel rod is secured strongly between the supports as shown in the figure below is heated, determine the stress induced in it due to 25°C rise in temperature. Take the coefficient of thermal expansion and Young's modulus of elasticity of steel as α=17×10^{-6}/°C and E=200 GPa, respectively. (**Ans.** 0.0902 MPa (Compressive))

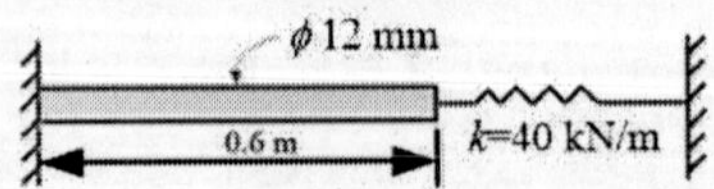

1.8 Consider two bars of different materials, brass and steel are held rigidly at B and C initially at a temperature of 20 °C separated by a gap δ=2.5 mm. Both the bars have the same diameter d=12 mm. The length of the brass bar is L_b=0.8 m and that of the steel bar is L_s= 1 m. If the temperature of the entire system is increased to 120 °C, which causes a free expansion greater than that required to close the gap, determine the thermal stress induced in the bars. Take the coefficient of thermal expansion of brass and steel as α_b = 18×10^{-6}/°C and

α_s= 12×10^{-6}/°C and their Young's moduli of elasticity are 100 GPa and 200 GPa. If there is no gap initially between the bars, then what is the value of stress induced? Compare your results with the previous result. What conclusion you can draw from your comparison? (**Ans.** 10.77 MPa (compressive), 203.08 MPa (compressive))

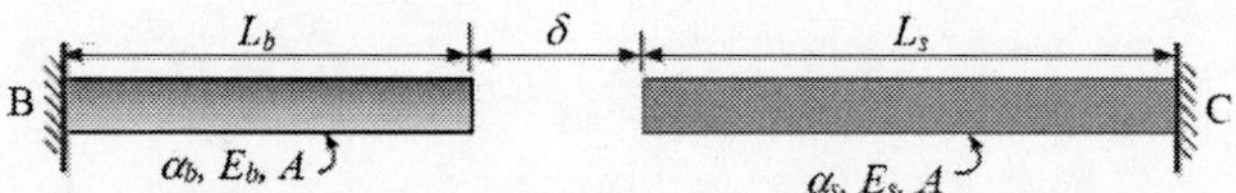

1.9 A compound bar is constructed using three steel bars of diameter 3 mm and two aluminium bars of diameter 2 mm. Assuming the initial length of all the individual bars to be same, determine the stresses in each of the bars when the compound bar is subjected to an axial tensile load of 1 kN. Take the Young's modulus of elasticity of steel as 200 GPa and that of the aluminium as 70 GPa. (**Ans.** σ_{steel}=42.72 MPa, σ_{Al}=14.96 MPa)

1.10 Calculate the strain energy stored in a steel bar of length 3 m and diameter 20 mm is subjected to an axial pull of 80 kN. Evaluate the strain energy stored in the bar. Take the Young's modulus of elasticity of steel as 200 GPa. If an equivalent square bar of same material of equal length has to store the same amount of energy, then what should the cross-sectional dimension of the equivalent bar subjected to the same axial pull. (**Ans.**152.79 J/m^3, 17.72 mm)

Unit 2

Compound Stresses and Strains

UNIT SPECIFICS

The following topics are covered in this unit:

- General state of stress at a point- stress tensor;
- Two-dimensional stress system- plane stress;
- Transformation of stresses;
- Principal stresses, principal directions and maximum in-plane shear stress;
- Mohr's circle of stress and stress ellipse;
- State of strain at a point;
- Two-dimensional strain system- plane strain;
- Strain transformation equations;
- Mohr's circle of strain and ellipse of strain;
- Relationship among various elastic constants.

All the topics are discussed in a lucid manner along with their engineering applications. For student's practice, a moderate number of multiple choice questions, short and long answer type questions and numerical problems are also given.

RATIONALE

Evaluation of stresses and strains in simple one-dimensional problems such as axially loaded bars was introduced in Unit 1. However, the combined loading situations is the most common in any engineering structure or machine elements. This requires the understanding of stresses and strains from three-dimensional point of view and their generalization to two-dimensions for the purpose of analysis. This particular aspect is considered in this unit.

PRE-REQUISITIES

Engineering Mechanics

Understanding of simple stresses and strains

UNIT OUTCOMES

After completing this unit students will be able to

U2-O1: understand the concept of state of stress and strain at a point in three-dimensions.

U2-O2: understand the concept of plane stress and plane strain problems.

U2-O3: evaluate stresses and strains on any plane using stress transformation equations and Mohr's circle.

U2-O4: evaluate principal stresses/strains and their orientation for plane problems.

U2-O5: understand the relationship between stresses and strains- generalized Hooke's law.

U2-O6: understand the relationship among different elastic constants.

Course Outcomes	Expected Mapping with Course Outcomes - CE (1- Weak Correlation; 2- Medium correlation; 3- Strong Correlation)			
	CO-1	CO-2	CO-3	CO-4
U2-O1	3	2	-	-
U2-O2	3	2	-	-
U2-O3	2	3	3	-
U2-O4	3	3	2	-
U2-O5	3	2	-	-
U2-O6	3	-	-	-

Course Outcomes	Expected Mapping with Course Outcomes - ME (1- Weak Correlation; 2- Medium correlation; 3- Strong Correlation)	
	CO-1	CO-2
U2-O1	3	3
U2-O2	3	3
U2-O3	3	3
U2-O4	3	3
U2-O5	3	3
U2-O6	2	2

2.1 Introduction

In Unit 1, problems of simple stresses and strains were covered. For example, when a bar is subjected to an axial load, it introduces only normal stress along the axis of the bar. No other component of stress is involved. As a result, longitudinal and transverse normal strains are introduced, but no shear strain. Hence, it is a case of simple stress and strain. Consider another example. Two plates are held together by a lap joint with the help of a rivet. In the lap joint, the bottom surface of one plate overlaps the top surface of another plate up to some length; overall length is the sum of lengths of the plate minus overlap length. A cylindrical rivet with a head is inserted through the holes in the plate and its other end is plastically deformed to make a head. Thus, the plates get locked with each other through the rivet. When a tensile load is applied on the plates, the loads on the pin act normal to its cylindrical axis.

Thus, the pin is subjected to shear force, which tends to displace the upper half of the pin with respect to the lower half. It is a case in which shear stress dominates. Thus, we have considered the cases, in which only one type of stress (either normal or shear) dominates at a point. In this unit, compound stresses and strains, involving more than one kind of stresses and strains acting simultaneously, will be taken up. The generation of compound stresses and strains in structural or machine members is fairly common.

2.2 General state of stress at a point

The stress vector, *i.e.*, traction, at a point is a function of the coordinates of the point and the plane passing through that point. Through a point of interest in a loaded body, an infinite number of cutting planes can be imagined, as shown in Fig. 2.1. Here, at point P, three cutting planes with outward normal $\hat{n}_1$, $\hat{n}_2$ and $\hat{n}_3$ are represented. There can be innumerable such planes. One can evaluate the intensity of the internal forces at the point of interest P on all planes. Thus, one obtains an infinite set of stress vectors acting at P. The set of stress vectors thus obtained at a point is called as the state of stress at a point. However, it can be shown that the state of stress at a point is completely described by three stress vectors acting on three mutually orthogonal planes. As a vector comprises three components in a three-dimensional space, the stress tensor is described by 9 components.

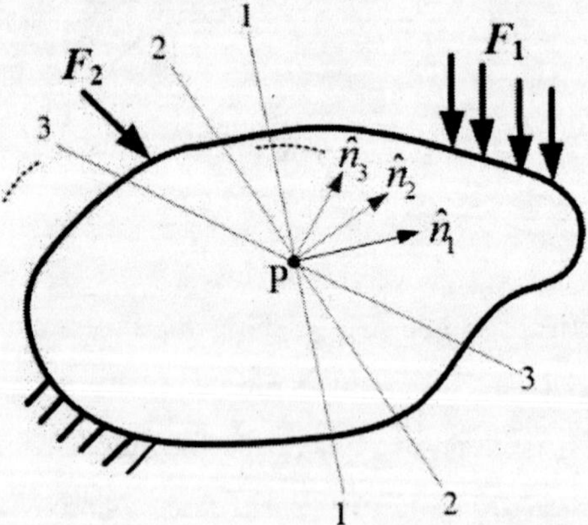

Fig. 2.1 Set of infinite planes imagined through a point in a loaded body (dashed lines indicate the existence of an infinite number of hypothetical cutting planes.)

2.2.1 State of stress at a point in three-dimensions

Consider a point P in a loaded solid, which is in the form of a sphere in its deformed state in three-dimensional Cartesian (x, y, z) reference frame as shown in Fig. 2.2 (a). The spherical shape of the body has been chosen for illustration purposes only. In fact, a deformed body may adopt any shape. The subsequent discussion is valid for all such shapes. Consider three cutting planes in such a way that their outwards normal vectors are along the three Cartesian directions x, y, and z, respectively. The plane whose normal is along the x direction is called the x-plane, the plane whose normal is along the y direction is called the y-plane, and the plane whose normal is along the z direction is called the z-pane. The resultant of the distributed internal force on the x-plane enclosing an infinitesimal area ΔA_x is $\Delta \vec{F}_x$. The force $\Delta \vec{F}_x$ can be resolved into three components, one perpendicular to the plane ΔF_{xx}, along the x- direction and two along the plane, ΔF_{xy}, ΔF_{xz}, along the y and z- directions, respectively. Now, the traction $\vec{t}_x$ on the x-plane is given by

$$\vec{t}_x = \lim_{\Delta A_y \to 0} \frac{\Delta \vec{F}_x}{\Delta A_x}. \tag{2.1}$$

The components of traction $\vec{t}_x$ along the x-direction is the normal stress component on the x-plane and can be expressed as

$$\sigma_{xx} = \lim_{\Delta A_x \to 0} \frac{\Delta F_{xx}}{\Delta A_x}. \tag{2.2}$$

Similarly, the components of $\vec{t}_x$ along y and z- directions are the shear stress components on the x-plane and are given by

$$\tau_{xy} = \lim_{\Delta A_x \to 0} \frac{\Delta F_{xy}}{\Delta A_x}, \tag{2.3}$$

$$\tau_{xz} = \lim_{\Delta A_x \to 0} \frac{\Delta F_{xz}}{\Delta A_x}. \tag{2.4}$$

In Eqs. (2.2) –(2.4), the first suffix to the stress components refers to the plane, and the second suffix refers to the direction along which it is acting. If the resultants of the distributed internal forces on the y and z-plane are $\Delta\vec{F}_y$ and $\Delta\vec{F}_z$ acting on infinitesimal areas ΔA_y and ΔA_z, respectively, then the traction at a point on the y and z-plane can be expressed as

$$\vec{t}_y = \lim_{\Delta A_y \to 0} \frac{\Delta\vec{F}_y}{\Delta A_y}, \tag{2.5}$$

$$\vec{t}_z = \lim_{\Delta A_z \to 0} \frac{\Delta\vec{F}_z}{\Delta A_z}. \tag{2.6}$$

Further, resolving $\Delta\vec{F}_y$ along x, y, and z-directions, the normal and shear components of $\vec{t}_y$ are given by

$$\tau_{yx} = \lim_{\Delta A_y \to 0} \frac{\Delta F_{yx}}{\Delta A_y}, \tag{2.7}$$

$$\sigma_{yy} = \lim_{\Delta A_y \to 0} \frac{\Delta F_{yy}}{\Delta A_y}, \tag{2.8}$$

$$\tau_{yz} = \lim_{\Delta A_y \to 0} \frac{\Delta F_{yz}}{\Delta A_y}. \tag{2.9}$$

Similarly, resolving $\Delta\vec{F}_z$ along x, y, and z-directions, the normal and shear components of $\vec{t}_z$ are given by

$$\tau_{zx} = \lim_{\Delta A_z \to 0} \frac{\Delta F_{zx}}{\Delta A_z}, \tag{2.10}$$

$$\tau_{zy} = \lim_{\Delta A_z \to 0} \frac{\Delta F_{zy}}{\Delta A_z}, \tag{2.11}$$

$$\sigma_{zz} = \lim_{\Delta A_z \to 0} \frac{\Delta F_{zz}}{\Delta A_z}. \tag{2.12}$$

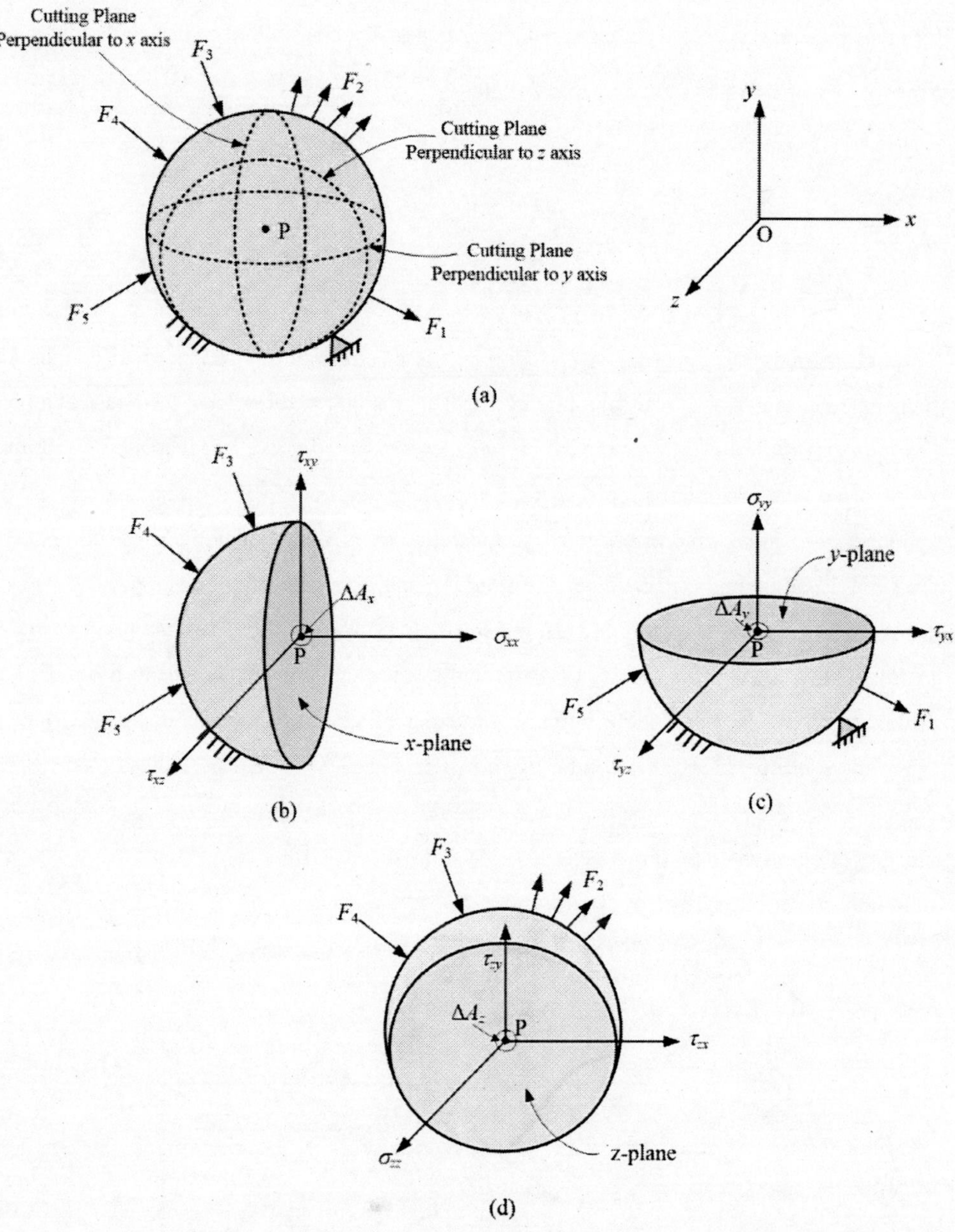

Fig. 2.2 Stress components acting on x, y, and z planes at a point in a three-dimensional space

It can be shown that the state of stress at point P can be completely described by the three tractions acting on three mutually perpendicular planes containing the point P given by Eqs. (2.1), (2.5) & (2.6) or by their components, *i.e.*, the nine stress components given by Eqs. (2.2) – (2.4), (2.7) – (2.12). The normal and shear stress components acting on three mutually perpendicular x, y and z planes are shown in Figs. 2.2 (b), (c), and (d), respectively, by revealing the respective planes considering imaginary cuts in the sphere perpendicular to the x, y, and z axes. The state of stress at a point of interest can be completely represented by the following matrix notation:

$$[\sigma]=\begin{bmatrix} \sigma_{xx} & \tau_{xy} & \tau_{xz} \\ \tau_{yx} & \sigma_{yy} & \tau_{yz} \\ \tau_{zx} & \tau_{zy} & \sigma_{zz} \end{bmatrix}. \tag{2.13}$$

Equation (2.13) represents the components of stress tensor acting on three mutually perpendicular x, y, and z- planes in three Cartesian x, y, and z- directions; the stress at a point is a tensor of order two. This can also be represented by using indices, ij as a subscript to σ, *i.e.*, σ_{ij}. Here, the first index i represents the x, y, and z planes on which the stresses are acting, and the second index j represents the x, y, and z directions along which the stress components are acting. For example, expanding σ_{ij} on the x-plane, one gets components σ_{xx}, σ_{xy}, and σ_{xz}. Often the symbol τ is used to represent the shear stress. Hence, the stress components σ_{xy}, σ_{xz} in Eq. (2.13) are written as τ_{xy}, τ_{xz}. By slicing out a cubical element from a solid of an arbitrary shape surrounding the point P, the state of stresses given by Eq. (2.13) can be represented on the faces of the cube as shown in Fig. 2.3. When the indices to the stress components are equal, *i.e.*, the plane and the direction of stresses coincides, sometimes they are simply represented by only one index. Thus, the normal stress components σ_{xx}, σ_{yy}, σ_{zz} can be simply represented by σ_x, σ_y, σ_z.

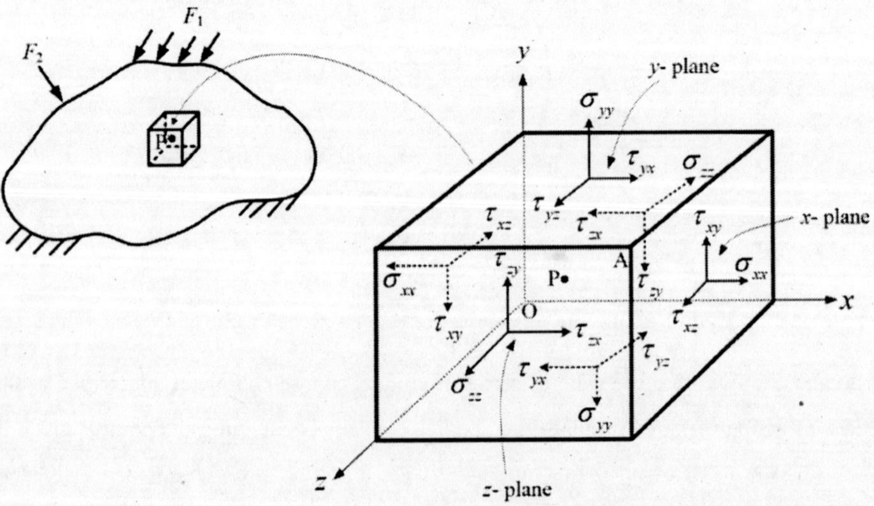

Fig. 2.3 State of stress at a point P represented on a cube element

2.2.2 Symmetry of stress tensor

Referring back to Eq. (2.13) which represents the stress tensor in matrix notation, we see that the total number of stress components at a point is 9, with three normal stress components– $\sigma_{xx}, \sigma_{yy}, \sigma_{zz}$ and six shear stress components– $\tau_{xy}, \tau_{xz}, \tau_{yx}, \tau_{yz}, \tau_{zx}, \tau_{zy}$. Now, it can be shown that this stress tensor is symmetric, *i.e.*, $[\sigma]=[\sigma]^T$ in the absence of unbalanced moments due to body forces. To prove this, consider an infinitesimal parallelepiped element surrounding the point P. The isolated parallelepiped element $\Delta x \Delta y \Delta z$ with the stress components on three faces are shown in Fig. 2.4. The stress components on the hidden faces are not shown, but they will be just opposite to corresponding opposite faces.

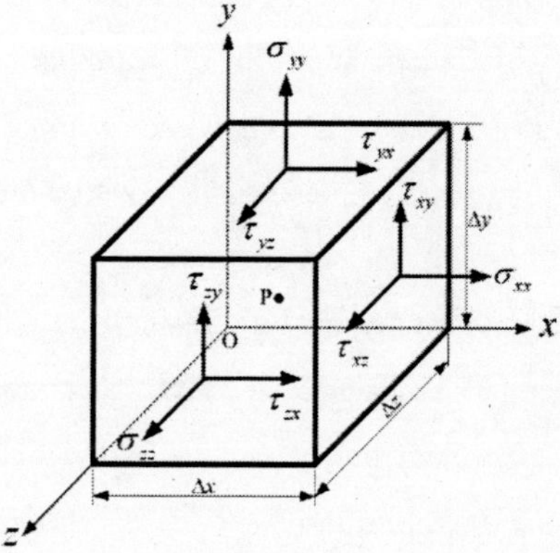

Fig. 2.4 A parallelepiped element isolated from a loaded solid with the stress components.

The moment about z-axis provides

$$M_z = \tau_{xy}\Delta y\Delta z(\Delta x) - \tau_{yx}\Delta x\Delta z(\Delta y) = (\tau_{xy} - \tau_{yx})\Delta x\Delta y\Delta z. \tag{2.14}$$

The moment due to body forces will contain higher order terms; hence neglected. In equilibrium, the moment M_z must vanish. Hence,

$$\tau_{xy} = \tau_{yx} \tag{2.15}$$

Similarly, by taking the moments about x and y- axis and using the condition of equilibrium, it can be shown that

$$\tau_{yz} = \tau_{zy}, \quad \tau_{xz} = \tau_{zx}. \tag{2.16}$$

In view of Eqs. (2.15) and (2.16), the stress tensor is symmetric. Thus, the stress tensor in symmetric form can be presented in the matrix form as

$$[\sigma]=\begin{bmatrix}\sigma_{xx} & \tau_{xy} & \tau_{zx}\\ \tau_{xy} & \sigma_{yy} & \tau_{yz}\\ \tau_{zx} & \tau_{yz} & \sigma_{zz}\end{bmatrix}. \tag{2.17}$$

Equation (2.17) reveals that there are six independent stress components at a point, $\sigma_{xx}, \sigma_{yy}, \sigma_{zz}, \tau_{xy}, \tau_{yz}$ and τ_{zx}.

2.2.3 Sign convention for stress components

For a stress component, we specify two things, the plane on which it acts and its direction. A plane *i* is described as the plane whose outward normal is directed along the ith direction. If the outward normal to the plane *i* is directed in the positive *i* direction, then the plane *i* is considered as a positive plane and if the outward normal to the plane *i* is directed in the negative *i* direction, then the plane *i* is considered as a negative plane. A positive stress component is one that acts on a positive plane in the positive direction or on a negative plane in the negative direction. Otherwise, the stress component is taken as negative. For example, let us consider a point P enclosed by an infinitesimal cube element ABCDEFGH in an arbitrary solid with reference to Cartesian (*x*, *y*, *z*) axes as shown in Fig. 2.5. Now, the faces ABCD and EFGH of the cube element are *x*-plane as the outward normal drawn to these faces are directed along the *x*-axis. Similarly, the faces EADH and FBCG are *y*-planes, and faces, EABF and HDCG, are *z*-planes. The outward normal to the face ABCD points to the positive *x*- direction and thus, it is designated as the positive *x* plane. On the other hand, the face EFGH is designated as the negative *x* plane as the outward normal to it points to the negative *x* direction. Similarly, EADH, and FBCG are the positive and negative *y* planes, respectively, and EABF, and HDCG are the positive and negative *z* planes, respectively. The positive and negative *x*, *y* and *z* planes are shown in Fig. 2.5 (a). The positive and negative stress components on these planes are depicted in Fig. 2.5 (b) and (c). For the purpose of understanding, the stresses on the positive *x*, *y*, and *z*-planes are represented by solid (black, red, and green coloured) arrows, and the stresses on the negative planes are shown by the corresponding dotted arrows.

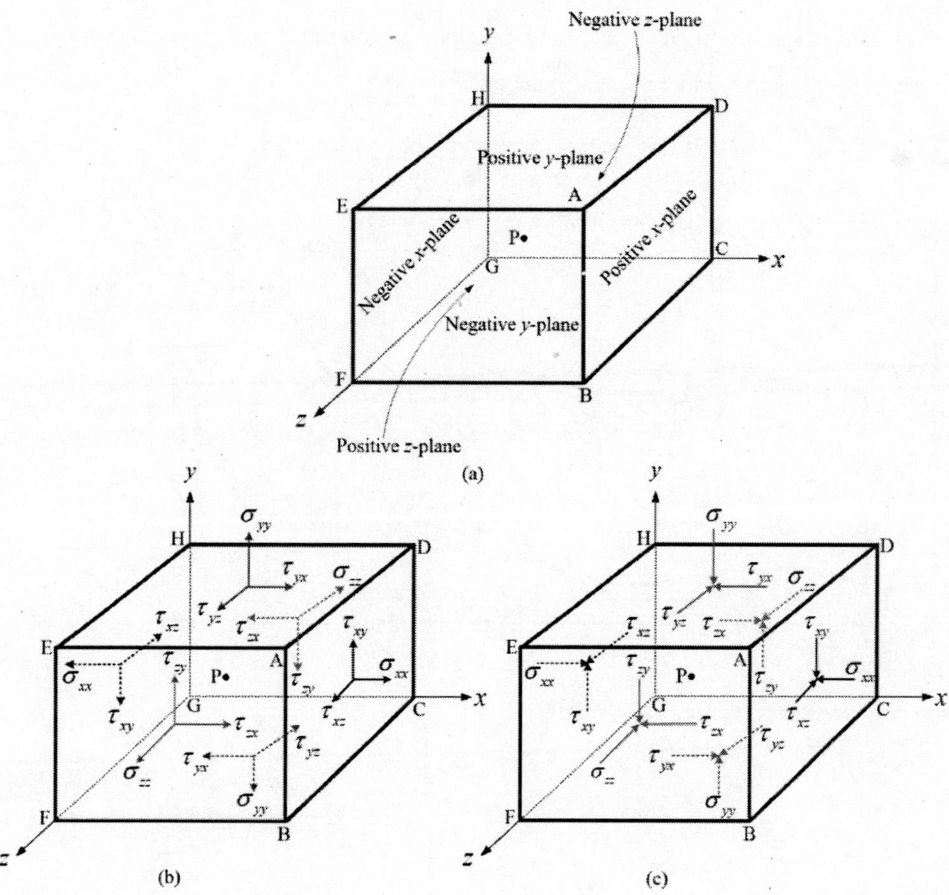

Fig. 2.5 (a) Positive and negative *x*, *y* and *z*-planes, (b) positive stresses on the planes and (c) negative stresses on the planes.

2.2.4 Cauchy's law: State of stress on an arbitrary plane

Cauchy's law states that there exists a Cauchy stress tensor [σ]which maps the normal to a surface to the traction vector acting on that surface, according to

$$\begin{aligned} \vec{t}_x &= \sigma_{xx}n_x + \tau_{xy}n_y + \tau_{xz}n_z, \\ \vec{t}_y &= \tau_{yx}n_x + \sigma_{yy}n_y + \tau_{yz}n_z, \\ \vec{t}_z &= \tau_{zx}n_x + \tau_{zy}n_y + \sigma_{zz}n_z, \end{aligned} \tag{2.18}$$

where n_x, n_y, n_z represents the components of the unit normal $\hat{n}$ to any arbitrary plane with respect to (*x*, *y*, *z*). Cauchy stress is force divided by the deformed area in the limit when the area goes to zero. Equation (2.18) dictates that the state of stress on an arbitrary plane can be completely represented by the three traction components acting on three mutually perpendicular planes or by their nine components.

2.3 Two-Dimensional Stress System- Stress at a point on a plane

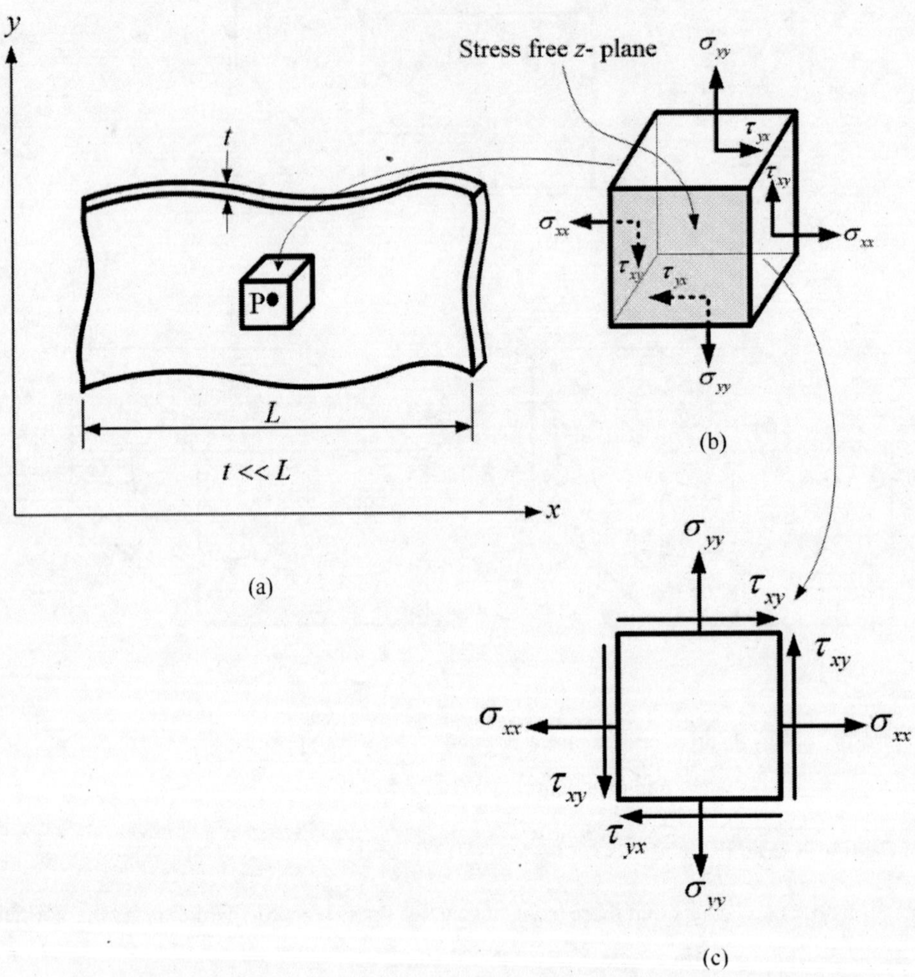

Fig. 2.6 Two-dimensional stress system (state of plane stress at a point)

Let us consider a solid continuum in the form of a thin plate in the x-y plane, as shown in Fig. 2.6 (a). As the plate is thin, its dimension in the z-direction, *i.e.*, thickness t is very small as compared to its length, L; it is reasonable to assume that the variation of stress in the z-direction at a point P within the loaded continuum is negligible or uniform. The state of stress at point P will be functions of x and y only. It is also assumed that the z-planes are unloaded or stress-free. Thus, the components of stress acting on any z-plane within the interior of the continuum are zero, *i.e.*, $\sigma_{zz}=\tau_{zx}=\tau_{zy}=0$. The state of stress at point P is then represented by the four components, σ_{xx}, τ_{xy}, σ_{yy}, and τ_{yx}, and is shown in a cube element (shown exaggerated) sliced out from the continuum in Fig. 2.6 (b). In Fig. 2.6 (c), a two-dimensional view is shown, which is the view of the cube element with the stress components when looked normal to the z-plane from a far distance apart. In view of the symmetry of the stress components ($\tau_{xy}=\tau_{yx}$), there are only three independent stress components acting on the plane and can be given by

$$[\sigma]=\begin{bmatrix}\sigma_{xx} & \tau_{xy}\\ \tau_{xy} & \sigma_{yy}\end{bmatrix}. \tag{2.19}$$

The state of stress given by Eq. (2.19) represents the two-dimensional stress system or the state of stress at a point on a plane. The two-dimensional stress system is an approximation to the generalized three-dimensional stress state often used for solving many problems, such as thin plate, or thin disk (very short cylinder) under different loading conditions, where one of the dimensions is negligibly small compared to the other two dimensions.

2.4 Transformation of Stress Components

The stress at a point is a tensor of order two, and its components get changed from one coordinate frame to the other when rotated with respect to the original coordinate system. It is noteworthy that the stress at the point of interest does not change; only its components get changed. This section discusses how the components of stress change to a rotated frame with respect to the given coordinate frame. It is of interest to engineers on many occasions when they need to evaluate stresses along different loading axes. As an example, the loading axes on an aircraft is shown in Fig. 2.7. The fuselage axes x-y are oriented along the thrust and lift of the aircraft, respectively. By knowing the thrust and lift forces acting on the aircraft, one can evaluate the stress components on any element taken on the fuselage of the aircraft, along x and y. If one is interested to know the components of stress along the wing axes x'-y', which are not oriented along the loading axes, but rotated at some angle θ with respect to the loading axes, then the transformation of the stress components is needed. Thus, the transformation of stresses plays an important role in many practical applications. In order to develop an understanding of the transformation of stresses, first, the simplest case of stress acting on an inclined plane in an axially loaded member is described.

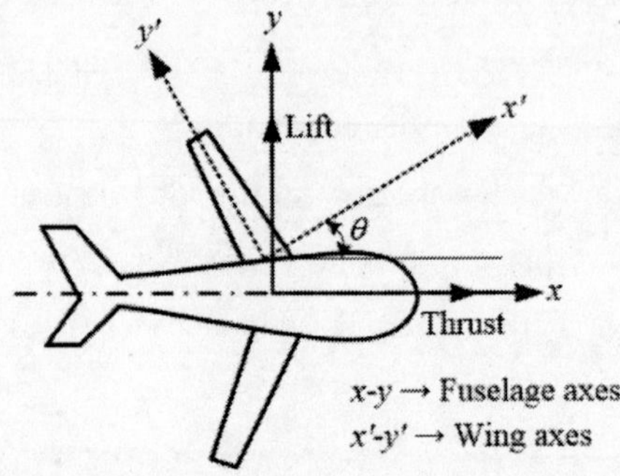

Fig. 2.7 Example of loading axes on an aircraft

2.4.1 The simplest case of stress transformation: stresses on an inclined plane in uniaxial loading

The transformation rules can be directly developed using the equations of static equilibrium. Let us consider the simplest case of a prismatic member of cross-sectional area A subjected to a uniaxial load P, as shown in Fig. 2.8 (a). With reference to the x-y Cartesian frame of reference, the only stress component acting on a vertical plane chosen at any arbitrary location slightly away from the load application points is $\sigma_{xx}=P/A$. Now, an imaginary cut is taken along an inclined plane oriented at an angle θ with respect to a vertical plane. A free-body diagram is then constructed by slicing out an element containing a vertical plane as well as the inclined plane, as shown in Fig. 2.8 (b). On the vertical plane, the stress component σ_{xx} is acting. We are interested in evaluating the stresses on the inclined plane- the component $\sigma_{x'x'}$ normal to the plane and the component $\tau_{x'y'}$ along the plane in the new coordinate system x'-y', which gets rotated by an angle θ with respect to the x-y coordinate system.

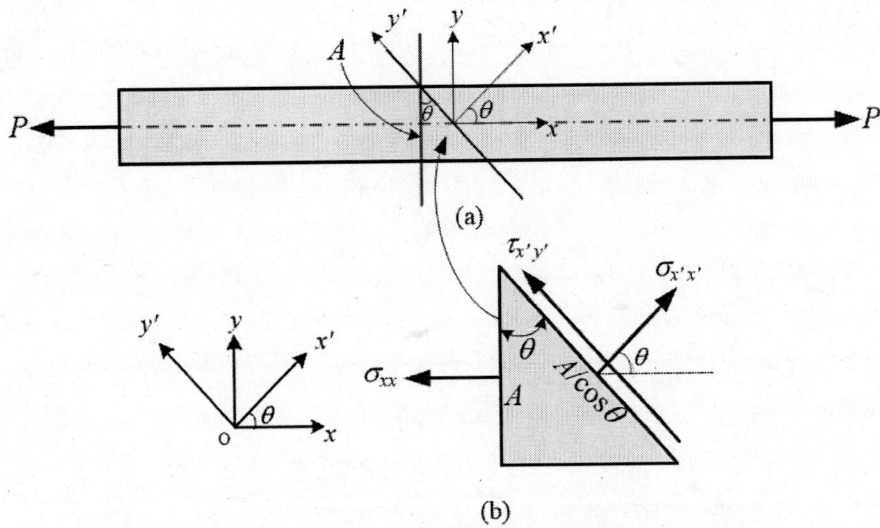

Fig. 2.8 Stresses on an inclined plane in an axially loaded member

It is to be noted that the area on which the transformed stresses $\sigma_{x'x'}$ and $\tau_{x'y'}$ are acting, *i.e.*, the inclined area normal to the x'-axis is different from that of the area normal to the x-axis. The area A normal to the x-axis when gets rotated by angle θ, it is transformed to $(A/\cos\theta)$. Writing the equation of static equilibrium in the x' direction, one obtains

$$\sigma_{x'x'}\left(\frac{A}{\cos\theta}\right) - \sigma_{xx}A\cos\theta = 0,$$

$$\sigma_{x'x'} = \sigma_{xx}\cos^2\theta. \tag{2.20}$$

Similarly, the equation of static equilibrium in the y' direction provides

$$\sigma_{xx}A\sin\theta + \tau_{x'y'}\left(\frac{A}{\cos\theta}\right) = 0,$$

$$\tau_{x'y'} = -\sigma_{xx}\sin\theta\cos\theta = -\frac{1}{2}\sigma_{xx}\sin 2\theta. \tag{2.21}$$

Equations (2.20) and (2.21) are the transformation equations that relate the stress components acting on the inclined plane to the uniaxial stress component.

2.4.2 Transformation of two-dimensional stress system

The transformation rules for a two-dimensional stress system can be developed in a similar way as discussed in Subsection 2.4.1. For this, consider an infinitesimal two-dimensional rectangular element surrounding a point P sliced out from a planar body (*e.g.*, a cantilever beam) as shown in Fig. 2.9 (a). The state of stress at point P can be conveniently represented by the normal stress components σ_{xx}, σ_{yy}, and the shear stress component τ_{xy}

acting on the x and y-planes of the rectangular element with reference to x-y coordinate system. Now, consider a plane a-a that cuts the rectangular element such that the outward normal drawn to plane a-a coincides with the x' axis oriented at an angle θ with respect to x axis. Rotating the y-axis by an angle θ, axis y' is drawn parallel to the plane a-a forming the new coordinate system x'-y'. The left cut part of the rectangular element by plane a-a, which is in the form of a right-angled triangle labeled as ABC, is now isolated from the rest of the elemental part, and a free body diagram is constructed as shown in Fig. 2.9 (b). The cut face AC, whose normal is oriented along x' axis, is referred to as the x' plane. The faces AB and BC are the x and y planes, respectively. Considering the area of the x' plane as dA, the areas of the x and y planes are evaluated as d$A\cos\theta$ and d$A\sin\theta$, respectively.

The transformed stresses on the x' plane are $\sigma_{x'x'}$ and $\tau_{x'y'}$. Resolving the normal and shear stresses acting on the x and y planes along x' and y' directions and then writing equations of static equilibrium, one will obtain the equations for the transformed stress components. The equation of static equilibrium in x' direction provides

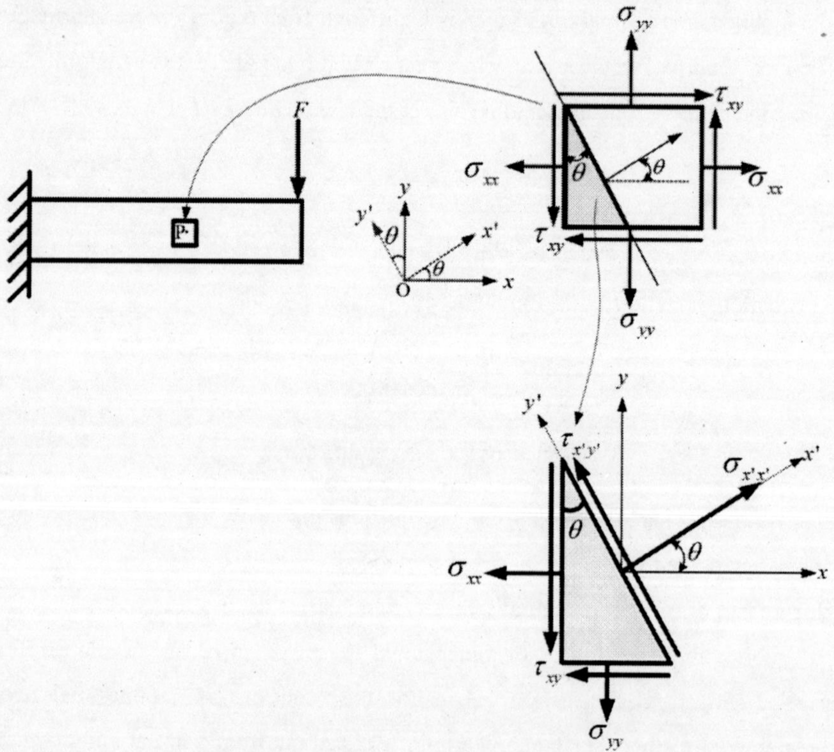

Fig. 2.9 Transformation of two-dimensional stress system

$$\sigma_{x'x'}\mathrm{d}A - \sigma_{xx}\left(\mathrm{d}A\cos\theta\right)\cos\theta - \tau_{xy}\left(\mathrm{d}A\cos\theta\right)\sin\theta - \tau_{xy}\left(\mathrm{d}A\sin\theta\right)\cos\theta - \sigma_{yy}\left(\mathrm{d}A\sin\theta\right)\sin\theta = 0,$$

$$\sigma_{x'x'} = \sigma_{xx}\cos^2\theta + \sigma_{yy}\sin^2\theta + \tau_{xy}\sin 2\theta,$$

$$= \sigma_{xx}\frac{1}{2}\left(1+\cos 2\theta\right) + \sigma_{yy}\frac{1}{2}\left(1-\cos 2\theta\right) + \tau_{xy}\sin 2\theta,$$

$$\sigma_{x'x'} = \frac{1}{2}\left(\sigma_{xx}+\sigma_{yy}\right) + \frac{1}{2}\left(\sigma_{xx}-\sigma_{yy}\right)\cos 2\theta + \tau_{xy}\sin 2\theta. \tag{2.22}$$

Similarly, by writing the equation of static equilibrium, one obtains

$$\tau_{x'y'}\mathrm{d}A + \sigma_{xx}\left(\mathrm{d}A\cos\theta\right)\sin\theta - \sigma_{yy}\left(\mathrm{d}A\sin\theta\right)\cos\theta - \tau_{xy}\left(\mathrm{d}A\cos\theta\right)\cos\theta + \tau_{xy}\left(\mathrm{d}A\sin\theta\right)\sin\theta = 0,$$

$$\tau_{x'y'} = -\sigma_{xx}\cos\theta\sin\theta + \sigma_{yy}\sin\theta\cos\theta + \tau_{xy}\cos^2\theta - \tau_{xy}\sin^2\theta,$$

$$\tau_{x'y'} = \left(\sigma_{yy}-\sigma_{xx}\right)\sin\theta\cos\theta + \tau_{xy}\left(\cos^2\theta - \sin^2\theta\right),$$

$$\tau_{x'y'} = -\frac{1}{2}\left(\sigma_{xx}-\sigma_{yy}\right)\sin 2\theta + \tau_{xy}\cos 2\theta. \tag{2.23}$$

Equations (2.22) and (2.23) provide the transformed stress components $\sigma_{x'x'}$ and $\tau_{x'y'}$ on the x' plane with reference to the stress components on the x plane. If one wants to obtain the stress components on the y' plane, one can imagine a cutting plane such that its outward normal is aligned with the y' axis, which is oriented at an angle of (θ+90°) with respect to the x-axis. Now, replacing θ by (θ+90°) in the expression of $\sigma_{x'x'}$, the expression for normal stress $\sigma_{y'y'}$ on the y' plane is obtained as

$$\sigma_{y'y'} = \frac{1}{2}\left(\sigma_{xx}+\sigma_{yy}\right) - \frac{1}{2}\left(\sigma_{xx}-\sigma_{yy}\right)\cos 2\theta - \tau_{xy}\sin 2\theta. \tag{2.24}$$

The expression for shear stress component $\tau_{x'y'}$ on the y' plane remains the same as obtained in Eq. (2.23) due to the symmetry of the stress tensor. The representative of the transformed two-dimensional stress system in rectangular element rotated with respect to the original element is shown in Fig. 2.10.

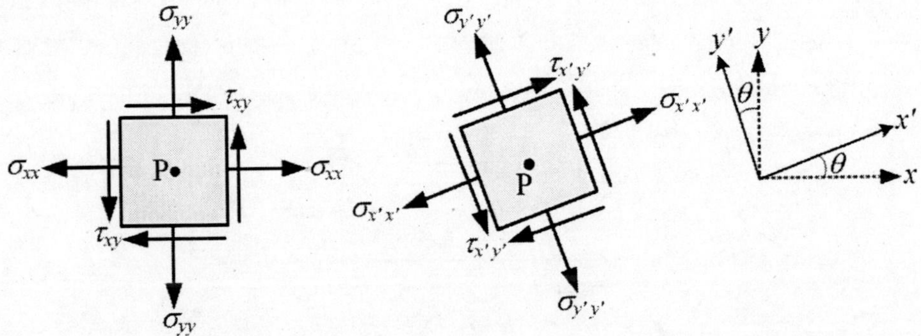

Fig. 2.10 Representation of the transformed two-dimensional stress components

Using Eqs. (2.22)–(2.24), the stress components acting on the x' and y' planes can be expressed in matrix form as

$$\begin{bmatrix} \sigma_{x'x'} & \tau_{x'y'} \\ \tau_{x'y'} & \sigma_{y'y'} \end{bmatrix} = \begin{bmatrix} \sigma_{xx}\cos^2\theta + \sigma_{yy}\sin^2\theta + \tau_{xy}\sin 2\theta & (\sigma_{yy} - \sigma_{xx})\sin\theta\cos\theta + \tau_{xy}\cos 2\theta \\ (\sigma_{yy} - \sigma_{xx})\sin\theta\cos\theta + \tau_{xy}\cos 2\theta & \sigma_{xx}\sin^2\theta + \sigma_{yy}\cos^2\theta - \tau_{xy}\sin 2\theta \end{bmatrix}.$$

(2.25)

Rearranging the right-hand side of Eq. (2.25), one can write

$$\begin{bmatrix} \sigma_{x'x'} & \tau_{x'y'} \\ \tau_{x'y'} & \sigma_{y'y'} \end{bmatrix} = \begin{bmatrix} \cos\theta & -\sin\theta \\ \sin\theta & \cos\theta \end{bmatrix} \begin{bmatrix} \sigma_{xx} & \tau_{xy} \\ \tau_{xy} & \sigma_{yy} \end{bmatrix} \begin{bmatrix} \cos\theta & \sin\theta \\ -\sin\theta & \cos\theta \end{bmatrix}, \tag{2.26}$$

where $\begin{bmatrix} \cos\theta & -\sin\theta \\ \sin\theta & \cos\theta \end{bmatrix}$ is the rotation matrix, in which the first row provides the direction cosine of x with respect to coordinate system x'-y'. The second row provides the direction cosine of y with respect to the coordinate system x'-y'. Denoting the stress matrix in the transformed coordinate system x'-y' as $[\sigma']$, the direction cosine matrix as $[\alpha]$ and the stress matrix in the original coordinate system x-y as $[\sigma]$, Eq. (2.26) in matrix notation can be expressed as

$$[\sigma'] = [\alpha][\sigma][\alpha]^{\mathrm{T}}, \tag{2.27}$$

where $[\alpha]^{\mathrm{T}}$ denotes the transpose of matrix $[\alpha]$. Equation (2.27) is the transformation rule for stress and can be extended to transform stress components in three dimensions as well. If we assume $\boldsymbol{\sigma}$ to be any tensor of order two in Eq. (2.27), it turns out to be the generalized transformation rule for any tensor quantity of order two with respect to two Cartesian coordinate systems. As stress transforms according to Eq. (2.27), the state of stress at a point is termed as the tensor of order two.

Example 2.1 Two wooden pieces of thickness 1 cm are glued together, as shown in the figure, to make a rectangular block of 1 cm × 5 cm × 30 cm. The two ends of the block are pulled by a force of 5 kN. What should be the minimum shear strength of the glue so that wooden pieces do not separate?

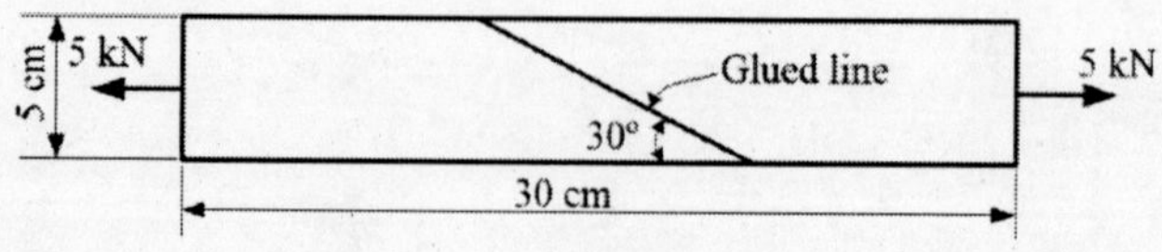

Solution

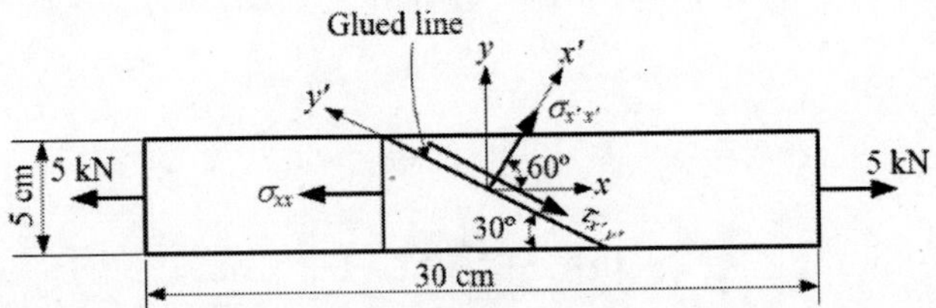

Choosing the x axis normal to the cross-section of the glued rectangular block and y axis parallel to its cross-section, the normal stress acting on the vertical plane is evaluated as

$$\sigma_{xx} = \frac{5\times1000}{(1\times5)\times10^2} = 10\,\text{MPa}.$$

The inclined plane is taken along the x' direction, and the y' direction is taken along its normal, which makes an angle θ=60° with x axis. Now, using transformation Eq. (2.21), the shear stress acting along the glued line is obtained as

$$\tau_{x'y'} = \frac{1}{2}\sigma_{xx}\sin 2\theta = \frac{1}{2}\times10\times\sin(2\times60°) = 4.33\,\text{MPa}.$$

Therefore, the minimum shear strength of the glue should be 4.33 MPa.

Example 2.2 The plane state of stress at a point acting on two mutually perpendicular planes is given by σ_{xx}=20 MPa, τ_{xy}= −10 MPa and σ_{yy}=10 MPa in the Cartesian (x, y) coordinate system. When this set of coordinate axes is rotated counter-clockwise by an angle 30° to form a new coordinate system (x', y'), evaluate the components of stress in this new coordinate system.

Solution

Given, σ_{xx}=20 MPa, τ_{xy}= −10 MPa, σ_{yy}=10 MPa and θ=30°.

Now, using transformation Eqs. (2.22) – (2.24), the components of stress in the (x', y') coordinate system are obtained as

$$\sigma_{x'x'} = \frac{1}{2}(\sigma_{xx}+\sigma_{yy}) + \frac{1}{2}(\sigma_{xx}-\sigma_{yy})\cos 2\theta + \tau_{xy}\sin 2\theta,$$

$$= \frac{1}{2}(20+10) + \frac{1}{2}(20-10)\cos(2\times30°) + (-10)\sin(2\times30°) = 8.84\,\text{MPa}.$$

$$\tau_{x'y'} = -\frac{1}{2}(\sigma_{xx} - \sigma_{yy})\sin 2\theta + \tau_{xy}\cos 2\theta,$$

$$= -\frac{1}{2}(20-10)\sin(2\times 30°) + (-10)\cos(2\times 30°) = -9.33\,\text{MPa}.$$

$$\sigma_{y'y'} = \frac{1}{2}(\sigma_{xx} + \sigma_{yy}) - \frac{1}{2}(\sigma_{xx} - \sigma_{yy})\cos 2\theta - \tau_{xy}\sin 2\theta,$$

$$= \frac{1}{2}(20+10) - \frac{1}{2}(20-10)\cos(2\times 30°) - (-10)\sin(2\times 30°) = 21.16\,\text{MPa}.$$

2.5 Concept of principal planes, principal stresses, and principal directions

In order to understand the concept of principal stresses, principal plane, and principal directions, let us consider a plane with normal $\hat{n}$, and the components of its direction cosines with respect to Cartesian (x, y, z) axes are taken as n_x, n_y and n_z. Further, we consider that only normal stress σ_n acts on this plane. If $\vec{t}_n$ is the traction acting on this plane, then its components in the directions of x, y and z in terms of the direction cosines can be written as $(t_n)_x = \sigma_n n_x, (t_n)_y = \sigma_n n_y$ and $(t_n)_z = \sigma_n n_z$, which are nothing but the normal stress components along x, y and z. Using Cauchy's stress relation from Eq. (2.18), one can write

$$\begin{Bmatrix} \sigma_n n_x \\ \sigma_n n_y \\ \sigma_n n_z \end{Bmatrix} = \begin{bmatrix} \sigma_{xx} & \tau_{xy} & \tau_{zx} \\ \tau_{xy} & \sigma_{yy} & \tau_{yz} \\ \tau_{zx} & \tau_{yz} & \sigma_{zz} \end{bmatrix} \begin{Bmatrix} n_x \\ n_y \\ n_z \end{Bmatrix}. \tag{2.28}$$

From Eq. (2.28), we get

$$\sigma_n n_x = \sigma_{xx} n_x + \tau_{xy} n_y + \tau_{zx} n_z, \tag{2.29a}$$

$$\sigma_n n_y = \tau_{xy} n_x + \sigma_{yy} n_y + \tau_{yz} n_z, \tag{2.29b}$$

$$\sigma_n n_z = \tau_{zx} n_x + \tau_{yz} n_y + \sigma_{zz} n_z. \tag{2.29c}$$

The above set of equations can be rearranged to get the following equation in matrix form:

$$\begin{bmatrix} \sigma_{xx} - \sigma_n & \tau_{xy} & \tau_{zx} \\ \tau_{xy} & \sigma_{yy} - \sigma_n & \tau_{yz} \\ \tau_{zx} & \tau_{yz} & \sigma_{zz} - \sigma_n \end{bmatrix} \begin{Bmatrix} n_x \\ n_y \\ n_z \end{Bmatrix} = \begin{Bmatrix} 0 \\ 0 \\ 0 \end{Bmatrix}. \tag{2.30}$$

Equation (2.30) can be thought of as simultaneous equations in n_x, n_y and n_z. To evaluate the unknowns n_x, n_y, and n_z, Eq. (2.30) neds to be solved such that it satisfies the following condition:

$$n_x^2 + n_y^2 + n_z^2 = 1. \tag{2.31}$$

For a non-trivial solution of Eq. (2.30), the determinant of the coefficients of n_x, n_y, and n_z should be zero. Thus,

$$\begin{vmatrix} \sigma_{xx} - \sigma_n & \tau_{xy} & \tau_{zx} \\ \tau_{xy} & \sigma_{yy} - \sigma_n & \tau_{yz} \\ \tau_{zx} & \tau_{yz} & \sigma_{zz} - \sigma_n \end{vmatrix} = 0. \tag{2.32}$$

Evaluating the determinant in Eq. (2.32), one obtains a cubic equation of the following form:

$$\sigma_n^3 - I_{1\sigma}\sigma_n^2 - I_{2\sigma}\sigma_n - I_{3\sigma} = 0, \tag{2.33}$$

where

$$I_{1\sigma} = \sigma_{xx} + \sigma_{yy} + \sigma_{zz}, \tag{2.34a}$$

$$I_{2\sigma} = \frac{1}{2}\left\{\left(\sigma_{xx}{}^2 + \sigma_{yy}{}^2 + \sigma_{zz}{}^2 + 2\tau_{xy}{}^2 + 2\tau_{yz}{}^2 + 2\tau_{zx}{}^2\right) - \left(\sigma_{xx} + \sigma_{yy} + \sigma_{zz}\right)^2\right\}, \tag{2.34b}$$

$$I_{3\sigma} = \begin{vmatrix} \sigma_{xx} & \tau_{xy} & \tau_{zx} \\ \tau_{xy} & \sigma_{yy} & \tau_{yz} \\ \tau_{zx} & \tau_{yz} & \sigma_{zz} \end{vmatrix} = \sigma_{xx}\left(\sigma_{yy}\sigma_{zz} - \tau_{yz}{}^2\right) - \tau_{xy}\left(\tau_{xy}\sigma_{zz} - \tau_{yz}\tau_{zx}\right) + \tau_{zx}\left(\tau_{xy}\tau_{yz} - \sigma_{yy}\tau_{zx}\right). \tag{2.34c}$$

The solution of the cubic Eq. (2.33) provides three real roots, and let us denote the roots as σ_1, σ_2 and σ_3. The values of σ_1, σ_2, and σ_3 are the stresses acting on the three mutually perpendicular planes in the deformed configuration where the stresses are wholly normal, and shear components are zero. The three mutually perpendicular planes on which the traction or stress components are wholly normal and free of shear are called the *principal planes*. The normal stresses σ_1, σ_2, and σ_3 acting on the principal planes are called the *principal stresses*, and the normal to the principal planes are referred to as the *principal directions* (of stress).

2.6 Principal invariants of stress

The quantities $I_{1\sigma}$, $I_{2\sigma}$, and $I_{3\sigma}$ defined in Eqs. (2.34a) – (2.34c) are called as the principal invariants of stress, because they do not change under the change of coordinate system. The quantity $I_{1\sigma}$ is called as the first principal invariant, $I_{2\sigma}$ is called as the second principal invariant and $I_{3\sigma}$ is called as the third principal invariant of stress.

We have evaluated $I_{1\sigma}$, $I_{2\sigma}$, and $I_{3\sigma}$ in Eqs. (2.61a) – (2.61c) choosing the Cartesian coordinate system (x, y, z). Now, if we choose a new coordinate system (x', y', z'), the corresponding stress components acting on the x', y' and z' plane are designated as $\sigma_{x'x'}, \tau_{x'y'}, \tau_{x'z'}, \tau_{y'x'}$, $\sigma_{y'y'}, \tau_{y'z'}$, $\tau_{z'x'}, \tau_{z'y'}$ and $\sigma_{z'z'}$. The values of $I_{1\sigma}$, $I_{2\sigma}$, and $I_{3\sigma}$ in the new coordinate system can be expressed in a similar way as in Eqs. (2.34a) – (2.34c) in terms of the above stress components. One will see that the values of $I_{1\sigma}$, $I_{2\sigma}$, and $I_{3\sigma}$ evaluated using the stress components in (*x*, *y*, *z*) system and that in the (x', y', z') system remain the same. Thus, $I_{1\sigma}$, $I_{2\sigma}$, and $I_{3\sigma}$ are termed as invariants.

As an example, the invariance of $I_{1\sigma}$ can be easily verified from the two-dimensional (plane stress) transformation Eqs. (2.22) and (2.24). If we add the quantities on the left-hand side and right-hand side of Eqs. (2.22) and (2.24), we get

$$\sigma_{x'x'} + \sigma_{y'y'} = \sigma_{xx} + \sigma_{yy}, \tag{2.35}$$

where the left-hand side indicates the value of the first invariant of stress in (x', y') the coordinate system, and the right-hand side indicates the value of the first invariant of stress in (*x*, *y*) coordinate system. Thus, Eq. (2.35) verifies the invariance if I_σ under the change of coordinate system. As $I_{1\sigma}$, $I_{2\sigma}$, and $I_{3\sigma}$ are invariants, it can be inferred from Eq. (2.33) that the principal stresses at a point remain the same irrespective of the reference axes system.

2.7 The Maximum and minimum normal stresses

We have evaluated the normal stress $\sigma_{x'x'}$ on the x' plane oriented at any angle θ in Subsection 2.4.2. Now, we shall look into the position of the planes where the normal stresses are maximum or minimum, and correspondingly we will obtain the values of the maximum and minimum normal stresses.

For maximum or minimum normal stress:

$$\frac{d\sigma_{x'x'}}{d\theta} = 0. \tag{2.36}$$

Substituting for $\sigma_{x'x'}$ from Eq. (2.22) in Eq. (2.36), we get

$$-2\sin 2\theta \frac{1}{2}\left(\sigma_{xx} - \sigma_{yy}\right) + 2\tau_{xy}\cos 2\theta = 0. \tag{2.37}$$

The solution of Eq. (2.37) provides the orientation $\theta = \theta_p$ of the planes of maximum or minimum normal stress as

$$\tan 2\theta_p = \frac{\tau_{xy}}{\frac{1}{2}\left(\sigma_{xx} - \sigma_{yy}\right)}. \tag{2.38}$$

Equation (2.38) provides two values of $2\theta_p$— one is $2\theta_{p_1} = 2\theta_p$, and the other is $2\theta_{p_2} = 2\theta_p + 180°$. As the values of $2\theta_{p_1}$ and $2\theta_{p_2}$ are 180° apart, the values of θ_{p_1} and θ_{p_2}

will be 90° apart. The graphical representation of Eq. (2.38) is shown in Fig. 2.11 (a) when the orientation of the plane is at $2\theta_{p_1}$, and it is shown in Fig. 2.11 (b) when the orientation of the plane is at $2\theta_{p_2} = 2\theta_p + 180°$ in (σ, τ) reference axes.

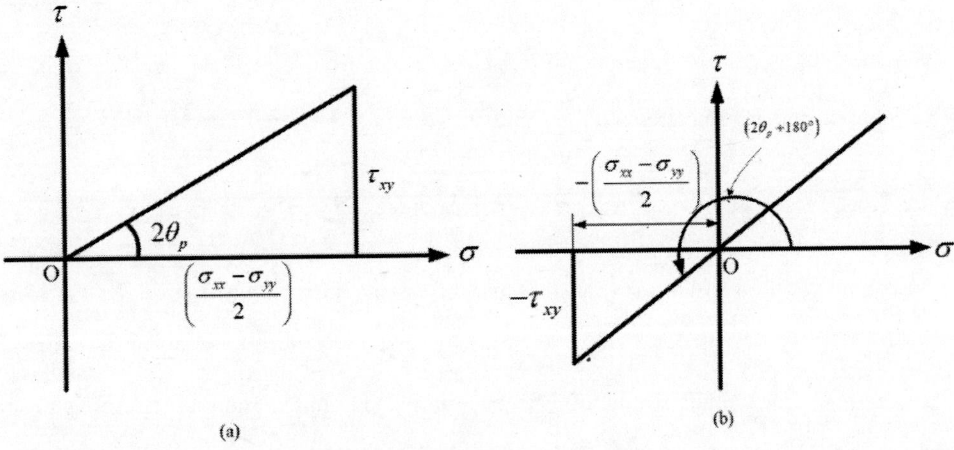

Fig. 2.11 Graphical representation of the orientation of the plane of maximum and minimum normal stress

From Fig. 2.11 (a), one can write

$$\sin 2\theta_p = \frac{\tau_{xy}}{\sqrt{\left(\frac{\sigma_{xx}-\sigma_{yy}}{2}\right)^2 + \tau_{xy}^2}}, \tag{2.39}$$

$$\cos 2\theta_p = \frac{\left(\frac{\sigma_{xx}-\sigma_{yy}}{2}\right)}{\sqrt{\left(\frac{\sigma_{xx}-\sigma_{yy}}{2}\right)^2 + \tau_{xy}^2}}. \tag{2.40}$$

Similarly, from Fig. 2.11 (b),

$$\sin 2\theta_{p_2} = \sin\left(2\theta_p + 180^\circ\right) = -\sin 2\theta_p = -\frac{\tau_{xy}}{\sqrt{\left(\frac{\sigma_{xx}-\sigma_{yy}}{2}\right)^2 + \tau_{xy}^2}}, \tag{2.41}$$

$$\cos 2\theta_p = \cos\left(2\theta_p + 180^\circ\right) = -\cos 2\theta_p = -\frac{\left(\frac{\sigma_{xx}-\sigma_{yy}}{2}\right)}{\sqrt{\left(\frac{\sigma_{xx}-\sigma_{yy}}{2}\right)^2 + \tau_{xy}^2}}. \tag{2.42}$$

Now, substituting the values of $\sin 2\theta_p$ and $\cos 2\theta_p$ from Eqs. (2.39) and (2.40) in Eq. (2.22), the normal stress on the plane θ_{p_1} can be evaluated as

$$\sigma_{\theta_{p_1}} = \frac{\sigma_{xx}+\sigma_{yy}}{2} + \sqrt{\left(\frac{\sigma_{xx}-\sigma_{yy}}{2}\right)^2 + \tau_{xy}^2}. \tag{2.43}$$

Upon substitution of the values of $\sin 2\theta_{p_2}$ and $\cos 2\theta_{p_2}$ from Eqs. (2.41) and (2.42) in Eq. (2.22) provide the normal stress on the plane θ_{p_2} as

$$\sigma_{\theta_{p_2}} = \frac{\sigma_{xx}+\sigma_{yy}}{2} - \sqrt{\left(\frac{\sigma_{xx}-\sigma_{yy}}{2}\right)^2 + \tau_{xy}^2}. \tag{2.44}$$

Equation (2.43) will provide the value of the maximum normal stress on the plane θ_{p_1}, and the normal stress provided by Eq. (2.44) will be the minimum one oriented at $\theta_{p_2} = \theta_p + 90°$. Denoting the values of the maximum and minimum normal stresses as σ_1 and σ_2, we can rewrite Eqs. (2.43) and (2.44) as

$$\sigma_1 = \frac{\sigma_{xx}+\sigma_{yy}}{2} + \sqrt{\left(\frac{\sigma_{xx}-\sigma_{yy}}{2}\right)^2 + \tau_{xy}^2}, \tag{2.45}$$

$$\sigma_2 = \frac{\sigma_{xx}+\sigma_{yy}}{2} - \sqrt{\left(\frac{\sigma_{xx}-\sigma_{yy}}{2}\right)^2 + \tau_{xy}^2}. \tag{2.46}$$

In order to ascertain that Eq. (2.45) provides the maximum and Eq. (2.46) provides the minimum, a double derivative test is needed. However, one can visualize it intuitively also. Combining Eqs. (2.45) and (2.46), one can also express the maximum and minimum normal stresses as

$$\sigma_{1,2} = \frac{\sigma_{xx}+\sigma_{yy}}{2} \pm \sqrt{\left(\frac{\sigma_{xx}-\sigma_{yy}}{2}\right)^2 + \tau_{xy}^2}. \tag{2.47}$$

It can be shown that the maximum and minimum normal stresses are also the principal stresses. Interestingly one obtains the value of $\tan 2\theta$ by setting $\tau_{x'y'} = 0$ in Eq. (2.23) as

$$\tan 2\theta = \frac{\tau_{xy}}{\frac{1}{2}\left(\sigma_{xx}-\sigma_{yy}\right)}, \tag{2.48}$$

which coincides with Eq. (2.38), indicates that the planes of the maximum and minimum normal stresses coincide with the planes on which the shear stress vanishes. Thus, the planes on which the maximum and minimum normal stresses are acting are called as the principal planes and the corresponding stresses are referred as the principal stresses.

2.8 The Maximum In-plane Shear Stress

For the condition of maximum shear stress,

$$\frac{d\tau_{x'y'}}{d\theta} = 0. \tag{2.49}$$

Using the value of $\tau_{x'y'}$ from Eq. (2.23) in Eq. (2.49), one gets the orientation of the plane of maximum shear stress as

$$\tan 2\theta_s = -\frac{\left(\dfrac{\sigma_{xx} - \sigma_{yy}}{2}\right)}{\tau_{xy}}. \tag{2.50}$$

Equation (2.50) provides two values of θ_s denoted as $\theta_{s_1} = \theta_s$ and $\theta_{s_2} = \theta_s + 90^\circ$ in a similar way as obtained for θ_p from Eq. (2.38).

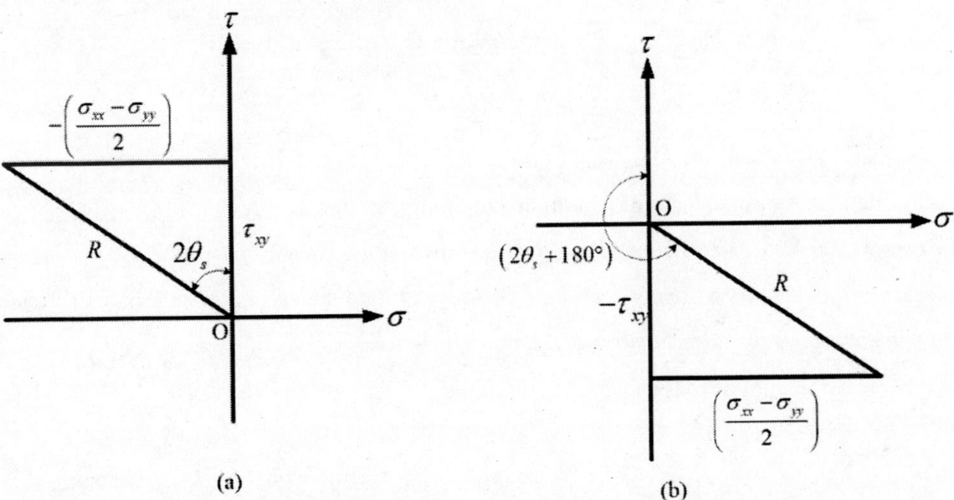

Fig. 2.12 Graphical representation of orientations of the maximum in-plane shear stress

The geometrical form of Eq. (2.50) can be represented in Fig. 2.12 (a) and (b) using (σ, τ) coordinate axes. Referring to Fig. 2.12 (a) and (b), one can write

$$R = \sqrt{\left(\frac{\sigma_{xx} - \sigma_{yy}}{2}\right)^2 + \tau_{xy}^2}, \tag{2.51}$$

$$\cos 2\theta_{s_1} = \frac{\tau_{xy}}{R}, \quad \sin 2\theta_{s_1} = -\frac{\sigma_{xx} - \sigma_{yy}}{2R}, \tag{2.52}$$

$$\cos 2\theta_{s_2} = -\frac{\tau_{xy}}{R}, \quad \sin 2\theta_{s_2} = \frac{\sigma_{xx} - \sigma_{yy}}{2R}. \tag{2.53}$$

Substituting the values of θ_{s_1} and θ_{s_2} from Eqs. (2.52) and (2.53) in Eq. (2.23), the magnitude of the maximum in-plane shear stress is obtained as

$$|\tau_{\max}| = \pm\sqrt{\left(\frac{\sigma_{xx} - \sigma_{yy}}{2}\right)^2 + \tau_{xy}^2}. \tag{2.54}$$

Comparison of Eq. (2.50) with Eq. (2.38) provides

$$\tan 2\theta_s = -\frac{1}{\tan 2\theta_p} = -\cot 2\theta_p,$$

$$\tan 2\theta_s = \tan\left(90^\circ + 2\theta_p\right),$$

$$2\theta_s = 90^\circ + 2\theta_p,$$

$$\theta_s = 45^\circ + \theta_p. \tag{2.55}$$

Equation (2.55) shows that the plane of maximum shear stress forms an angle of 45° with the principal planes or the planes of maximum and minimum normal stresses.

Example 2.3 The state of stress at a point is shown in the figure. Determine the normal and shear stresses acting on the vertical plane. Also, determine the values of the principal stresses and maximum in-plane shear stress at the point.

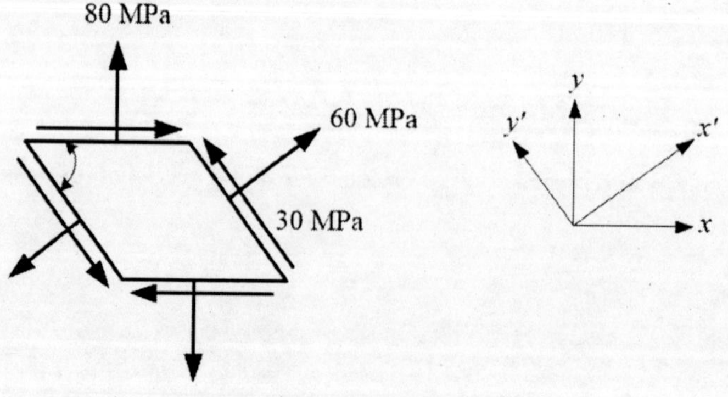

Solution

Referring to the figure,

$$\sigma_{yy} = 80\,\text{MPa},\ \sigma_{x'x'} = 60\,\text{MPa},\ \tau_{x'y'} = 30\,\text{MPa}.$$

Now, using transformation Eqs. (2.23)

$$\tau_{x'y'} = -\frac{1}{2}(\sigma_{xx} - \sigma_{yy})\sin 2\theta + \tau_{xy}\cos 2\theta,$$

$$30 = -\frac{1}{2}(\sigma_{xx} - 80)\sin(2\times 45°) + \tau_{xy}\cos(2\times 45°),$$

$$-\frac{1}{2}(\sigma_{xx} - 80) = 30,$$

$$\sigma_{xx} = 20\,\text{MPa}.$$

From the transformation relation given by Eq. (2.22) and substituting the value of σ_{xx},

$$\sigma_{x'x'} = \frac{1}{2}(\sigma_{xx} + \sigma_{yy}) + \frac{1}{2}(\sigma_{xx} - \sigma_{yy})\cos 2\theta + \tau_{xy}\sin 2\theta,$$

$$60 = \frac{1}{2}(20+80) + \frac{1}{2}(20-80)\cos(2\times 45°) + \tau_{xy}\sin(2\times 45°),$$

$$\tau_{xy} = 10\,\text{MPa}.$$

Thus, the normal and shear stresses acting on the vertical plane are σ_{xx}=20 MPa, and τ_{xy}=10 MPa.

The principal stresses acting at the point are evaluated using Eqs. (2.45) and (2.46) as

$$\sigma_1 = \frac{\sigma_{xx} + \sigma_{yy}}{2} + \sqrt{\left(\frac{\sigma_{xx} - \sigma_{yy}}{2}\right)^2 + \tau_{xy}^2} = \frac{20+80}{2} + \sqrt{\left(\frac{20-80}{2}\right)^2 + 10^2} = 81.62\,\text{MPa},$$

$$\sigma_2 = \frac{\sigma_{xx} + \sigma_{yy}}{2} - \sqrt{\left(\frac{\sigma_{xx} - \sigma_{yy}}{2}\right)^2 + \tau_{xy}^2} = \frac{20+80}{2} - \sqrt{\left(\frac{20-80}{2}\right)^2 + 10^2} = 18.38\,\text{MPa}.$$

Using Eq. (2.54), the maximum in-plane shear stress at the point is obtained as

$$\tau_{\max} = \sqrt{\left(\frac{\sigma_{xx} - \sigma_{yy}}{2}\right)^2 + \tau_{xy}^2} = \sqrt{\left(\frac{20-80}{2}\right)^2 + 10^2} = 31.62\,\text{MPa}.$$

2.9 Mohr's Circle of Stress

In 1895, Otto Mohr, a German civil engineer, suggested a graphical approach to study the transformation of plane stress, known as the Mohr's circle of stress. The construction of Mohr's circle can be interpreted from the transformation equations discussed in Subsection 2.4.2 to obtain the variation of stress components as a function of the orientation of the plane in which it is acting.

2.9.1 Interpretation of Mohr's circle from two-dimensional transformation equations

The transformation Eq. (2.22) can be rewritten in the following form:

$$\left\{\sigma_{x'x'}-\left(\frac{\sigma_{xx}+\sigma_{yy}}{2}\right)\right\}=\left(\frac{\sigma_{xx}-\sigma_{yy}}{2}\right)\cos 2\theta+\tau_{xy}\sin 2\theta. \tag{2.56}$$

Now, squaring the left-hand side and right-hand side of Eqs. (2.56) & (2.23) and summing them up, one obtains

$$\left\{\sigma_{x'x'}-\left(\frac{\sigma_{xx}+\sigma_{yy}}{2}\right)\right\}^2+\left(\tau_{x'y'}\right)^2=\left(\frac{\sigma_{xx}-\sigma_{yy}}{2}\right)^2+\left(\tau_{xy}\right)^2. \tag{2.57}$$

Equation (2.57) can be represented in the following form:

$$(x-a)^2+y^2=b^2 \tag{2.58}$$

which is an equation of a circle with centre at ($+a$, 0) and radius b in the (x, y) coordinate system. Thus, Eq. (2.58) can be interpreted as an equation of a circle with centre at $\left(+\frac{\sigma_{xx}+\sigma_{yy}}{2},0\right)$ and radius $b=\sqrt{\left(\frac{\sigma_{xx}-\sigma_{yy}}{2}\right)^2+\left(\tau_{xy}\right)^2}$ in the $\left(\sigma_{x'x'},\tau_{x'y'}\right)$ reference frame. This circle is termed as the Mohr's circle. The construction of Mohr's circle is discussed in Subsection 2.9.3. In constructing the Mohr's circle, the reference axes is taken as (σ, τ) instead of $\left(\sigma_{x'x'},\tau_{x'y'}\right)$ as we can obtain the state of stress on any plane passing through a point of interest in a planar stressed body. Further, the students often get confused with the sign of shear stress, whether the positive shear stress axis τ to be taken in the upward direction or in the downward direction. To clarify this, a discussion on the sign convention of shear stress is provided in Subsection 2.4.2.

2.9.2 Sign convention of shear stress in constructing Mohr's circle

Convention of shear stress may differ from book to book. In this book, the convention is that on an x-plane (with normal along the positive x-axis), the shear force acting along positive y-axis provides a positive shear stress. Assume now the situation in which only σ_{xx} is non-zero. Other components are zero. From Eq. (2.21), it is seen that shear stress on a plane inclined at an angle θ from the x-plane will be equal to the radius of Mohr circle multiplied by sin2θ, but with a negative sign. However, graphically we shall interpret the y-coordinate of point (b, 2θ) in the polar coordinate on the circle given by Eq. (2.58) as the shear stress. Thus, there is sign difference in analytical formula and graphical interpretation. To resolve this conflict, it is customary to show positive value of τ_{xy} as negative value in the Mohr's circle. However, while marking point (σ_{yy}, τ_{yx}), positive shear stress is shown as positive value only. This can be understood from Eq. (2.23). Here, if only non-zero component is σ_{yy}, then that shear stress on a plane inclined at an angle θ from the x-plane will be equal to the radius of the Mohr circle multiplied by sin2θ, with no negative sign.

2.9.3 Construction of Mohr's circle

Let the state of stress at a point in a two-dimensional solid is given by the components σ_{xx}, σ_{yy} and τ_{xy} in the Cartesian (x, y) reference axes. This state of stress can be conveniently represented on a rectangular element surrounding the point of interest, as shown in Fig. 2.13.

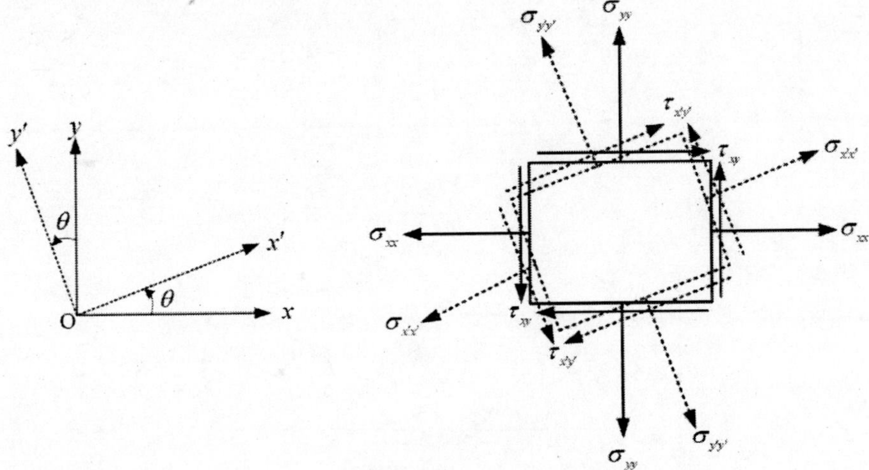

Fig. 2.13 State of plane stress in physical space represented on a rectangular element

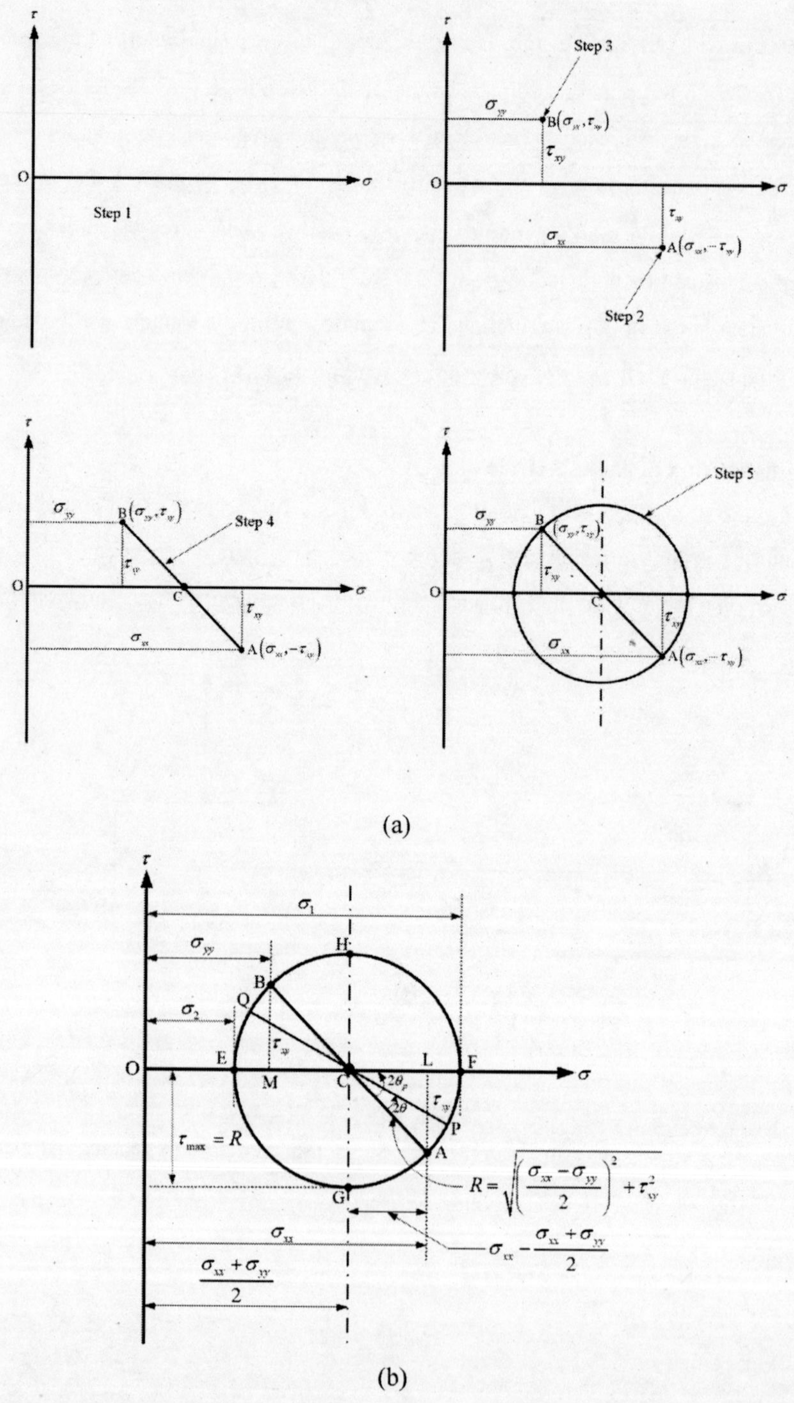

Fig. 2.14 Method for constructing Mohr's Circle: (a) Steps involved in constructing the Mohr's circle, (b) The Mohr's circle of stress for plane stress showing all the steps together.

One can evaluate the state of stress on any plane passing through the point of interest by constructing a Mohr's circle using the interpretation discussed in Section 2.9.1. The different steps involved in the construction of Mohr's circle are shown in Fig. 2.14 (a), and the corresponding description is outlined in the following:

Step 1: Choose the positive normal stress axis along the positive x-direction and positive shear stress along the negative y- direction.

Step 2: Locate the point A (σ_{xx}, $-\tau_{xy}$) representing the positive normal and positive shear stress components acting on the x-plane.

Step 3: Locate the point B (σ_{yy}, τ_{xy}) representing the positive normal and positive shear stress components acting on the y-plane.

Step 4: Join the points A and B intersecting the σ-axis at point C.

Step 5: Taking point C as the centre and CA or CB as the radius, draw the circle. The circle thus drawn is the Mohr's circle of stress. It is to be noted that the positive value of shear stress obtained from Mohr's circle will have a tendency to rotate the element clockwise.

A typical Mohr's circle is drawn in Fig. 2.14 (b) following the above steps showing all its features.

2.9.4 Observation from Mohr's circle

The main observations from the Mohr's circle (refer Fig. 2.14) are as follows:

(i) It is observed that at the points E and F, which are the intercepts of the Mohr's circle with the σ-axis, the value of the shear stress is zero. Thus, the planes represented by points E and F are referred as the principal planes, oriented at an angle of $2\theta_p$ and ($2\theta_p$+180°), respectively, in the Mohr's circle with reference to the plane represented by point A. Correspondingly, the values of the normal stresses on these planes are the principal stresses. The maximum principal stress is indicated by the distance measured from the vertical axis to the point F and is denoted by σ_1. The minimum principal stress is indicated by the distance measured from the vertical axis to point E and is denoted by σ_2. In the physical stressed body, if we rotate the element by an angle θ_p in the counter clockwise direction, the line drawn at angle of θ_p with the x-axis gives the normal to the principal plane where σ_1 acts. Similarly, the line drawn at an angle of (θ_p+90°) with x-axis gives the normal to the principal plane where σ_2 acts.

(ii) If one is interested to obtain the stresses on some other plane at any angle θ with x-plane, another diameter, say PQ can be drawn oriented at an angle 2θ from AB. The coordinate of the points P and Q will provide the state of stress on the desired planes.

(iii) The end points of the vertical diameter, G and H indicates the magnitude of the maximum shear stress. The line GH is perpendicular to the line of principal stress EF. Thus, the plane of maximum shear stress is oriented at an angle of 45° to the plane of principal stress. The magnitude of maximum shear stress is given by the radius of the Mohr's circle (CG, CH or CA etc.), which is

$$R = \frac{\sigma_1 - \sigma_2}{2} = \sqrt{\left(\frac{\sigma_{xx} - \sigma_{yy}}{2}\right)^2 + \left(\tau_{xy}\right)^2}. \tag{2.59}$$

(iv) If $\sigma_1 = \sigma_2$, Mohr's circle reduces to a point. This indicates that no shear stress τ_{xy} acts on the x and y planes, and the normal stresses acting on these planes are of equal magnitudes, $\sigma_{xx} = \sigma_{yy}$.

(v) If $\sigma_{xx} + \sigma_{yy} = 0$, *i.e.*, the first principal invariant of stress is zero, the centre of the Mohr's circle coincides with the origin of σ-τ coordinate axes. This results in a state of pure shear in the body. This indicates that the magnitudes of the maximum and the minimum principal stresses are equal and of opposite signs, *i.e.*, $\sigma_1 = -\sigma_2$. Moreover, σ_1 and σ_2 represent the radius of the Mohr's circle, and hence they are equal to the magnitude of the maximum shear stress. This situation corresponds to the state of pure shear in the element.

Know More

Example 2.4 The plane state of stress at a point acting on two mutually perpendicular planes are given by σ_{xx}=20 MPa, τ_{xy}= −10 MPa and σ_{yy}=10 MPa in the Cartesian (x, y) coordinate system. This set of coordinate axes is rotated counter-clockwise by an angle 30° to form a new coordinate system (x', y'). Evaluate the components of stress in the new coordinate system. Also, find the principal stresses and the maximum in-plane shear stress at the point. What is the value of normal stress on the plane of maximum shear stress?

Solution

Construction of Mohr's circle:

In the σ-τ coordinate axes, by plotting the normal and shear stresses acting on the x and y planes, points A (20, 10) and B (10, –10) are obtained. Points A and B are joined by a line that intersects the σ axis at point C. Now, taking C as centre and AC or BC as the radii, the Mohr's circle for the present case is constructed as shown in the figure.

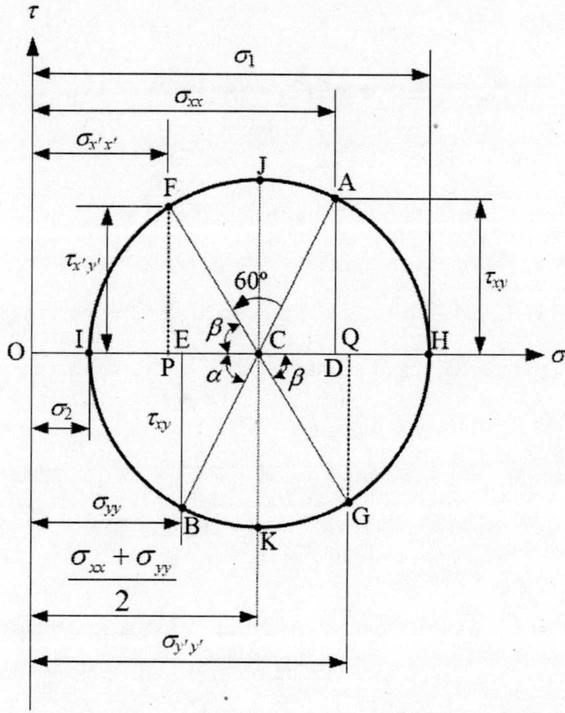

Determination stress components in the rotated (x′, y′) coordinate system:

In the Mohr's circle, $OD=\sigma_{xx}=20$ MPa, $OE=\sigma_{yy}=10$ MPa, $AD=BE=\tau_{xy}=-10$ MPa. The centre of the circle is located at $\left(\dfrac{\sigma_{xx}+\sigma_{yy}}{2},0\right)$. Therefore,

$OC=\dfrac{\sigma_{xx}+\sigma_{yy}}{2}=\dfrac{20+10}{2}=15\,\text{MPa}$, and $CE=OC-OE=15-10=5$ MPa.

The radius of Mohr's circle,

$R=CF=CG=\sqrt{CE^2+BE^2}=\sqrt{5^2+10^2}=11.18\,\text{MPa}.$

Since the x-y axes rotated by an angle 30° counter-clockwise, a radial line CF must be drawn on σ-τ plane at an angle $2\times30°=60°$ counter-clockwise from the radial line CA (θ=0°). Point F represents the x' plane. The radial line CF is extended to intersect the periphery of the Mohr's circle at point G, which represents the y' plane and is at an angle of (60°+180°) counter-clockwise from the radial line CA. It is required to determine the normal and shear stress components on planes F, and G. Let us drop perpendiculars FP and GQ from F and G, respectively, on σ axis. OP will measure the normal stress on the x' plane, and OQ will measure the normal stress on the y' plane. The corresponding shear stress on the planes is given by either FP or GQ.

Let $\angle BCE = \alpha$.

Now, $\alpha = \tan^{-1}\left(\frac{EB}{CE}\right) = \tan^{-1}\left(\frac{10}{5}\right) = \tan^{-1}(2) = 63.43°$.

Also, let $\angle FCP = \beta$.

From Mohr's circle, $\beta = 180° - \alpha - 60° = 56.57°$.

From Mohr's circle, the normal stress acting on the x' plane is obtained as

$$\sigma_{x'x'} = OC - CP = 15 - CF\cos\beta = 15 - 11.18\cos(56.57°) = 8.84\,\text{MPa}.$$

The shear stress component $\tau_{x'y'}$ can be obtained as

$$\tau_{x'y'} = -FP = -CF\sin\beta = -11.18\sin(56.57°) = -9.33\,\text{MPa}.$$

The normal stress acting on the y' plane from Mohr's circle is evaluated as

$$\sigma_{y'y'} = OQ = OC + CQ = 15 + CG\cos\beta = 15 + 11.18\cos(56.57°) = 21.16\,\text{MPa}.$$

Determination of principal stresses:

In the Mohr's circle, the measure of OH and OI will provide the magnitudes of the maximum principal stress (σ_1) and minimum principal stress (σ_2), respectively. Thus,

$$\sigma_1 = OH = OC + CH = 15 + R = 15 + 11.18 = 26.18\,\text{MPa},$$
$$\sigma_2 = OI = OC - CI = 15 - R = 15 - 11.18 = 3.82\,\text{MPa}.$$

Determination of the maximum in-plane shear stress:

From Mohr's circle, the maximum in-plane shear stress occurs on planes J and K. The magnitude of the maximum in-plane shear stress is given by the radial lines, either CJ or CK, which is equal to the radius of the Mohr's circle, *i.e.*,

$$|\tau_{max}| = R = 11.18\,\text{MPa}.$$

Normal stress on the plane of maximum in-plane shear stress:

Referring to the Mohr's circle, the value of the normal stress on the plane of maximum in-plane shear stress is given by the measure of the line OC, which is evaluated as 15 MPa.

2.10 Ellipse of Stress and Its Applications

In general, the state of stress at a point is the set of infinite stress vectors or traction acting on infinite planes passing through the point of interest. If one traces out the end points of all the normal components of stress vectors at a point on all the planes, it results into an ellipse in a two-dimensional stress space, and this ellipse is called the stress ellipse. Thus, a stress ellipse can be defined as the locus of the normal stress vector on the set of infinite planes passing through the point in a planar body where the state of stress is desired.

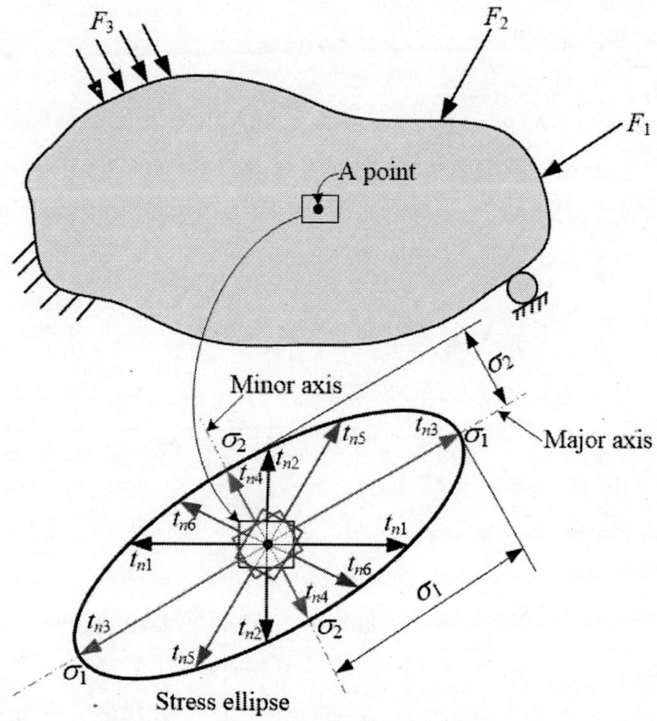

Fig. 2.15 Representation of stress ellipse

A representative stress ellipse is shown in Fig. 2.15 by considering a point in a loaded arbitrary solid. The point is enclosed by an infinitesimal two-dimensional element (shown by the black rectangle) with a pair of mutually perpendicular planes. These planes will pass through the point considered when the area of the element shrinks to zero. By rotating the infinitesimal element to different orientations around the point of interest, one can think of an infinite number of pairs of planes through that point in the limit when the area of each rotated element shrunk to zero. As an example, in Fig. 2.15, six pairs of such planes are considered (shown by the black, green, and blue rectangles). The normal components of traction or stress vector acting on the pair of planes in the black rectangle are represented by t_{n1} and t_{n2}. Similarly, the normal components of traction acting on the pair of mutually perpendicular planes in the green and blue rectangles are represented by t_{n3}, t_{n4}, and t_{n5}, t_{n6}, respectively. The equal magnitude of the respective normal component of traction must also act on the corresponding opposite plane of the rectangular element considered in order to keep the element in equilibrium. Now, if the end points of the normal components of traction t_{n1}, t_{n2}, t_{n3}, t_{n4}, t_{n5}, and t_{n6} are joined by a smooth curve, an ellipse is emerged out. This ellipse represents the stress ellipse.

The stress ellipse is a useful mental tool for the geometric representation of the state of stress at a point. The stress ellipse can be applied to determine the following:

a) The normal stress on any plane passing through the point of interest.
b) The length of the major axis of the stress ellipse measured from the point will provide the maximum principal stress σ_1.
c) The length of the minor axis of the stress ellipse measured from the point will provide the minimum principal stress σ_2.

There is another version of the stress ellipse that provides the magnitude of the entire traction vector, but it will not be discussed here.

2.11 Equations of Equilibrium

In a loaded continuum solid body, stress is a function of its positional coordinates. If one is interested to determine the variation of the stress components as function of position within the interior of the body, certain set of governing differential equations needs to be solved. These equations are called equilibrium equations. In order to develop the equilibrium equations, let us consider a two-dimensional differential element of size $\Delta x \Delta y$. The two x-faces are separated by a differential length Δx and the two y-faces are separated by a differential length Δy. Now, one should appreciate that the stress components on the two x-faces and on the two y-faces of the differential element may be different and varies as a function of their positional coordinate. The stress components on the x-face change as one moves from location x to location $x+\Delta x$ on the differential element. Similarly, the stress components on the y-face change as one move from location y to location $y+\Delta y$. At location x, the value of the normal stress on the x-face is σ_{xx}, *i.e.*, $f(x)=\sigma_x$. Now, at location $(x+\Delta x)$, the value of normal stress as a function of $(x+\Delta x)$ can be obtained by Taylor's series expansion approximated up to the first order term as Δx is extremely small. Thus, the value of normal stress at location $x+\Delta x$ on the x-face is $\sigma_{xx}+\frac{\partial \sigma_{xx}}{\partial x}\Delta x$. Similarly, the values of other stress components on the x and y-faces when they change their position are obtained and shown on the differential element in Fig. 2.16. The body force components per unit volume in the x and y directions are shown as b_x and b_y, respectively.

Taking the thickness of the element to be unity, the area of each face can be obtained by multiplying its length by unit thickness. Now, writing the equation of static equilibrium for forces acting in the x-direction,

$$-\sigma_{xx}(\Delta y\times 1)+\left(\sigma_{xx}+\frac{\partial\sigma_{xx}}{\partial x}\Delta x\right)(\Delta y\times 1)-\tau_{xy}(\Delta x\times 1)+\left(\tau_{xy}+\frac{\partial\tau_{xy}}{\partial y}\Delta y\right)(\Delta x\times 1)+b_x(\Delta x\times\Delta y\times 1)=0,$$

$$\frac{\partial\sigma_{xx}}{\partial x}\Delta x\Delta y+\frac{\partial\tau_{xy}}{\partial y}\Delta y\Delta x+b_x\Delta x\Delta y=0,$$

$$\frac{\partial\sigma_{xx}}{\partial x}+\frac{\partial\tau_{xy}}{\partial y}\Delta y\Delta x+b_x=0. \tag{2.60}$$

Similarly, the force equilibrium equation in the y-direction provides

$$\frac{\partial\tau_{xy}}{\partial x}+\frac{\partial\sigma_{yy}}{\partial y}+b_y=0. \tag{2.61}$$

Equations (2.60) and (2.61) are the differential equations of equilibrium in two-dimensions in the presence of body force components.

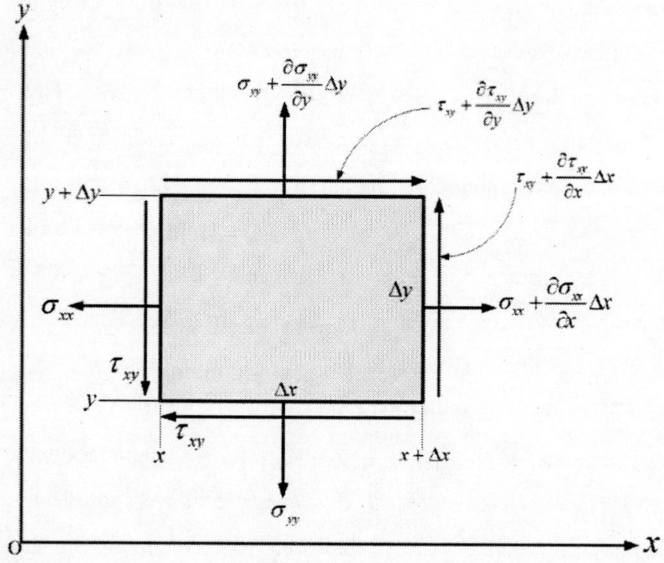

Fig. 2.16 Equilibrium of a two-dimensional differential element subjected to stress

2.12 Two Dimensional Stress-Strain System

In this section, first, the general state of strain at a point will be introduced. Then the concept of a two-dimensional plane strain system will be developed. Finally, the stress-strain relations in two-dimensions will be established, also called as the constitutive relations or generalized Hooke's law.

2.12.1 Introduction to the general state of strain at a point

One can imagine an infinite number of differently oriented lines through a point in any arbitrary body. When the body deforms, all these lines passing through the point of interest will also undergo deformation providing an infinite set of normal strains and associated shear strains in the limit when the length of all the line elements shrunk to zero. These infinite set of strains represents the state of strains at a point in general. Just like stress, the state of strain at a point can be completely represented by three normal strain components ε_{xx}, ε_{yy}, ε_{zz} (or ε_x, ε_y, ε_z) in three mutually perpendicular *x*, *y*, *z* directions and six associated shear strain components γ_{xy}, γ_{yx}, γ_{yz}, γ_{zy}, γ_{xz}, γ_{zx} in these directions in a three-dimensional Cartesian coordinate system. However, due to symmetry, $\gamma_{xy}=\gamma_{yx}$, $\gamma_{yz}=\gamma_{zy}$ and $\gamma_{xz} = \gamma_{zx}$. Thus, the state of strain at a point can be characterized by six independent strain components. It is also a tensor of order two, similar to stress. Please note that the indices used for the strain components do not have the same connotation as in stress. In stress, the first index referred to the plane of stress, and the second index referred to the stress direction. However, in the case of strain, the first index refers to the orientation of the infinitesimal line element under consideration and the second index denotes the direction of its displacement (deformation). For example, the strain component ε_{xx} means a line element oriented along the *x* direction gets displaced in the *x* direction. Similarly, γ_{xy} means a line element along the *x* direction deforms in the *y* direction to have an angular deformation. Like stress, the strain at a point is also a function of its position and orientation.

2.12.2 Two-dimensional strain system: Plane strain

A two-dimensional strain system or plane strain represents a situation where all the deformations take place in a given plane. For example, if we consider an element the *x-y* plane of original dimension $\Delta x \Delta y$ keeping its lower left corner fixed, the general deformation takes place (shown by dotted line) in the plane as shown in Fig. 2.17. The extensions in the *x* and *y* directions are taken as Δu and Δv, respectively, and cause the normal strains in the plane as

$$\varepsilon_{xx} = \frac{\Delta u}{\Delta x}, \quad \varepsilon_{yy} = \frac{\Delta v}{\Delta y}. \tag{2.62}$$

The total shear strain in the element is given by

$$\gamma_{xy} = \frac{\pi}{2} - \left\{ \frac{\pi}{2} - (\alpha + \beta) \right\} = \alpha + \beta. \tag{2.63}$$

Thus, the only non-zero strain components on this plane are ε_{xx}, ε_{yy}, and γ_{xy}, and all other strain components are zero, *i.e.*, $\varepsilon_{zz} = \gamma_{zy} = \gamma_{xz} = 0$. By convention, $\alpha = \beta$. Thus, the change in the angle with respect to the x and y axes are given by

$$\alpha = \beta = \frac{\gamma_{xy}}{2}. \tag{2.64}$$

In representing the strain components in matrix notation, the shear strain components are taken according to Eq. (2.64), and the state of plane strain at a point can be written as

$$[\varepsilon] = \begin{bmatrix} \varepsilon_{xx} & \frac{\gamma_{xy}}{2} \\ \frac{\gamma_{xy}}{2} & \varepsilon_{yy} \end{bmatrix}. \tag{2.65}$$

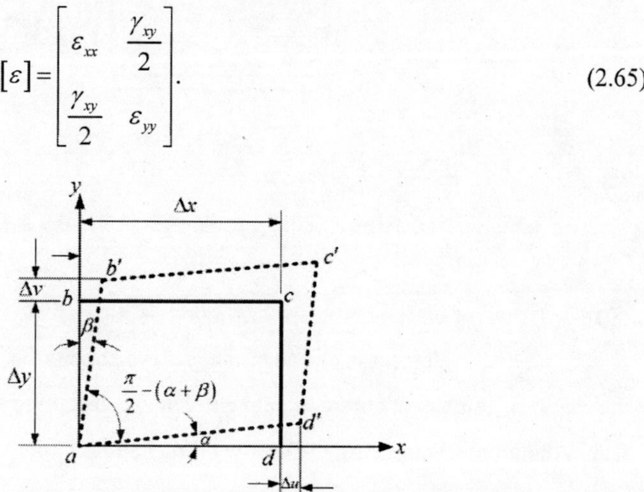

Fig. 2.17 General deformation of an element in two-dimensions

It is to be noted that the plane strain does not connote plane stress or vice-versa, although they represent their corresponding components on a plane. The reason for this is attributed to Poisson's effect. For example, if we consider an element subjected to plane stress (σ_{zz}=0), the stress components σ_{xx} and σ_{yy} cause corresponding normal strains ε_{xx} and ε_{yy} in the x and y directions. Moreover, there also exists an associated normal strain in the z direction ε_{zz} due to Poisson's effect. Hence, it does not imply the condition of plane strain. The plane stress and plane strain conditions coincide when the Poisson's ratio (v) is zero.

2.12.3 Stress-strain relations in two-dimensions

Let us consider a two-dimensional stressed element, as shown in Fig. 2.18. The original dimensions of the element along the x and y directions are Δx and Δy, respectively. The normal stresses σ_{xx} and σ_{yy} acting on the x and y face cause net changes to the original dimensions Δx and Δy causing normal strains ε_{xx} and ε_{yy}. The shear stress τ_{xy} causes shear deformation of the element, inducing shear strain γ_{xy}. We shall now consider the effects of the normal stresses σ_{xx} and σ_{yy} separately, and then the corresponding effects will be added following the superposition principle to obtain the net effect due to the simultaneous action of the normal stresses in the x and y directions.

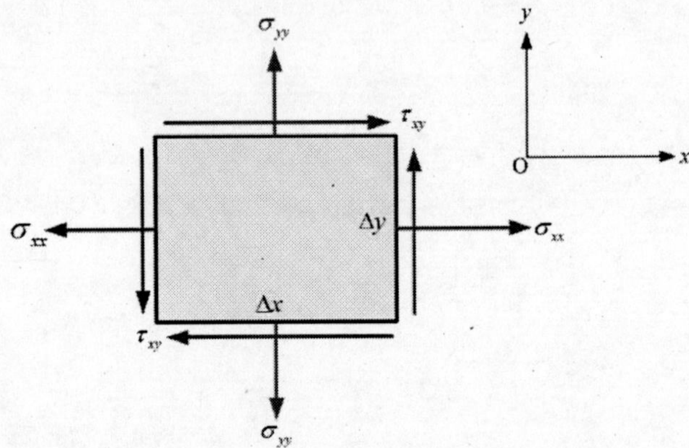

Fig. 2.18 A two-dimensional element under the action of σ_{xx}, σ_{yy}, and τ_{xy}.

Case 1: When the element is under the action of σ_{xx} only

When the element is considered under the action of σ_{xx} only, it will cause an extension in Δx and an equivalent contraction in Δy. Thus, considering the induced stress in the element within the proportional limit, the tensile normal strain in the x direction due to σ_{xx} is given by

$$\varepsilon_{xx}^{1} = \frac{\sigma_{xx}}{E}, \tag{2.66}$$

where E is the Young's modulus of elasticity of the element. The compressive normal strain in the y direction due to σ_{xx} is obtained using the definition of Poisson's ratio given by

$$\varepsilon_{yy}^{1} = -\nu\frac{\sigma_{xx}}{E}, \tag{2.67}$$

where ν is the Poisson's ratio.

Case 2: When the element is under the action of σ_{yy} only

When the element is considered under the action of σ_{yy} only, it will cause an extension in Δy and an equivalent contraction in Δx. Thus, similar to case 1, the tensile normal strain in the y direction and the compressive normal strains in the x direction due to σ_{yy} are obtained as

$$\varepsilon_{yy}^{2} = \frac{\sigma_{yy}}{E}, \tag{2.68}$$

$$\varepsilon_{xx}^2 = -\nu \frac{\sigma_{yy}}{E}. \tag{2.69}$$

Now, using the superposition principle, the net normal strain in the x direction due to the simultaneous action of σ_{xx} and σ_{yy} is obtained as

$$\varepsilon_{xx} = \varepsilon_{xx}^1 + \varepsilon_{xx}^2 = \frac{\sigma_{xx}}{E} + \left(-\nu \frac{\sigma_{yy}}{E}\right),$$

$$\varepsilon_{xx} = \frac{1}{E}\left(\sigma_{xx} - \nu\sigma_{yy}\right). \tag{2.70}$$

Similarly, the net normal strain in the y direction due to the simultaneous action of σ_{xx} and σ_{yy} is obtained as

$$\varepsilon_{yy} = \varepsilon_{yy}^1 + \varepsilon_{yy}^2 = -\nu \frac{\sigma_{xx}}{E} + \frac{\sigma_{yy}}{E},$$

$$\varepsilon_{yy} = \frac{1}{E}\left(\sigma_{yy} - \nu\sigma_{xx}\right). \tag{2.71}$$

Considering the element is under the action of shear stress τ_{xy}, the shear strain component is given by

$$\gamma_{xy} = \frac{\tau_{xy}}{G}, \tag{2.72}$$

where G is the shear modulus or modulus of rigidity. Eq. (2.70) – (2.72) provide the stress-strain relations in two-dimensions. These equations are also called as generalized Hooke's law or constitutive relations in two-dimensions.

Instead of a two-dimensional element, if we consider a cube element subjected to tensile normal stresses σ_{xx}, σ_{yy}, σ_{zz} and shear stresses τ_{xy}, τ_{yz}, τ_{zx} in Cartesian (x, y, z) coordinate system, then following the same procedure as above and considering the Poisson's effect in the z-direction, the stress-strain relations or generalized Hooke's law in three-dimensions can be derived as

$$\varepsilon_{xx} = \frac{1}{E}\left\{\sigma_{xx} - \nu\left(\sigma_{yy} + \sigma_{zz}\right)\right\}, \tag{2.73}$$

$$\varepsilon_{yy} = \frac{1}{E}\left\{\sigma_{yy} - \nu\left(\sigma_{xx} + \sigma_{zz}\right)\right\}, \tag{2.74}$$

$$\varepsilon_{zz} = \frac{1}{E}\left\{\sigma_{zz} - \nu\left(\sigma_{xx} + \sigma_{yy}\right)\right\}, \tag{2.75}$$

$$\gamma_{xy} = \frac{\tau_{xy}}{G}, \ \gamma_{yz} = \frac{\tau_{yz}}{G}, \ \gamma_{zx} = \frac{\tau_{zx}}{G}. \tag{2.76}$$

From Eq. (2.75), it can be easily inferred that for plane strain case (ε_{zz}=0), one will always have a non-zero normal stress component in the z direction given by

$$\sigma_{zz} = \nu\left(\sigma_{xx} + \sigma_{yy}\right). \tag{2.77}$$

Similarly, for the case of plane stress (σ_{zz}=0), there is a non-zero normal strain component in the z direction given by

$$\varepsilon_{zz} = -\frac{\nu}{E}\left(\sigma_{xx} + \sigma_{yy}\right). \tag{2.78}$$

Know More

Example 2.5 In a plane stress problem, σ_{xx}=10 MPa, σ_{yy}=4 MPa, τ_{xy}=2 MPa. Find out all six components of strain, if E=200 GPa, G=66.67 GPa and ν=0.5.

Solution

For plane stress, $\sigma_{zz}=\tau_{zx}=\tau_{yz}=0$. Given that σ_{xx}=10 MPa, σ_{yy}=4 MPa, τ_{xy}=2 MPa, E=200 GPa and ν=0.5. Using Eqs. (2.70)–(2.72), the normal strain components ε_{xx}, ε_{yy}, and shear strain component γ_{xy} are obtained as

$$\varepsilon_{xx} = \frac{1}{E}\left(\sigma_{xx} - \nu\sigma_{yy}\right) = 4\times10^{-5}\ \text{MPa},$$

$$\varepsilon_{yy} = \frac{1}{E}\left(\sigma_{yy} - \nu\sigma_{xx}\right) = -0.5\times10^{-5}\ \text{MPa},$$

$$\gamma_{xy} = \frac{\tau_{xy}}{G} = 3\times10^{-5}\ \text{MPa}.$$

From Eq. (2.78), the normal strain component ε_{zz} is obtained as

$$\varepsilon_{zz} = -\frac{\nu}{E}\left(\sigma_{xx} + \sigma_{yy}\right) = -3.5\times10^{-5}\ \text{MPa}.$$

As for plane stress, $\tau_{zx}=\tau_{yz}=0$, the shear strain components $\gamma_{zx}=\gamma_{yz}=0$.

2.13 Transformation equations for two-dimensional strain system

The strain at appoint is a tensor of order two and in a two-dimensional space, it has four components. The components of strain at a point changes under the transformation of the coordinate frame. However, the strain tensor itself does not change at that point. As strain at a point is a tensor, it follows the transformation rule given by Eq. (2.27). Here, we will develop the transformation equations for a two-dimensional strain system using Eq. (2.27), which can be rewritten in terms of strain tensor $[\varepsilon]$ as

$$[\varepsilon'] = [\alpha][\varepsilon][\alpha]^{\mathrm{T}}. \tag{2.79}$$

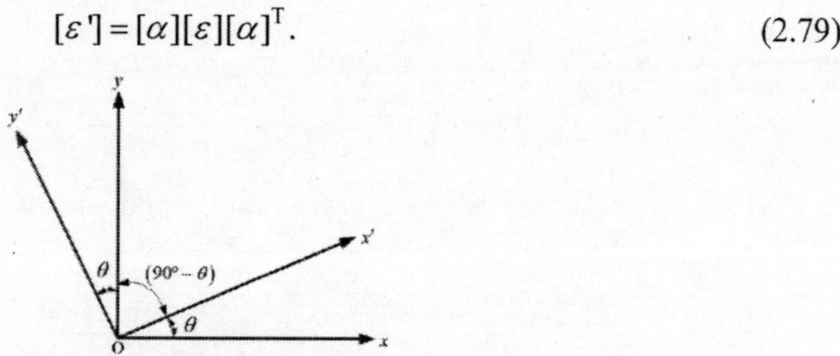

Fig. 2.19 The transformed coordinate system x'-y' with respect to x-y.

Let the components of plain strain in x-y Cartesian coordinate system be ε_{xx}, ε_{yy}, and γ_{xy}. Now, the coordinate system is rotated by an angle θ, and the transformed coordinate system is named as x'-y'. The transformed components of strain in the x'-y' are taken as $\varepsilon_{x'x'}$, $\varepsilon_{y'y'}$ and $\gamma_{x'y'}$. The rotated coordinate system with respect to the original coordinate system is shown in Fig. 2.19. Referring to Fig. 2.19, the direction cosine matrix of (x, y) with respect to (x', y') can be written as

$$[\alpha] = \begin{bmatrix} \cos\theta & \cos(90^\circ + \theta) \\ \cos(90^\circ - \theta) & \cos\theta \end{bmatrix} = \begin{bmatrix} \cos\theta & -\sin\theta \\ \sin\theta & \cos\theta \end{bmatrix}. \tag{2.80}$$

The stress component in the x-y coordinate in matrix notation is given by Eq. (2.65). The transformed strain components in the rotated x'-y' coordinate in matrix notation can be expressed as

$$[\varepsilon'] = \begin{bmatrix} \varepsilon_{x'x'} & \dfrac{\gamma_{x'y'}}{2} \\ \dfrac{\gamma_{x'y'}}{2} & \varepsilon_{y'y'} \end{bmatrix}. \tag{2.81}$$

Now, using expressions for $[\varepsilon]$, $[\alpha]$, and $[\varepsilon']$ from Eqs. (2.65), (2.80), and (2.81) in Eq. (2.79), one obtains the transformation relations for strains as

$$\varepsilon_{x'x'} = \frac{1}{2}(\varepsilon_{xx} + \varepsilon_{yy}) + \frac{1}{2}(\varepsilon_{xx} - \varepsilon_{yy})\cos 2\theta + \frac{\gamma_{xy}}{2}\sin 2\theta, \tag{2.82}$$

$$\varepsilon_{y'y'} = \frac{1}{2}(\varepsilon_{xx} + \varepsilon_{yy}) - \frac{1}{2}(\varepsilon_{xx} - \varepsilon_{yy})\cos 2\theta - \frac{\gamma_{xy}}{2}\sin 2\theta, \tag{2.83}$$

$$\frac{\gamma_{x'y'}}{2} = -\frac{1}{2}(\varepsilon_{xx} - \varepsilon_{yy})\sin 2\theta + \frac{\gamma_{xy}}{2}\cos 2\theta. \tag{2.84}$$

2.13.1 The maximum and minimum normal strains

Using the condition for maximum or minimum normal strain, $\frac{d\varepsilon_{x'x'}}{d\theta} = 0$, the direction of the maximum or minimum normal strain is obtained as

$$\tan 2\theta_p = \frac{\frac{\gamma_{xy}}{2}}{\frac{1}{2}(\varepsilon_{xx} - \varepsilon_{yy})}. \tag{2.85}$$

Equation (2.85) will provide two values of θ_p: $\theta_{p_1} = 2\theta_p$, $\theta_{p_2} = 2\theta_p + 180°$. Now, following the same procedure as for stress in Section 2.7, the values of the maximum normal strain corresponding to the direction θ_{p_1} and the minimum normal strain corresponding to the direction θ_{p_2} are obtained as

$$\varepsilon_{max} = \frac{\varepsilon_{xx} + \varepsilon_{yy}}{2} + \sqrt{\left(\frac{\varepsilon_{xx} - \varepsilon_{yy}}{2}\right)^2 + \left(\frac{\gamma_{xy}}{2}\right)^2}, \tag{2.86}$$

$$\varepsilon_{min} = \frac{\varepsilon_{xx} + \varepsilon_{yy}}{2} - \sqrt{\left(\frac{\varepsilon_{xx} - \varepsilon_{yy}}{2}\right)^2 + \left(\frac{\gamma_{xy}}{2}\right)^2}. \tag{2.87}$$

2.13.2 The maximum in-plane shear strain

Using the condition for maximum shear strain $\frac{d\gamma_{x'y'}}{d\theta} = 0$, the direction of the maximum in-plane shear strain is obtained as

$$\tan 2\theta_s = -\frac{\frac{1}{2}(\varepsilon_{xx} - \varepsilon_{yy})}{\frac{\gamma_{xy}}{2}}. \tag{2.88}$$

From Eq. (2.88), one can obtain two values of θs: $\theta_{s_1} = 2\theta_{s_1}, \theta_{s_2} = 2\theta_{p_1} + 180°$. Now, following the similar procedure as in Section 2.8, one obtains the magnitude of the maximum in-plane shear strain as

$$\left|\left(\frac{\gamma}{2}\right)_{\max}\right| = \pm\sqrt{\left(\frac{\varepsilon_{xx} - \varepsilon_{yy}}{2}\right)^2 + \left(\frac{\gamma_{xy}}{2}\right)^2}. \tag{2.89}$$

2.14 Principal Strains and Principal Axes of Strain

It can be seen from Eq. (2.84) that when $\gamma_{x'y'}$=0, it provides the directions of the maximum and minimum normal strains given by Eq. (2.85). This indicates that in the directions given by Eq. (2.85), the strains are wholly normal, and there is no associated shear strain. Such directions (of strain) along which only normal strains occur without any associated shear strain are referred as the principal directions or principal axes of strain. It is to be noted that principal axes of strains exist in the initial configuration of the element. This means that the axes remain perpendicular in their deformed configuration producing no shear deformation. The strains induced along the principal axes of strain are called the principal strains. Hence, the maximum and minimum normal strains given by Eqs. (2.86) and (2.87) are also the expressions of the maximum and minimum principal strains, respectively. Denoting the maximum principal strain by ε_1 and the minimum principal strain by ε_2, they can be expressed as

$$\varepsilon_1 = \frac{\varepsilon_{xx} + \varepsilon_{yy}}{2} + \sqrt{\left(\frac{\varepsilon_{xx} - \varepsilon_{yy}}{2}\right)^2 + \left(\frac{\gamma_{xy}}{2}\right)^2}, \tag{2.90}$$

$$\varepsilon_2 = \frac{\varepsilon_{xx} + \varepsilon_{yy}}{2} - \sqrt{\left(\frac{\varepsilon_{xx} - \varepsilon_{yy}}{2}\right)^2 + \left(\frac{\gamma_{xy}}{2}\right)^2}. \tag{2.91}$$

Know More

Example 2.6 The state of strain at a point in plane strain with respect to the Cartesian (*x*, *y*) coordinate system are given by

$$[\varepsilon]=\begin{bmatrix}6\times10^{-4} & 2\times10^{-4}\\ 2\times10^{-4} & -4\times10^{-4}\end{bmatrix}.$$

Now, if the axes system is rotated by an angle of 35° clockwise to form a new coordinate system (x', y'), then determine the state of strain at that point in the new coordinate system. Also, find the principal strains at the point and their orientations. What are the maximum in-plane shear strain at the point and its orientation?

Solution

Given, $\varepsilon_{xx}=6\times10^{-4}$, $\varepsilon_{yy}=-4\times10^{-4}$, $\dfrac{\gamma_{xy}}{2}=2\times10^{-4}$ and $\theta=-35°$.

Now, using the transformation relations given by Eqs. (2.82) – (2.84), the state of strain at the point in the (x', y') coordinate system is evaluated as

$$\varepsilon_{x'x'}=\frac{1}{2}\left(\varepsilon_{xx}+\varepsilon_{yy}\right)+\frac{1}{2}\left(\varepsilon_{xx}-\varepsilon_{yy}\right)\cos 2\theta+\frac{\gamma_{xy}}{2}\sin 2\theta,$$

$$=\frac{1}{2}(6-4)\times10^{-4}+\frac{1}{2}(6+4)\times10^{-4}\cos\{2\times(-35°)\}+\left(2\times10^{-4}\right)\sin\{2\times(-35°)\}=0.83\times10^{-4}.$$

$$\varepsilon_{y'y'}=\frac{1}{2}\left(\varepsilon_{xx}+\varepsilon_{yy}\right)-\frac{1}{2}\left(\varepsilon_{xx}-\varepsilon_{yy}\right)\cos 2\theta-\frac{\gamma_{xy}}{2}\sin 2\theta,$$

$$=\frac{1}{2}(6-4)\times10^{-4}-\frac{1}{2}(6+4)\times10^{-4}\cos\{2\times(-35°)\}-\left(2\times10^{-4}\right)\sin\{2\times(-35°)\}=1.17\times10^{-4}.$$

$$\frac{\gamma_{x'y'}}{2}=-\frac{1}{2}\left(\varepsilon_{xx}-\varepsilon_{yy}\right)\sin 2\theta+\frac{\gamma_{xy}}{2}\cos 2\theta,$$

$$=-\frac{1}{2}(6+4)\times10^{-4}\sin\{2\times(-35°)\}+\left(2\times10^{-4}\right)\cos\{2\times(-35°)\}=5.38\times10^{-4}.$$

The principal strains at the point are evaluated using Eqs. (2.90) and (2.91) as

$$\varepsilon_1 = \frac{\varepsilon_{xx}+\varepsilon_{yy}}{2} + \sqrt{\left(\frac{\varepsilon_{xx}-\varepsilon_{yy}}{2}\right)^2 + \left(\frac{\gamma_{xy}}{2}\right)^2},$$

$$= \frac{(6-4)}{2}\times 10^{-4} + \sqrt{\left\{\frac{(6+4)\times 10^{-4}}{2}\right\}^2 + \left(2\times 10^{-4}\right)^2} = 6.38\times 10^{-4},$$

$$\varepsilon_2 = \frac{\varepsilon_{xx}+\varepsilon_{yy}}{2} - \sqrt{\left(\frac{\varepsilon_{xx}-\varepsilon_{yy}}{2}\right)^2 + \left(\frac{\gamma_{xy}}{2}\right)^2},$$

$$= \frac{(6-4)}{2}\times 10^{-4} - \sqrt{\left\{\frac{(6+4)\times 10^{-4}}{2}\right\}^2 + \left(2\times 10^{-4}\right)^2} = -4.38\times 10^{-4}.$$

The orientations of the principal strains are given by Eq. (2.85). Thus, we get

$$\tan 2\theta_p = \frac{\frac{\gamma_{xy}}{2}}{\frac{1}{2}\left(\varepsilon_{xx}-\varepsilon_{yy}\right)} = \frac{2\times 10^{-4}}{\frac{1}{2}(6+4)\times 10^{-4}} = \frac{2}{5},$$

$$2\theta_p = 21.8°,\ \ 21.8°+180° = 201.8°,$$

$$\theta_p = 10.9°,\ \ 100.9°.$$

The magnitude of maximum in-plane shear strain at the point is evaluated using Eq. (2.89) as

$$\left(\frac{\gamma}{2}\right)_{max} = \sqrt{\left\{\frac{(6+4)\times 10^{-4}}{2}\right\}^2 + \left(2\times 10^{-4}\right)^2} = 5.38\times 10^{-4}.$$

Equation (2.88) provides the orientation of the maximum in-plane shear strain as

$$\tan 2\theta_s = -\frac{\frac{1}{2}\left(\varepsilon_{xx}-\varepsilon_{yy}\right)}{\frac{\gamma_{xy}}{2}} = -\frac{\frac{1}{2}(6+4)\times 10^{-4}}{2\times 10^{-4}} = -\frac{5}{2},$$

$$2\theta_s = -68.2°,\ \ -68.2°+180° = 111.8°,$$

$$\theta_s = -34.1°,\ \ 55.9°.$$

Example 2.7 At a point in plane strain, the volumetric strain is 5×10^{-4}. One principal strain is 3×10^{-4}. Determine the other non-zero principal strain.

Solution

The volumetric strain (ε_V) at a point is given by (Refer Eq. (1.34) of Unit 1)

$$\varepsilon_V = \varepsilon_{xx} + \varepsilon_{yy} + \varepsilon_{zz}.$$

For the plane strain case, ε_{zz}=0. Thus, the volumetric strain

$$\varepsilon_V = \varepsilon_{xx} + \varepsilon_{yy}.$$

Given, $\varepsilon_V = 5\times10^{-4}$. Therefore,

$$\varepsilon_{xx} + \varepsilon_{yy} = 5\times10^{-4}.$$

One principal strain is given as 3×10^{-4}. Let's take this principal strain as ε_1. Now, using Eq. (2.90),

$$\varepsilon_1 = \frac{\varepsilon_{xx} + \varepsilon_{yy}}{2} + \sqrt{\left(\frac{\varepsilon_{xx} - \varepsilon_{yy}}{2}\right)^2 + \left(\frac{\gamma_{xy}}{2}\right)^2},$$

$$3\times10^{-4} = \frac{5\times10^{-4}}{2} + \sqrt{\left(\frac{\varepsilon_{xx} - \varepsilon_{yy}}{2}\right)^2 + \left(\frac{\gamma_{xy}}{2}\right)^2},$$

$$\sqrt{\left(\frac{\varepsilon_{xx} - \varepsilon_{yy}}{2}\right)^2 + \left(\frac{\gamma_{xy}}{2}\right)^2} = 0.5\times10^{-4}.$$

Now, substituting the above value in Eq. (2.91), one obtains the other non-zero principal strain as

$$\varepsilon_2 = \frac{5\times10^{-4}}{2} - \left(0.5\times10^{-4}\right) = 2\times10^{-4}.$$

Alternative method: Expressing the volumetric strain in terms of the principal strains, we get

$$\varepsilon_1 + \varepsilon_2 = 5\times10^{-4}.$$

If one of the principal strain $\varepsilon_1 = 3\times10^{-4}$, then the other non-zero principal strain can be obtained from the above equation as $\varepsilon_2 = 3\times10^{-4}$.

2.15 Mohr's Circle of Strain

The transformation relations for stresses and strains are mathematically similar as can be seen from Sections 2.7 and 2.13. Thus, a Mohr's circle of strain can be interpreted from the transformation equations of strain similar to Eq. (2.57) as

$$\left\{\varepsilon_{x'x'} - \left(\frac{\varepsilon_{xx} + \varepsilon_{yy}}{2}\right)\right\}^2 + \left(\frac{\gamma_{x'y'}}{2}\right)^2 = \left(\frac{\varepsilon_{xx} - \varepsilon_{yy}}{2}\right)^2 + \left(\frac{\gamma_{xy}}{2}\right)^2. \quad (2.92)$$

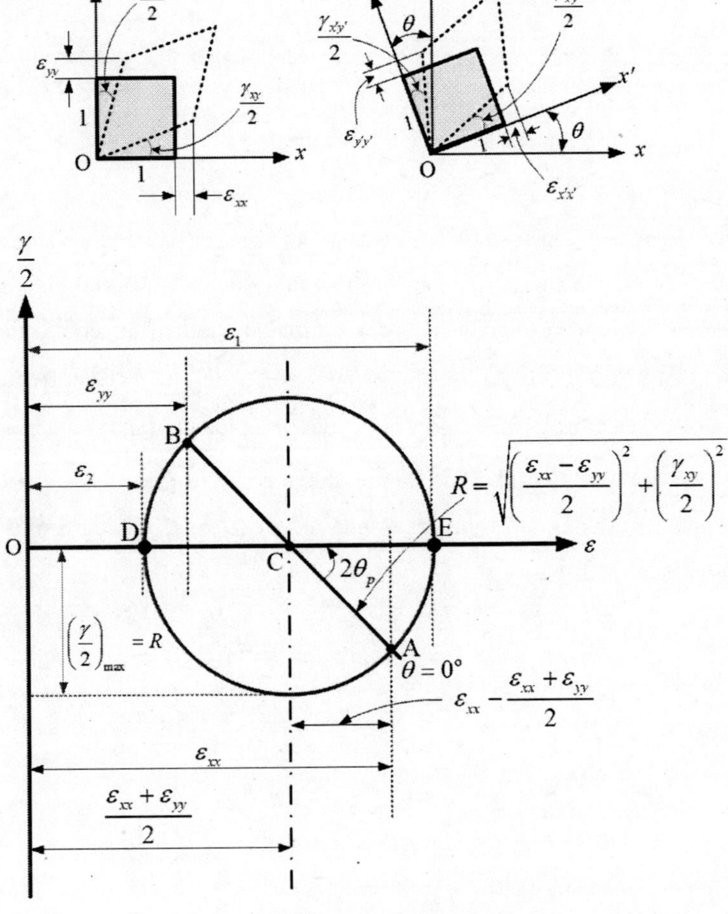

Fig. 2.20 Mohr's circle of strain

Equation (2.92) represents a circle with centre at $\left(+\frac{\varepsilon_{xx}+\varepsilon_{yy}}{2}, 0\right)$ and radius,

$$R=\sqrt{\left(\frac{\varepsilon_{xx}-\varepsilon_{yy}}{2}\right)^2+\left(\frac{\gamma_{xy}}{2}\right)^2}. \tag{2.93}$$

The construction procedure for Mohr's circle of strain and observations that can be made from it are similar to that for Mohr's circle of stress, as discussed in Section 2.9. The Mohr's circle of strain can be used to solve problems involving the transformation of strain components in two-dimensions. A Mohr's circle constructed using Eq. (2.92) in $(\varepsilon, \gamma/2)$ space is shown in Fig. 2.20. The components of strain in the original x-y coordinate system and in the transformed coordinate system x'-y' are also shown on an element of unit dimension. The sign convention for shear strain is similar to that of shear stress.

Example 2.8 The state of plane strain at a point are given by the following components:

$$\varepsilon_{xx} = 8.5\times10^{-4},\ \varepsilon_{yy} = -3\times10^{-4},\ \gamma_{xy} = 5\times10^{-4}.$$

Determine the state of principal strains and their orientations at the point using Mohr's circle of strain.

Solution

To construct the Mohr's circle, we take the normal strain (ε) axis along the positive x-direction and the positive shear strain ($\gamma/2$) axis in the negative y-direction. This convention is taken, so that counter clockwise rotations of the infinitesimal element considered around the point of interest correspond to counter clockwise rotation around the circle, and vice-versa. Now, the points A (8.5×10^{-4}, 2.5×10^{-4}) and B(-3×10^{-4}, 2.5×10^{-4}) representing the deformation of the element in the x and y directions are plotted in the strain space, $(\varepsilon, \gamma/2)$. The point of intersection C of the line joining the points A and B on the ε axis locates the centre of the circle. Taking C as the centre and either AC or BC as the radius, the Mohr's circle of strain is constructed.

In the Mohr's circle, $OD = \varepsilon_{xx} = 8.5\times10^{-4}$, $OE = \varepsilon_{yy} = -3\times10^{-4}$, $AD = BE = \gamma_{xy}/2 = 2.5\times10^{-4}$.

Also,

$$OC = \frac{\varepsilon_{xx} + \varepsilon_{yy}}{2} = \frac{(8.5-3)}{2}\times10^{-4} = 2.75\times10^{-4},$$

$$CD = OD - OC = (8.5-2.75)\times10^{-4} = 5.75\times10^{-4}.$$

The radius of the Mohr's circle is

$$R = AC = \sqrt{CD^2 + AD^2}$$

$$= \sqrt{(5.75\times10^{-4})^2 + (2.5\times10^{-4})^2} = 6.27\times10^{-4}.$$

Now, the maximum principal strain ε_1 from Mohr's circle is obtained as

$$\varepsilon_1 = OF = OC + R = (2.75+6.27)\times10^{-4} = 9.02\times10^{-4}.$$

The Mohr's circle provides the minimum principal strain ε_2 as

$$\varepsilon_2 = -OG = -(R - OC) = -(6.27-2.75)\times10^{-4} = -3.52\times10^{-4}.$$

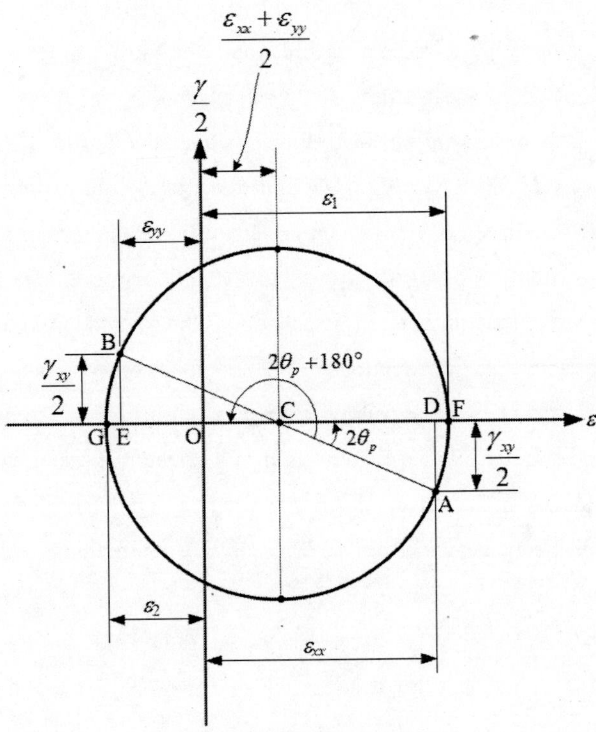

The direction of the maximum principal strain ε_1 is obtained by a counter-clockwise rotation of $2\theta_p$ from the reference radial line CA (θ=0°) to the line CF. Now, from Mohr's circle,

$$\tan 2\theta_p = \frac{AD}{CD} = \frac{2.5\times10^{-4}}{5.75\times10^{-4}} = \frac{2.5}{5.75},$$

$$2\theta_p = \tan^{-1}\left(\frac{2.5}{5.75}\right) = 23.50°,$$

$$\theta_p = 11.75°.$$

The direction of the minimum principal strain ε_2 is oriented at an angle of θ_p+90°=101.75°, counter-clockwise from the reference line CA to the line CG.

2.16 Ellipse of Strain

In a two-dimensional space, one can imagine an infinite number of lines passing through a point in a planar body oriented in different directions. It is the most convenient way in two-dimensions to imagine a circular element with the point of interest as the centre that encloses all the infinite set of radial lines of unit length before deformation. Now, if the circular element is subjected to homogeneous deformation, all the line elements of unit length passing through the centre of the circle will also undergo homogeneous deformation producing normal strains in the respective directions equal to its corresponding extension or contraction and associated shear strains. Now, if one traces out the end points of all the deformed lines, it provides an ellipse. This ellipse is called the ellipse of strain. The extension of the semi-major axis of the strain ellipse with respect to the unit radius of the undeformed circle provides the measure of the maximum principal strain, and the contraction of the semi-minor axis of the strain ellipse with respect to the unit radius of the undeformed circle provides the measure of the minimum principal strain. The orientation of the major and minor axes of the ellipse represents the directions of the principal axes of strain. A formal definition for the strain ellipse can be given as follows: The strain ellipse is the geometric representation of two-dimensional strain system at a point used to illustrate the magnitude and direction of the maximum and minimum principal strains, when a reference circle of unit radius is subjected to homogeneous deformation. A representative strain ellipse is shown in Fig. 2.21.

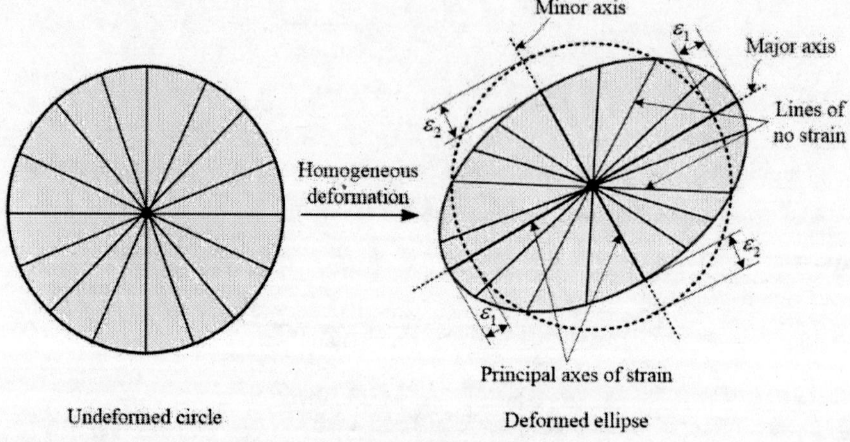

Fig. 2.21 Illustration of strain ellipse

2.17 Relationship Among Elastic Constants

In Unit 1, four elastic constants were introduced for homogeneous and isotropic material, *viz*., Young's modulus of elasticity (E), the modulus of rigidity or shear modulus (G), the bulk modulus (K) and the Poisson's ratio (v). Out of these four elastic constants, only two are independent. Knowing any two of the elastic constants, the other two can be obtained by establishing certain relationships among them. This section is devoted to establish the relationships among different elastic constants.

2.17.1 Relationship among *E*, *G* and ν

Let us consider a two-dimensional square element of side equal to unity in a bar subjected to axial tensile force *P* that deforms the element into a rectangle of sides $(1+\varepsilon_{xx})$ and $(1-\nu\varepsilon_{xx})$ as shown in Fig. 2.22 (a). Now, if the element is oriented at 45° to the axis of the bar, the elemental square is deformed into the shape of a rhombus and the axial load *P* causes a shear strain $\gamma_{x'y'}$ in the element as depicted in Fig. 2.22 (b). Further, the axial load *P* causes a uniaxial normal stress $\sigma_{xx}=P/A$ (*A* being the area of the *x* plane) in the element shown in Fig. 2.22 (a). When the element is rotated by an angle of 45° with respect to the axis of the bar, pure shear state exists in the bar (refer to Subsection 2.9.4, Point no. (v)) and the element is subjected to equal magnitudes of the maximum normal stress σ_1 and the minimum normal stress σ_2, directed in opposite sense as shown in Fig. 2.22 (b). Also, the magnitudes of the maximum and minimum normal stress are equal to the magnitude of the maximum shear stress induced in the element, *i.e.*, $\sigma_1 = -\sigma_2 = \tau_{max}$. The magnitude of the maximum shear stress induced in the element is obtained using Eq. (2.54) as

$$\tau_{max} = \frac{\sigma_{xx}}{2} = \frac{P}{2A} = \sigma_1 = -\sigma_2. \tag{2.94}$$

The maximum shear stress τ_{max} causes the shear strain $\gamma_{x'y'}$ in the element. Thus, it follows from the Hooke's law for shear stress and strain that $\gamma_{x'y'} = \gamma_{max}$. Let us now create a new element by cutting the square element diagonally, as shown in Fig. 2.22 (c). This new element deforms into a shape as shown in Fig. 2.22 (d), which has horizontal and vertical sides equal to $(1+\varepsilon_{xx})$ and $(1-\nu\varepsilon_{xx})$, respectively. The angle formed by the oblique and horizontal sides of the element is precisely half of one of the right angles of the square element. This angle deforms into the angle β, which must therefore be equal to half of $\left(\frac{\pi}{2} - \gamma_{max}\right)$. Thus,

$$\beta = \frac{\pi}{4} - \frac{\gamma_{max}}{2}. \tag{2.95}$$

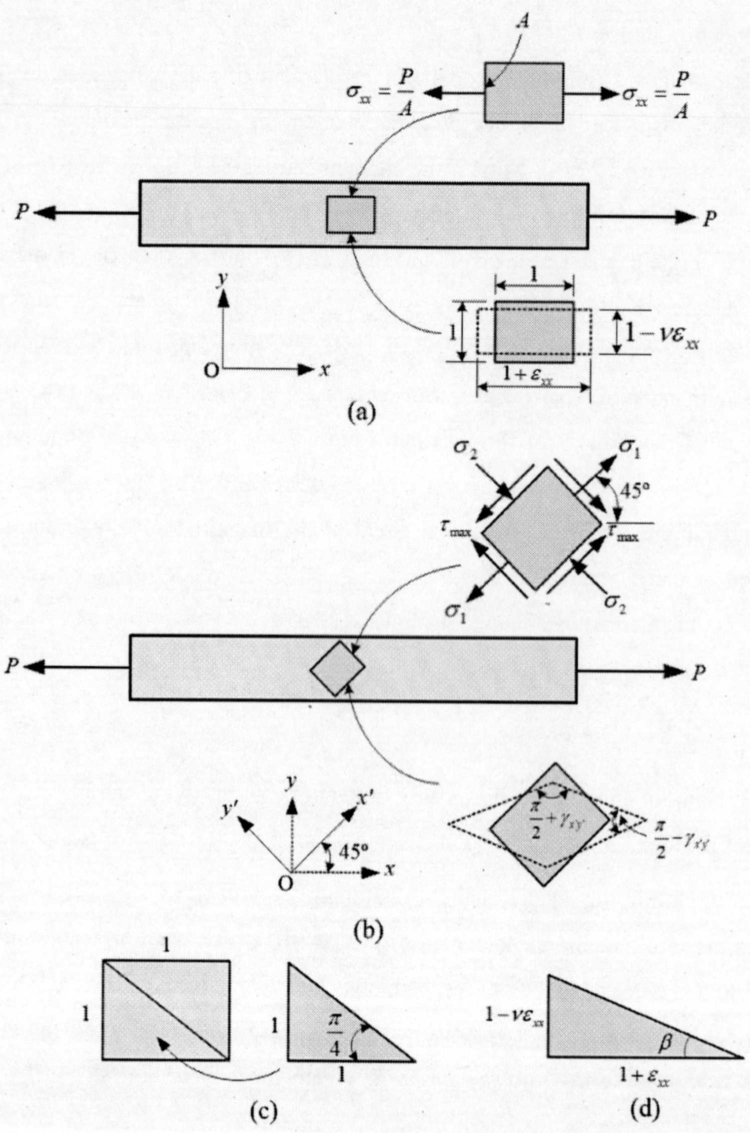

Fig. 2.22 Stress and strains in a square element considered in a uniaxially loaded bar when kept (a) horizontal, (b) rotated at 45° to the bar axis, (c) a new element is formed by cutting the square element diagonally, (d) deformation of the new element under axial loading.

Now,

$$\tan\beta = \tan\left(\frac{\pi}{4} - \frac{\gamma_{max}}{2}\right) = \frac{\tan\frac{\pi}{4} - \tan\frac{\gamma_{max}}{2}}{1 + \tan\frac{\pi}{4}\tan\frac{\gamma_{max}}{2}} = \frac{1 - \tan\frac{\gamma_{max}}{2}}{1 + \tan\frac{\gamma_{max}}{2}}. \tag{2.96}$$

As $\gamma_{max}/2$ is a very small angle, Eq. (2.96) reduces to

$$\tan\beta = \frac{1-\frac{\gamma_{max}}{2}}{1+\frac{\gamma_{max}}{2}}. \tag{2.97}$$

Also, referring to Fig. 2.22 (d), one can write

$$\tan\beta = \frac{1-\nu\varepsilon_{xx}}{1+\varepsilon_{xx}}. \tag{2.98}$$

From Eqs. (2.97) and (2.98),

$$\frac{1-\frac{\gamma_{max}}{2}}{1+\frac{\gamma_{max}}{2}} = \frac{1-\nu\varepsilon_{xx}}{1+\varepsilon_{xx}},$$

$$\gamma_{max} = \frac{(1+\nu)\varepsilon_{xx}}{1+\left(\frac{1-\nu}{2}\right)\varepsilon_{xx}}. \tag{2.99}$$

Since $\varepsilon_{xx} \ll 1$, Eq. (2.99) can be written as

$$\gamma_{max} = (1+\nu)\varepsilon_{xx}. \tag{2.100}$$

Using Hooke's law, in Eq. (2.100), one obtains

$$\frac{\tau_{max}}{G} = (1+\nu)\frac{\sigma_{xx}}{E}, \quad \frac{E}{G} = (1+\nu)\frac{\sigma_{xx}}{\tau_{max}},$$

$$\frac{E}{G} = (1+\nu)\frac{\frac{P}{A}}{\frac{P}{2A}},$$

$$E = 2G(1+\nu). \tag{2.101}$$

Equation (2.101) provides the relationship among the elastic constants *E*, *G* and *ν*.

2.17.2 Relationship among *E*, *K* and *ν*

In order to establish a relationship among *E*, *K* and *ν*, let us go back to Eq. (1.34) of Unit 1. Using Eq. (1.34), the dilatation or volumetric strain of the element under hydrostatic stress with the help of Hooke's law can be expressed as

$$\varepsilon_{xx}+\varepsilon_{yy}+\varepsilon_{zz}=\frac{\sigma_{xx}+\sigma_{yy}+\sigma_{zz}}{E}-\frac{2\nu\left(\sigma_{xx}+\sigma_{yy}+\sigma_{zz}\right)}{E},$$

$$\varepsilon_V=\left(\frac{1-2\nu}{E}\right)\left(\sigma_{xx}+\sigma_{yy}+\sigma_{zz}\right). \tag{2.102}$$

Now, for the special case dictated by Eq. (1.35), Eq. (2.102) can be expressed as

$$\varepsilon_V=-\left(\frac{1-2\nu}{E}\right)3p,$$

$$-\frac{p}{K}=-\left(\frac{1-2\nu}{E}\right)3p,$$

$$\frac{1}{K}=3\left(\frac{1-2\nu}{E}\right),$$

$$K=\frac{E}{3(1-2\nu)}, \tag{2.103}$$

which represents the relationship among the elastic constants E, K, and ν. Using Eqs. (2.101) and (2.103) it can be shown that the Poisson's ratio (ν) of material lies between –1 to 0.5. Also, using Eqs. (2.101) and (2.103), the following relationship among the elastic moduli E, G and K can be established:

$$E=\frac{9GK}{3K+G}. \tag{2.104}$$

Example 2.9 From the Mohr's circles of stress and strain for the case of pure shear and using the stress-strain relations, prove the relationship among the elastic constants E, G and ν given by Eq. (2.101).

Solution

A two-dimensional element subjected to a pure state of shear is shown in Fig. (a). For this case, the Mohr's circle of stress and strain can be constructed as shown in Figs. (b) and (c), respectively.

From the Mohr's circle of stress, the principal stresses, σ_1, σ_2 and shear stress, τ can be related as

$$\sigma_1=-\sigma_2=\tau. \tag{i}$$

Further, from Mohr's circle of strain, it is seen that

$$\varepsilon_1=-\varepsilon_2=\frac{\gamma}{2}, \tag{ii}$$

where ε_1, and ε_2 are the principal strains and γ is the shear strain. Using generalized Hooke's law (stress-strain relations) in two-dimensions, the principal strain ε_1 is related to principal stresses by

$$\varepsilon_1 = \frac{1}{E}(\sigma_1 - \nu\sigma_2). \tag{iii}$$

Hooke's law for shear stress provides

$$\tau = G\gamma. \tag{iv}$$

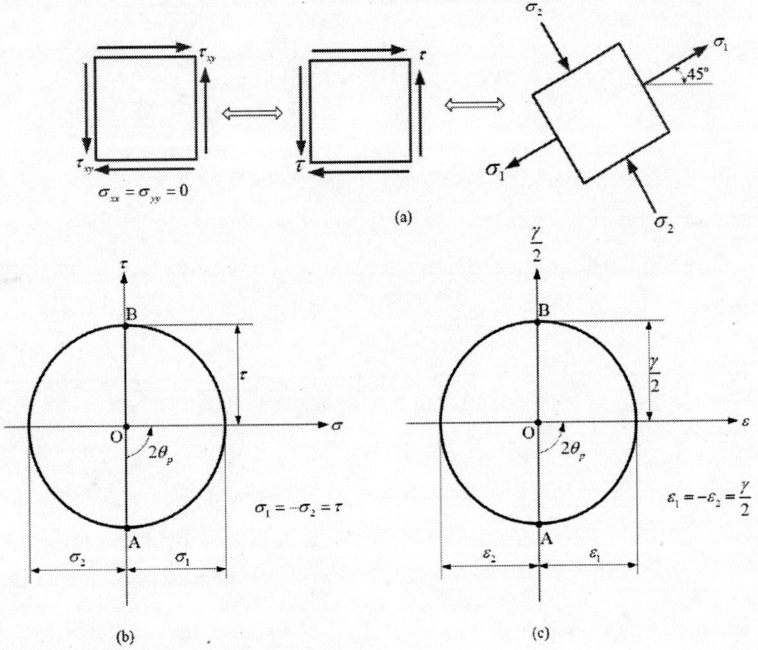

Using Eq. (ii) in Eq. (iv), one obtains

$$\varepsilon_1 = \frac{\tau}{2G}. \tag{v}$$

Now, substituting Eq. (i) and (v) in Eq. (iii), we get the following relationship among E, G and ν:

$$\frac{\tau}{2G} = \frac{1}{E}\{\tau - \nu(-\tau)\},$$
$$\frac{\tau}{2G} = \frac{\tau}{E}(1+\nu),$$
$$E = 2G(1+\nu),$$

which is same as given by Eq. (2.101).

Example 2.10 If the modulus of elasticity and shear modulus of a material are 206 GPa and 78 GPa, respectively, determine the Poisson's ratio of the material. What is the bulk modulus of the material?

Solution

Given, E=206 GPa, G=78 GPa.

Using Eq. (2.101), the Poisson's ratio (ν) of the material is obtained as

$$\nu = \frac{E}{2G} - 1 = \frac{206}{2 \times 78} - 1 = 0.32.$$

The bulk modulus of elasticity of the material can be evaluated using Eq. (2.103) as

$$K = \frac{E}{3(1-2\nu)} = \frac{206}{3(1-2\times 0.32)} = 190.74\,\text{GPa}.$$

2.18 Summary

In this unit, the concept of compound stresses and strains are introduced. The general state of stress at a point is discussed. It has been comprehended that the state of stress at a point can be completely represented by three traction vectors acting on three mutually perpendicular planes or by their nine components in a three-dimensional space, called a stress tensor. Due to the similarity of the stress tensor, the state of stress at a point can be described by six independent stress components, three normal stress, and three shear stress components. Then the three-dimensional state of stress at a point is reduced to a two-dimensional stress system to represent the stress components acting on a plane. The transformation rule for a two-dimensional plane stress system is developed, followed by the concepts of principal planes and principal stresses. It is also demonstrated that the problems involving the transformation of plane stress can be solved by a graphical method called Mohr's circle of stress. Another graphical representation of the state of stress at a point in two-dimensions is introduced, termed as the stress ellipse. The state of strain at a point is introduced, which is then reduced to the state of plane strain consisting of components of strain on a plane. The relationship between the two-dimensional stresses and strains is established for a linear elastic solid, followed by the development of transformation relations for plane strain and discussion on the concept of principal strains and principal axes of strain. Similar to Mohr's circle of stress, the Mohr's circle for two-dimensional strain is introduced, followed by the concept of an ellipse of strain. Towards the end, the relationships among various elastic constants are established. It is understood that out of four elastic constants, only two are independent. Knowing any two of the elastic constants, the other two can be obtained using the established relationships.

Know More

EXERCISES

Multiple Choice Questions

2.1 Stress at a point is a tensor of order

(a) zero (b) one

(c) two (d) three

2.2 Which of the following quantity is a tensor of second order?

(a) mass (b) velocity

(c) traction (d) strain

2.3 Under the transformation of coordinate axes,

(a) the stress tensor itself at a point changes without the change of its components

(b) the stress tensor itself at a point does not change, but its components get changed.

(c) the stress tensor at a point, as well as its components, remain the same

(d) both the stress tensor at a point as well as its components gets changed

2.4 Non-zero stress components at a point are $\sigma_{xx} = 30$ MPa, $\sigma_{yy} = 20$ MPa. The maximum shear stress is

(a) 5 MPa (b) 10 MPa

(c) 15 MPa (d) 20 MPa

2.5 In a plane stress situation, $\sigma_{xx} = 50\text{MPa}$, $\sigma_{yy} = -10\text{MPa}$, $\tau_{xy} = 40\text{MPa}$. The angle between the principle plane and the x-plane is

(a) 53.1°
(b) 36.9°
(c) 26.6°
(d) 18.5°

2.6 An isotropic material in plane strain is subjected to a shear strain of 0.0001 with respect to some coordinate system. All other components of strain are zero. Which one of the following statements is true?

(a) Principal stresses are zero.
(b) Both the in-plane principal stresses are equal.
(c) One in-plane principal stress is zero, and the other is non-zero.
(d) One in-plane principal stress is positive, and the other negative.

2.7 For the Mohr circle shown:

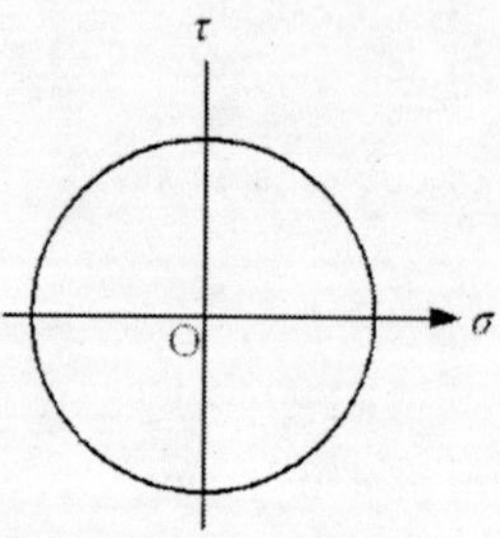

(a) The maximum principle stress is equal to the maximum shear stress.
(b) The maximum principle stress is equal to twice the maximum shear stress.
(c) The maximum principle stress is equal to half the maximum shear stress.
(d) The shear stress is positive on the x-plane and negative on the y-plane.

2.8 If the Mohr circle for strain reduces to a point, it indicates that

(a) volumetric strain is zero
(b) volumetric strain is negative

(c) there is no shear strain at any plane

(d) there is no normal strain at any plane

2.9 In a plane strain problem, the strain components are given as $\varepsilon_{xx}=0$, $\varepsilon_{yy}=8\times10^{-4}$, $\gamma_{xy}= 6\times10^{-4}$. Note that γ_{xy} is the engineering shear strain. The radius of the Mohr circle is

(a) 10^{-3}

(b) 5×10^{-4}

(c) 7.2×10^{-4}

(d) 3×10^{-4}

2.10 In a plane strain problem, the strain components are given as $\varepsilon_{xx}=0$, $\varepsilon_{yy}=8\times10^{-4}$, $\gamma_{xy}= 6\times10^{-4}$. The engineering shear strain component on a plane inclined at 45° to this plane is

(a) 3×10^{-4}

(b) 6×10^{-4}

(c) 10^{-3}

(d) 5×10^{-4}

2.11 A Mohr circle is centred at 10 MPa on the normal stress axis, and its diameter is 10 MPa. The shear stress on a plane with 13 MPa normal stress is

(a) 13.9 MPa

(b) 5 MPa

(c) 4 MPa

(d) 3 MPa

2.12 The Young's modulus of elasticity of steel is 210 GPa, and the Poisson's ratio is 0.29. The shear modulus is

(a) 110 MPa

(b) 105 GPa

(c) 81 GPa

(d) 71 GPa

2.13 For the data of Question 2.12, the bulk modulus is

(a) 113 MPa

(b) 167 GPa

(c) 210 GPa

(d) 403 MPa

2.14 If the yield strength of the material of Question 2.12 is 350 MPa, the percentage change in the volume of the specimen in a uni-axial tensile test, just before yielding, is

(a) 1% (b) 0.1%

(c) 0.09% (d) 0.07%

2.15 For an isotropic material, the number of independent elastic constants are

(a) 81 (b) 36

(c) 21 (d) 2

Answers of Multiple Choice Questions

2.1 (c), 2.2 (d), 2.3 (b), 2.4 (a), 2.5 (c), 2.6 (d), 2.7 (a), 2.8 (c), 2.9 (b), 2.10 (b), 2.11 (c), 2.12 (c), 2.13 (b), 2.14 (d), 2.15 (d)

Short and Long Answer Type Questions

Category I

2.1 What do you mean by state of stress at a point? How many independent components of stress are there at a point?

2.2 Why do engineers need the transformation equations of stress and strain?

2.3 What are the maximum normal and shear stress in an axially loaded bar and their orientations? What is the relation between them?

2.4 What is Mohr's circle? Draw the Mohr's circle of stress for any generic point on the tensile test specimen during loading.

2.5 What do you mean by state of pure shear? Explain with the help of Mohr's circle.

2.6 What are stress invariants? Why are they called invariants?

2.7 In a strained material, one of the principal stresses is twice the other at a given point. The maximum shear stress at the same point is τmax. What is the value of the maximum principal stress?

2.8 Suppose you are given a choice to load the material as per the following configurations of principal stresses. Which one would you prefer in order to keep the maximum normal stress as low as possible? Explain the logic.

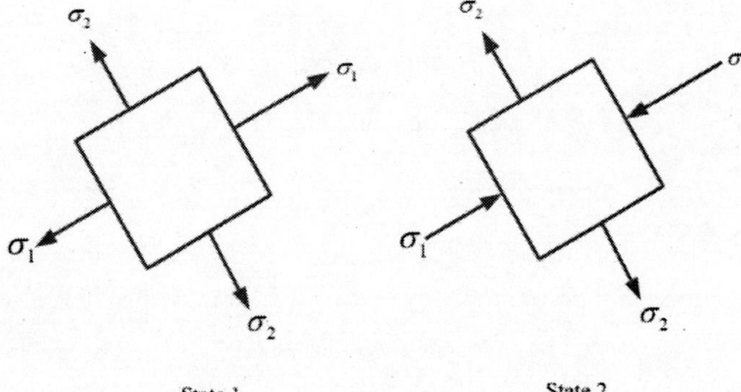

2.9 What is the value of shear stress on the planes of maximum and minimum normal stress at a point? Also, determine the value of the normal stress on the plane where the maximum in-plane shear stress occurs.

2.10 What do you mean by state of strain at a point?

2.11 What do you mean by state of plane stress and plane strain? Are they the same? Under what conditions do the state of plane stress and plane strain coincide?

2.12 What is the expression for ε_{zz} for a plane stress problem of an isotropic material? Also, write the expression for σ_{zz} for a problem of the plane strain of an isotropic material.

2.13 Draw the Mohr's circle of strain for any generic point on a tensile test specimen of circular cross-section subjected to deformation.

2.14 Under what condition, Mohr's circle of strain reduces to a point?

2.15 Using the transformation relations, show that the maximum in-plane shear strain occurs on a plane that is at an angle of 45° with respect to the plane of maximum normal strain.

2.16 Poisson's ratio is defined as the negative of the ratio of lateral strain to axial strain in a uniaxial loading. Argue that it should lie between -1 to 0.5.

Category II

2.17 Prove that the traction on any arbitrary plane can be completely represented by the three traction components acting on three mutually perpendicular planes or by their nine components.

2.18 Prove that for a two-dimensional stress system, the values of the principal stresses obtained from Mohr's circle are the same as those obtained mathematically by setting the derivatives of the stress transformation equations with respect to the transformation angle to zero.

2.19 Show that the elastic moduli E, G and K can be related as

$$E = \frac{9GK}{3K + G}.$$

2.20 Write short notes on the ellipse of stress and ellipse of strain.

Numerical Problems

2.1 The state of stress at a point in a body is shown on an infinitesimal rectangular element considered around the point as depicted in the figure in (x, y) coordinate system. Determine the normal, and shear stresses acting on a plane, the normal to which makes an angle of 40° with the x-axis. Solve the problem using transformation relations and constructing a Mohr's circle. (**Ans.** $\sigma_{x'x'}$=65.26 MPa, $\sigma_{y'y'}$= –15.26 MPa, $\tau_{x'y'}$=2.02 MPa)

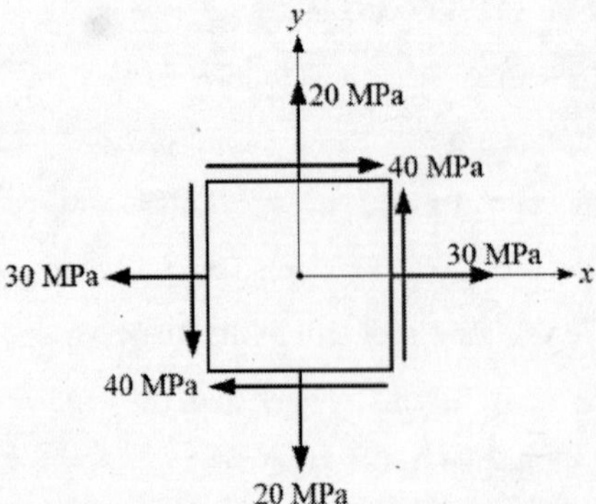

2.2 Draw the Mohr's circles for the following stress states and determine the magnitudes of the principal stresses and their orientations. Also, denote the principal stress state on a suitably rotated rectangular element.

a) σ_{xx}=35 MPa, σ_{yy} = –12 MPa, τ_{xy}=25 MPa. (**Ans.** σ_1=45.81 MPa, σ_2= –22.81 MPa, θ_p=23.38°, 113.38°)

b) σ_{xx}= – 40 MPa, σ_{yy} = –70 MPa, τ_{xy}= –50 MPa. (**Ans.** σ_1= –2.80 MPa, σ_2= –107.20 MPa, θ_p= –36.65°, 53.35°)

c) σ_{xx}= – 80 MPa, σ_{yy} = 60 MPa, τ_{xy}= – 45 MPa. (**Ans.** σ_1=73.22 MPa, σ_2= –93.21 MPa, θ_p=16.37°, 106.37°)

2.3 Consider a point on the wing of the aircraft and the state of stress at that point is shown in the figure on a rectangular element using the wing axes as the reference coordinate frame. Evaluate the stress components at that point using the fuselage axes as the coordinate frame or determine the stresses when the element is rotated back to align with the fuselage axe. (**Ans.** σ_{xx}=86.57 MPa, σ_{yy}=163.42 MPa, τ_{xy}=40.59 MPa)

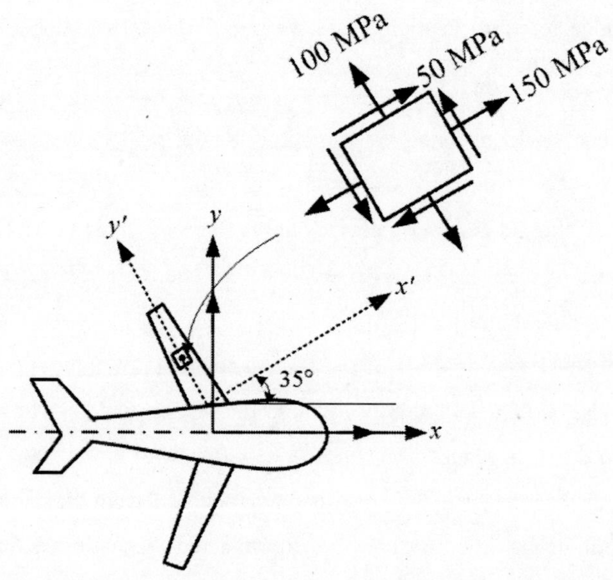

2.4. For the Problem 2.3, determine the principal stresses and their orientations. Also, find on which plane the maximum in-plane shear stress occurs and the magnitude of the maximum in-plane shear stress. (**Ans.** σ_1=180.89 MPa, σ_2=69.10 MPa, θ_p = – 23.28°, 66.72°, θ_s = 21.72°, 111.72°, τ_{max}=55.89 MPa)

2.5 If the material of the wing is of aluminium alloy with Young's modulus of elasticity E=71.7 GPa, and Poisson's ratio ν=0.28, using the data of Problem 2.4, determine the principal strains and the in-plane maximum shear strains at the point. (**Ans.** $\varepsilon_1=2.253\times10^{-3}$, $\varepsilon_2=2.573\times10^{-4}$, $\gamma_{max}=9.978\times10^{-4}$)

2.6 In a plane strain state at a point, the strains are $\varepsilon_{xx}=3.25\times10^{-6}$, $\varepsilon_{yy}=4.18\times10^{-6,}$ $\gamma_{xy}=1.44\times10^{-6}$ Evaluate the two principal strains and their orientations using Mohr's circle. Verify your results using the analytical equations. (**Ans.** $\varepsilon_1=4.572\times10^{-6}$, $\varepsilon_2=2.858\times10^{-6}$, θ_p= –28.57°, 61.43°)

2.7 Using the data of Problem 2.6, determine all the six stress components at the point, knowing that for the material, the shear modulus of elasticity G=80 GPa and Poisson's ratio ν=0.3. (**Ans.** σ_{xx}=1.03 MPa, σ_{yy}=1.18 MPa, σ_{zz}=0.66 MPa, τ_{xy}=0.12 MPa, $\tau_{yz}=\tau_{zx}$=0)

2.8 The state of plane strain at a point for isotropic material is represented on an infinitesimal rectangular element and is given by $\varepsilon_{xx}=-400\times10^{-6}$, $\varepsilon_{yy}=-650\times10^{-6,}$ $\gamma_{xy}=250\times10^{-6}$. Determine the state of strain at the point, when the element is rotated 22.5° clockwise from the above referred position. (**Ans.** $\varepsilon_{x'x'} = -540.41\times10^{-6}$, $\varepsilon_{y'y'} = -509\times10^{-6}$, $\gamma_{x'y'} = 352.21\times10^{-6}$)

2.9 In a tensile test, a rod of length 150 mm and diameter 30 mm is subjected to a tensile force of P=80 kN. This causes the rod to elongate to a length of 150.6 mm. If the deformation of the rod is linearly elastic and its shear modulus G=12 GPa, determine the Poisson's ratio of the material. Also, evaluate the change in diameter of the rod. (**Ans.** ν=0.18, Δd= – 0.0216 mm)

2.10 Consider a one-dimensional bar of cross-sectional area 350 mm^2 subjected to a uniaxial pull of 250 kN. Write a computer program to find the normal and shear stresses acting at any point on different planes as a function of θ (angle of inclination). Plot the variation of normal and shear stress at the point as a function of θ from the computer program and thereby obtain the maximum values of the normal and shear stress acting at the point.

Unit 3

Shear Force and Bending Moment Diagrams

UNIT SPECIFICS

The following topics are covered in this unit:

- Beams, their different types and types of loads act on them;
- Shear force, bending moment and their relationship;
- Construction of shear force and bending moment diagram for different statically determinate beams subjected to different kinds of loads.

Emphasis is given on the importance of shear force and bending moment diagrams in the design of beams used in many engineering structures. At the end, a moderate number of practice exercises are provided.

RATIONALE

Beams are the integral part of a plethora of engineering structures. Upon loading, they induce internal forces, *viz.*, shear force and bending moment. The evaluation of shear force and bending moment at every beam cross-section along its length is important to locate the point of maximum shear force and bending moment. This can be conveniently and more precisely obtained by plotting the shear force and bending moment diagrams for a given beam. This will serve as the foundation for the design of a beam. From this perspective, in this unit, it is attempted to introduce the shear force and bending moment diagram and the procedures for constructing them.

PRE-REQUISITIES

Engineering Mechanics

Understanding of internal forces.

UNIT OUTCOMES

After completing this unit, students will be able to

U3-O1: understand the concept of beam and their different types.

U3-O2: understand the concept of shear force, bending moment and their relationship.

U3-O3: evaluate reactive forces, shear force and bending moment at any point in a beam for different kinds of loading.

U3-O4: construct shear force and bending moment diagrams for different types of beams.

Course Outcomes	Expected Mapping with Course Outcomes - CE (1- Weak Correlation; 2- Medium correlation; 3- Strong Correlation)			
	CO-1	CO-2	CO-3	CO-4
U3-O1	3	-	-	-
U3-O2	3	-	-	-
U3-O3	3	-	-	1
U3-O4	3	-	-	1

Course Outcomes	Expected Mapping with Course Outcomes - ME (1- Weak Correlation; 2- Medium correlation; 3- Strong Correlation)	
	CO-1	CO-2
U3-O1	3	-
U3-O2	3	-
U3-O3	3	-
U3-O4	3	-

3.1 Introduction

One of the most commonly employed structural or mechanical elements in engineering systems is beam. This unit is solely devoted to understanding the concept of shear force and bending moment induced at the cross-sections of a beam and their variation along the length of the beam. Only planar beams are considered in this unit, which means the beam bends in a plane only and there is no displacement or force normal to the plane of bending. The unit begins with an introduction to beam and their different types, followed by a discussion on how to construct shear force and bending moment diagrams for different types of beams. The shear force and bending moment diagrams provide the information of magnitudes of shear force and bending moment at every beam cross-section along its length. Knowing the shear force and bending moment, bending and shear stresses in beams can be evaluated, which will be discussed later. From the shear force and bending moment diagrams, one can easily locate the position where the maximum shear force and bending moment occurs. This information is very useful to safeguard the structure against potential failure in service due to the externally applied loads. It is assumed here that the beams are made of prismatic sections and slender members with at least one axis of symmetry. A slender member is one whose length is much larger than any other dimensions used to describe the size of the member.

3.2 Beams and Different Types of Loads Acting Over a Beam Span

Beams are slender members that are designed to resist transversely applied loadings on it. Transversely applied loadings on the members are the forces and moments whose vector directions are perpendicular to the axis of the member. A typical beam is shown in Fig. 3.1 with forces and moments acting on it. Concentrated forces P_1, P_2, P_3, and P_4 are acting along the y-axis, perpendicular to the longitudinal x-axis. Mathematically, the downward forces P_3 and P_4 can be considered as negative forces. The moments M_{z1} and M_{z2} acting at points A and B are shown using two representations— (1) as a double arrow-head vector and (2) as an arc of a circle displaying its tendency to rotate.

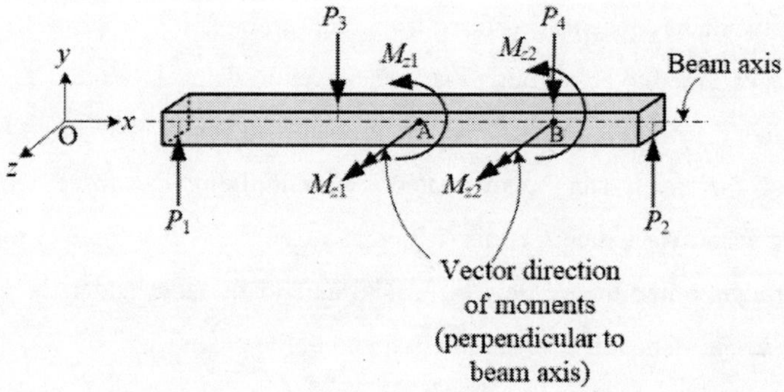

Fig. 3.1 A typical beam loaded with transverse forces and moment

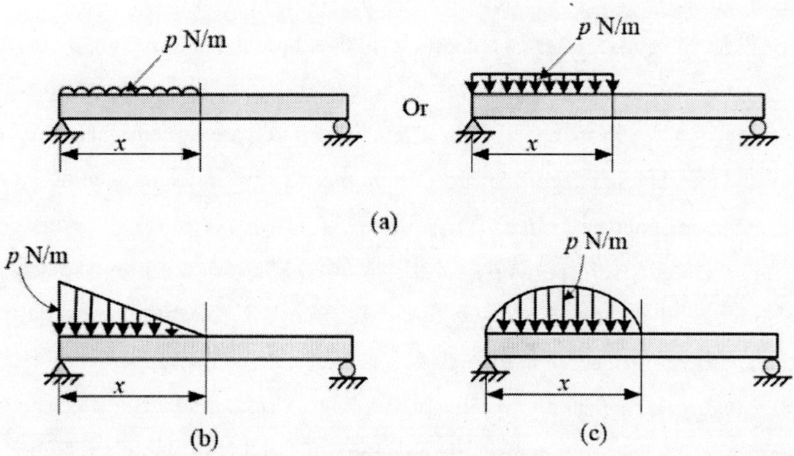

Fig. 3.2 Simply supported beam with (a) uniformly distributed load, (b) triangularly distributed load, and (c) elliptically distributed load over a span x

It is important to note that other than the concentrated loads, a beam member may also be subjected to distributed loads. In practice, all loads are applied over a finite area and thus distributed in nature. However, for analysis, if the area over which the loads are applied is very small, they can be assumed to act at a point and are called concentrated loads as depicted in Fig. 3.1. Distributed loads are considered to act over a certain part or over the entire span of the beam. If the loads are distributed over the span equally or uniformly, they are termed as uniformly distributed loads. In certain occasions, the distribution of loads may not be uniform, rather, they may vary linearly over the beam span, *e.g.*, trapezoidal or triangularly distributed loads. The loads may vary non-linearly also such as loads with the parabolic or elliptic distribution. A typical beam member subjected to different types of distributed loads over a span x are shown in Fig. 3.2. The distributed force system can suitably be reduced to an equivalent resultant concentrated force using the principle of composition of force, where the resultant is assumed to act through the vertical centroidal axis of the distributed load over the beam segment. In Fig. 3.2 (a), the resultant of the uniformly distributed load p N/m over the span x of the beam can be evaluated by multiplying the force intensity with the corresponding span over which it is distributed as px N. This px N force is supposed to act at a location through which the vertical centroidal axis of the area under the load-distribution curve passes, *i.e.*, at a span of $x/2$ from the left end of the beam.

3.3 Types of supports and Classification of Beams

There are three basic types of supports that are used to constrain the planar beams. They are pin or hinge supports, roller or pinned-on roller supports, and fixed supports as depicted in Figs. 3.3 (a), (b), and (c), respectively. The corresponding free-body diagrams are also shown in Fig. 3.3 with reference to the Cartesian coordinate system. The hinge support constrains the translational degrees of freedom in the x and y directions keeping the rotational degree of freedom about z axis free. Thus, the support provides two reactive forces R_x and R_y, in the x and y directions, respectively, as shown in Fig. 3.3 (a). A roller or pinned-on roller support provides the vertical reactive force R_y (Fig. 3.3 (b)) as it constrains only the translational degree of freedom in the y direction. If a beam end is supported by fixed support such as welded or joined rigidly by nuts and bolts to a rigid wall, then it constrains all the three degrees of freedom (two translational degrees of freedom in x and y directions and one rotational degree of freedom about z axis) at the support location when isolated. Thus, it provides three support reactions, two reactive forces in the x and y directions, and a reactive moment in the z-direction, as shown in Fig. 3.3 (c).

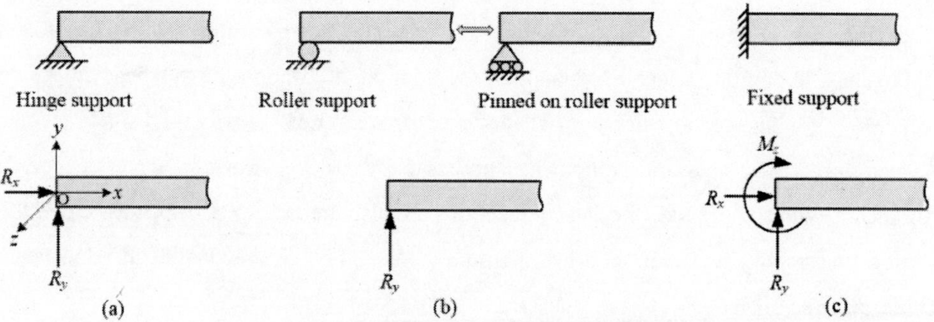

Fig. 3.3 Different types of supports

Based on the types of supports used to constrain the beams, they are classified into following types:

- *Simply supported beam*: When one end of the beam is supported by a pin or hinge support, and the other end is supported by a roller or pinned on roller support, then the beam is referred to as the simply supported beam.
- *Cantilever beam*: When one end of a beam is supported by a fixed support and the other end is kept free, then the beam is referred as the cantilever beam.
- *Overhanging beam*: When one or both of the ends of a beam are freely extended over the supports, then the beam is known as the overhanging beam.
- *Fixed beam*: When both the ends of a beam are supported by the fixed supports, then the beam is referred as the fixed beam or built-in beam. By construction, these types of beams are statically indeterminate.

All the above four types of beams are schematically shown in Fig. 3.4.

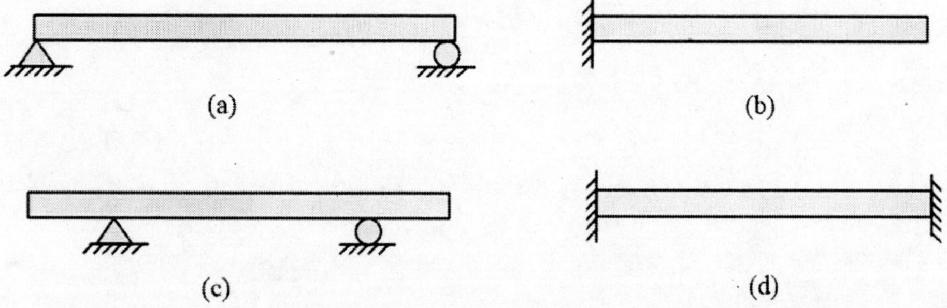

Fig. 3.4 Types of beams: (a) simply supported beam, (b) cantilever beam, (c) overhanging beam, and (d) fixed beam

Beams are the most versatile engineering components present in a plethora of engineering structures and also in nature. For example, beams are used in bridges to support the deck, in building structures to support the floor and to support the overhead cranes used in construction sites or in workshops. The wings of an aircraft, railway tracks, and elements of many other machines and equipment, such as the cantilever arm of a waterjet pipe-cutting machine and a coordinate measuring machine, are also the examples of beams. Often the axle of an automobile and even load-bearing body parts and bones are also idealized as beams for the purpose of analysis.

3.4 Concept of Shear Force and Bending Moment

Shear force and bending moment are the internal forces that are induced at the cross-sections of a beam when it is subjected to transversely applied forces and moments. The loadings on the beam tend to fail the member primarily by shearing, bending, or a combination of bending and shearing. Fig. 3.5 depicts the fracture due to shear and bending. In order to resist shear, the internal forces across the cross-sections of the beam are developed, which are termed as shear forces. To resist the bending, internal moments are developed at the beam cross-sections, which are termed as bending moments.

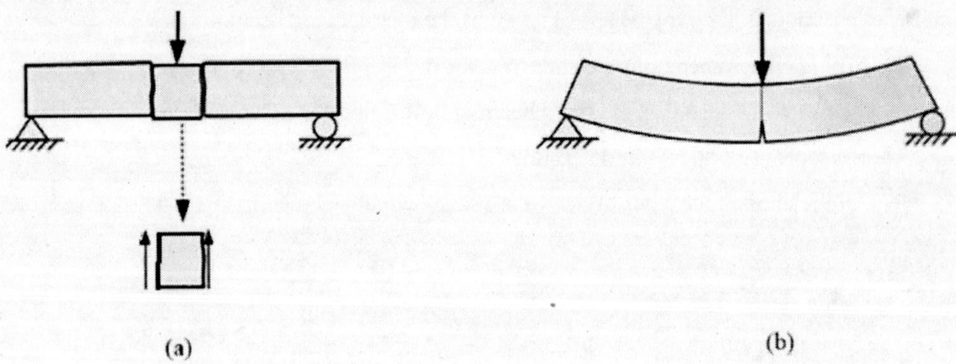

Fig. 3.5 Failure of beam (a) by shearing across its cross-sections and (b) by excessive bending

To reveal the shear force and bending moment at the cross-section of a beam, an imaginary cutting plane is visualized across the cross-section of interest. A free-body diagram is then constructed either of the beam segment left to the cutting plane or right to the cutting plane showing the shear force and bending moment at the cut cross-section. For example, let us consider a cut across the cross-section of a simply supported beam at a distance of x from the left support as shown in Fig. 3.6. Due to the transversely applied loads P_1 and P_2 on the beam, the cross-section of the beam is subjected to a shear force and a bending moment. Considering the curvature of the beam to be concave upwards, the horizontal zone above a certain level is subjected to compression, and the zone below that level is subjected to tension. The interface between these tensile and compressive zones is stress-free. Thus, the horizontal internal normal forces to the left and right of the cut section are distributed as compressive on the fibers above the stress-free level, and below it, they are distributed as tensile. This nature of distribution of internal normal force on the beam cross-section results in an internal moment, *i.e.*, bending moment $M(x)$ on each half of the beam segment. Similarly, the resultant of the distributed internal force parallel to the beam cross-section provides the shear force $V(x)$ on each half of the beam segment. The shear force $V(x)$ and bending moment $M(x)$ acting at the beam cross-section at a span of x keep both the beam segments to the left and right of the cutting plane in equilibrium.

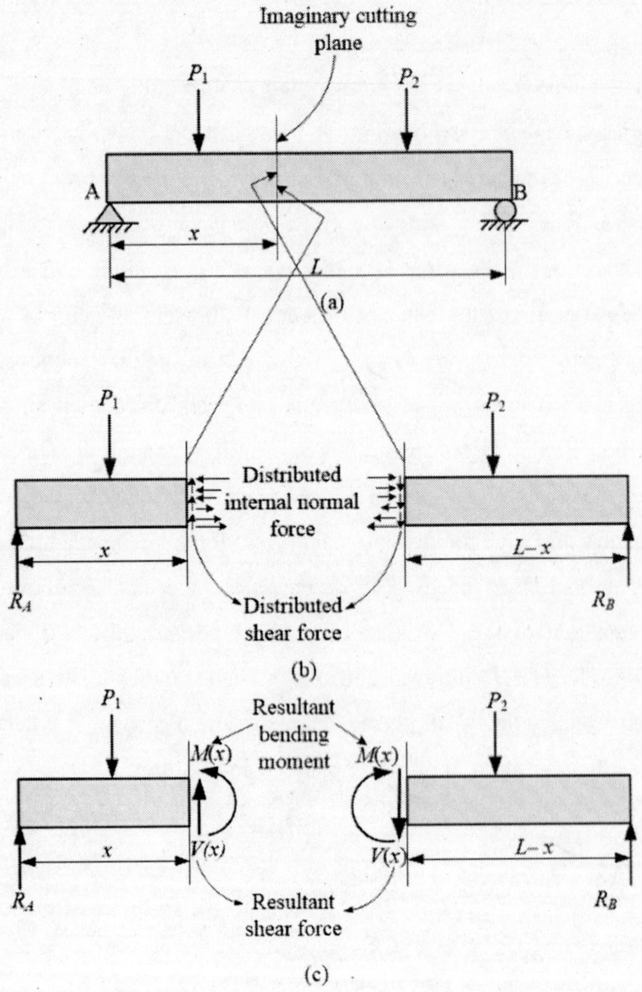

Fig. 3.6 Shear force and bending moment on the cross-section of a typical beam: (a) simply supported beam, (b) distribution of forces on a typical cross-section, and (c) resultant shear force and bending moment.

Shear forces can be defined as the algebraic sum of the transverse loads to the left or right of a cross-section considered over a beam span. The algebraic sum of these loads must restore the vertical equilibrium of the beam segments under consideration. Similarly, the bending moment can be defined as the sum of the moments about a beam cross-section produced by all external loads acting on the left or right of that section. Moments on a section are evaluated by multiplying the magnitude of the loads (both active and reactive forces) by the perpendicular distance from the line of action of the loads.

3.5 Sign Conventions for Shear Force and Bending Moment

A shear force is considered as positive if it acts downwards to the left of a section or acts upwards to the right of a section of the beam segment; here, the positive direction of x-axis is from left to right. Thus, the outward normal to the right side plane is along positive x-direction. Hence, right side plane can be considered as a positive plane and the left-hand side plane a negative plane. Positive y-direction is from down to up. Hence, a force acting on a positive plane in a positive direction provides a positive force. Similarly, a force acting on a negative plane (left side plane) in the negative direction (downward) provides a positive force. In other cases, the sign for shear force is taken as negative. The sign convention for shear forces acting on the sections of a beam segment is depicted in Fig. 3.7 (a). It can be seen from Fig. 3.7 (a) that a pair of positive shear forces acting on a beam segment tends to rotate it counterclockwise, whilst a pair of negative shear forces tend to rotate it clockwise.

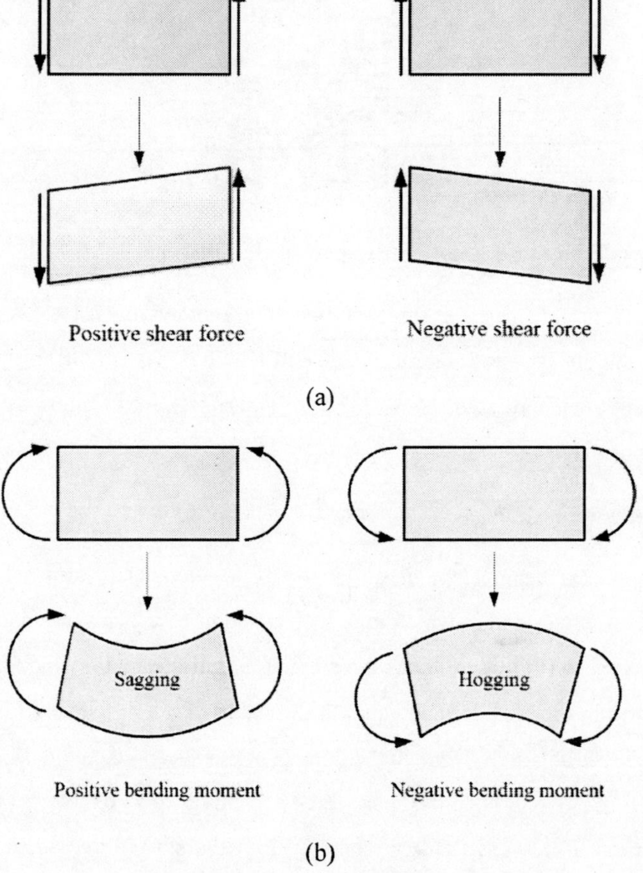

Fig. 3.7 Sign conventions for (a) shear force and (b) bending moment

If the bending moment is clockwise to the left of a beam section or counterclockwise to the right of a beam section, then it is considered as positive bending moment. On the other hand, if the bending moment is counterclockwise to the left of a beam section or clockwise to the right of a beam section, then the sign for the bending moment is taken as negative. The sign convention for bending moment acting on the sections of a beam segment is schematically represented in Fig. 3.7 (b). As depicted in Fig. 3.7 (b), the system of the positive bending moment causes the sagging of the beam segment, and conversely, the system of the negative bending moment causes the hogging of the beam segment. If the counterclockwise moment is taken as positive, then the sign convention for bending moment becomes similar to that of shear force; that is, a positive moment on a positive plane or negative moment on a negative plane provides a positive bending moment.

Know More

3.6 Load, Shear Force and Bending Moment Relationships

In this section, load, shear force, and bending moment are related for a beam segment subjected to different types of commonly applied loadings, *viz*., a uniformly distributed load, a point load and a concentrated moment. For this purpose, an infinitesimal beam element of length dx is considered.

Case 1: Beam segment subjected to a uniformly distributed load

A differential beam element of length dx is sliced out from the span of a beam subjected to distributed load q, which may be a function of x. The free body diagram of this beam element is shown in Fig. 3.8. As the element is infinitesimally small, it can be assumed that q is uniform in the element and equal to the value of the distributed load at x. As shown in Fig. 3.8, the shear force V on the left face of the beam element is considered to act downwards. Over the length dx, the shear force V changes to V+dV to act on the right face of the element directed upwards. By convention, both the shear forces acting on the left and right face of the element are positive. The bending moment over the length dx changes from M to M+dM, and they are taken as positive.

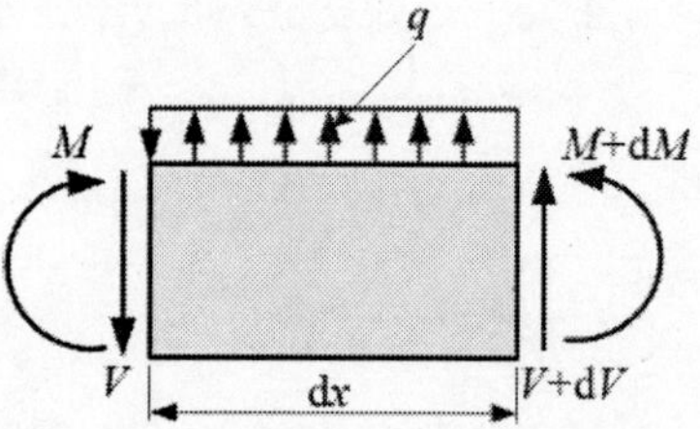

Fig. 3.8 Free body diagram of a beam element subjected to distributed load

Now, considering the vertical force equilibrium of the element, one obtains

$$q\mathrm{d}x + (V + \mathrm{d}V) - V = 0,$$

$$q\mathrm{d}x + \mathrm{d}V = 0,$$

$$\frac{\mathrm{d}V}{\mathrm{d}x} = -q. \tag{3.1}$$

Equation (3.1) provides the relationship between the shear force V and load q.

Taking the moment of all the loads about the left face of the element, the moment equilibrium equation can be written as

$$(M + \mathrm{d}M) - M + (V + \mathrm{d}V)\mathrm{d}x - q\mathrm{d}x\left(\frac{\mathrm{d}x}{2}\right) = 0, \tag{3.2}$$

Neglecting the product of the small quantities, Eq. (3.2) reduces to

$$\mathrm{d}M + V\mathrm{d}x = 0,$$

$$\frac{\mathrm{d}M}{\mathrm{d}x} = -V, \tag{3.3}$$

which represents the relationship between the shear force and the bending moment.

It is observed from Eq. (3.1) that if q=0, then dV/dx=0. Thus, the shear force is constant in that portion of the beam. Further, for constant q, dV/dx is also constant. This indicates that the shear force varies linearly over that span of the beam. Equation (3.1) also dictates that the change in shear force between two points in the beam is equal to the area of the loading diagram, *i.e.*, the plot of load q as a function of length coordinate x. It can be inferred from Eq. (3.3) that if the shear force is zero over a certain span of the beam, then the bending moment is constant over that span. For uniformly distributed or constant load q, upon integration of Eq. (3.1) with respect to x provides the linear shear force V. Substituting this shear force in Eq. (3.3) and then integrating, one can see that the bending moment over the beam span subjected to uniformly distributed load varies as a quadratic function of x.

Case 2: Beam segment subjected to a concentrated load

A beam element of infinitesimal length dx is sliced out from a beam such that it is subjected to a concentrated load P at the mid-span. The free body diagram of the element is shown in Fig. 3.9. On the section left to the concentrated load P, the positive shear force V and positive bending moment M change by finite values V_1 and M_1, respectively over the length dx to act on the section right to the concentrated load as shown in Fig. 3.9. It is to be noted that in Case 1, the shear force and bending moment from the left to the right section of the element changes by infinitesimally small values dV and dM as the element over the length dx was acted upon by distributed load. However, in the present case, as there is a point load acting on the small elemental length dx, there is a finite change of the shear force and bending moment from the left to the right section of the element.

The vertical force equilibrium provides,

$$V + V_1 - P - V = 0,$$

$$V_1 = P. \tag{3.4}$$

Thus, if a beam segment is subjected to only a concentrated load P, then the shear force V at the section left to the concentrated load changes to $V+P$ at the section right to that concentrated load.

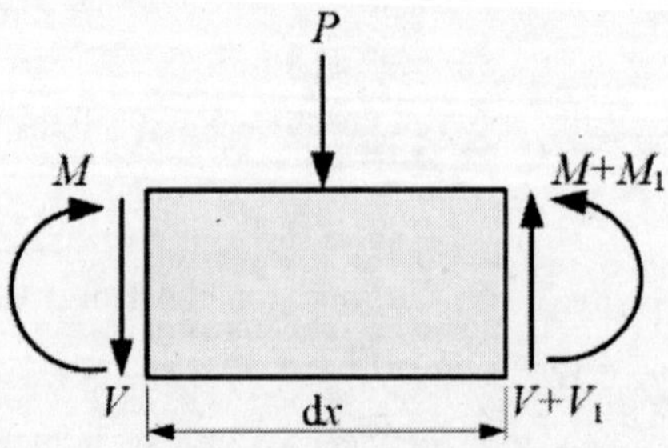

Fig. 3.9 Free body diagram of a beam element subjected to a point load

Taking the moment about the right section of the element and writing the equation of moment equilibrium, one obtains

$$M + M_1 - M + V\mathrm{d}x + P\frac{\mathrm{d}x}{2} = 0, \tag{3.5}$$

In Eq. (3.5), the last two terms can be neglected as they involve the multiplication of V and P with a very small quantity dx. Thus, Eq. (3.5) reduces to $M_1=0$. This indicates no change in bending moment from the left to the right of the concentrated load in the beam segment.

Case 3: Beam segment subjected to a concentrated moment

The free body diagram of a beam element of infinitesimal length dx subjected to a concentrated moment M_o sliced out from a beam is shown in Fig. 3.10. As the element is subjected to a concentrated moment, the bending moment M changes by a finite value M_1 from the left to the right of the concentrated moment. Let us assume that the shear force also changes by a finite value V_1 from the left to the right of the concentrated moment over the length dx. In a similar way as in Cases 1 and 2, writing the vertical force equilibrium and moment equilibrium equations, one obtains the changes in shear force and bending moment as

$$V_1 = 0, \quad M_1 = -M_0. \tag{3.6}$$

Thus, it can be concluded that if a portion of the beam is subjected to only concentrated moment, there is no change in shear force, but there is a reduction in bending moment by a value equal to the applied concentrated moment as one moves from the left to the right section of the beam segment.

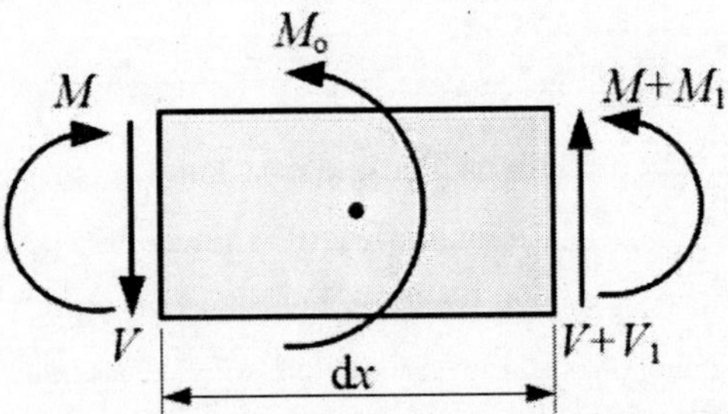

Fig. 3.10 Free body diagram of a beam element subjected to a concentrated moment

3.7 Shear Force and Bending Moment Diagram

The diagrams that describe the variation of shear force and bending moment acting at every cross-section of the beam along its length are called as shear force (SF) and bending moment (BM) diagrams. To construct the SF diagram, shear forces are plotted in ordinate against positional coordinate x along the length of the beam as abscissa. Similarly, the BM diagrams are constructed by plotting the bending moments in the ordinate as a function of the positional coordinate x along the length of the beam plotted in the abscissa. The abscissa and ordinate for constructing the SF and BM diagrams are shown in Fig. 3.11. The SF and BM diagrams serve as the basis for the initial design of beam structures as they provide the locations on the beam which are subjected to the maximum shear force and the maximum bending moment. This enables designers to evaluate the magnitudes of the maximum shear and bending stresses in the beam. Thus, appropriate measures for further strengthening the structure can be taken in its design stage to avoid failure.

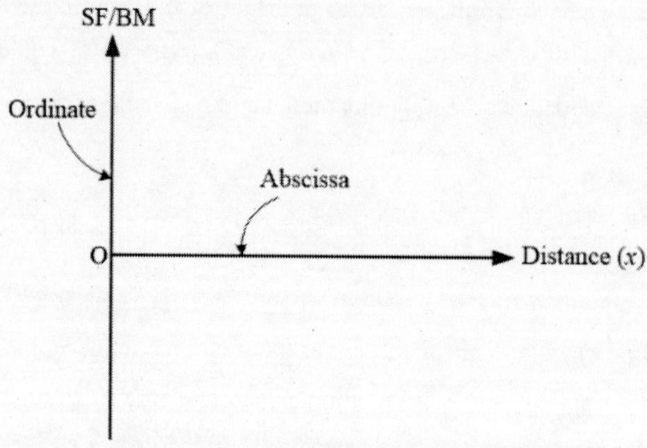

Fig. 3.11 Abscissa and ordinate for constructing the SF and BM diagrams

3.8 SF and BM Diagrams for Beams Subjected to Concentrated Loads Only

In this section, the procedure for the determination of shear force and bending moment at the cross-sections of different types of beams subjected to the simplest loading case, *i.e.*, concentrated load, is discussed. The values of shear force and bending moment are then plotted along the length of the beam to obtain the SF and BM diagrams. In the following subsections, the construction of SF and BM diagrams for statically determinate beams subjected to concentrated load is carried out.

3.8.1 SF and BM diagrams for simply supported beam carrying concentrated load

Let us consider a simply supported beam, as shown in Fig. 3.12 (a), subjected to a concentrated load P at distances of l_1 from the left support and l_2 from that of the right support. The free-body diagram of the beam is shown in Fig. 3.12 (b), attaching coordinate axes x-y. The reactions at the supports at A and B can be evaluated by using the equations of equilibrium. The force equilibrium equation in the x direction directly provides the horizontal reaction H_A=0 at the hinge support at A, as there is nothing to balance in that direction. By taking the moment of all the forces about point B and then writing the moment equilibrium equation, one obtains the vertical reaction R_A at A as

$$Pl_2 - R_A L = 0, \quad R_A = \frac{Pl_2}{L}. \tag{3.7}$$

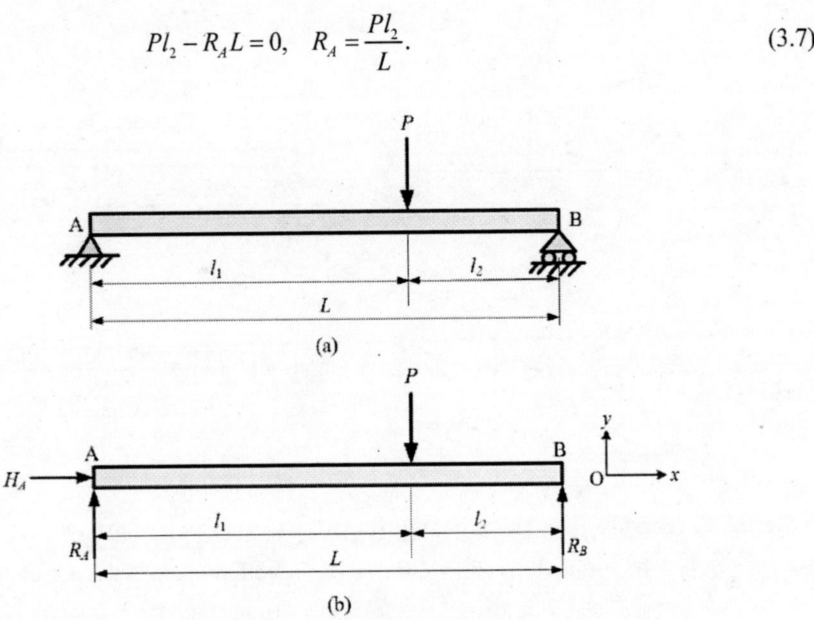

Fig. 3.12 A simply supported beam carrying a concentrated load: (a) schematic and (b) free body diagram

Using the equation of force equilibrium in the y direction and then substituting the value of R_A from Eq. (3.7), the vertical reaction R_B at the roller support at B as

$$R_A + R_B = P, \quad R_B = P - R_A, \quad R_B = P - \frac{Pl_2}{L},$$

$$R_B = \frac{P(L-l_2)}{L} = \frac{Pl_1}{L}. \tag{3.8}$$

To determine the shear force and bending moment in the beam portion to the left of the concentrated load P, *i.e.*, in the region $0 \leq x \leq l_1$, we take an imaginary cut in that region at a distance x from the left support. This reveals the shear force $V(x)$ and bending moment $M(x)$ at the cut section of the beam taken as positive, as shown in the free body diagram of the portion left to the cut section in Fig. 3.13 (a). Now, the force equilibrium equation in the y direction provides

$$V(x)+R_A=0, \qquad 0\leq x\leq l_1$$

$$V(x)=-R_A=-\frac{Pl_2}{L}. \tag{3.9}$$

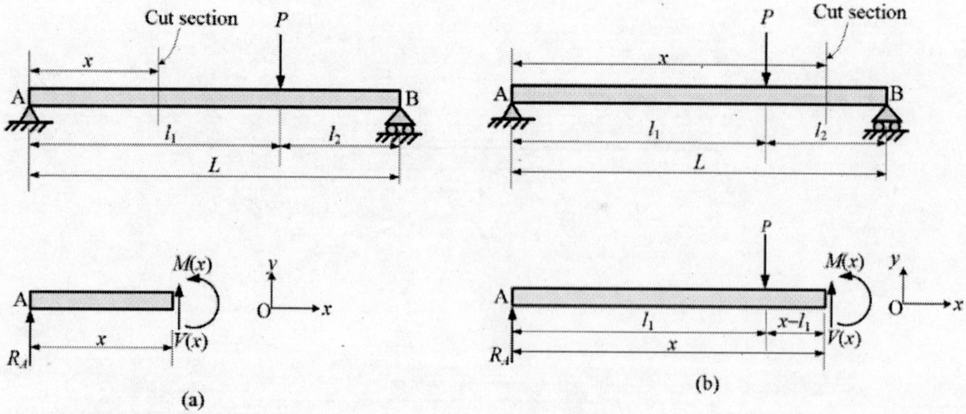

Fig. 3.13 Free body diagram of the beam portion (a) to the left of the cut section taken in the region $0 \leq x \leq l_1$ and (b) to the left of the cut section taken in the region $l_1 \leq x \leq L$.

Equation (3.9) indicates that the shear force in the beam portion to the left of the concentrated force P is constant and is negative. This means its direction should be reversed to that shown in the free body diagram (Fig. 3.13 (a)).

Taking the moment about the cut section and then writing the moment equilibrium equation, one obtains

$$M(x)-R_Ax=0, \qquad 0\leq x\leq l_1$$

$$M(x)=R_Ax=\frac{Pl_2}{L}x. \tag{3.10}$$

It can be inferred from Eq. (3.10) that the variation of bending moment in the region $0 \le x \le l_1$ is linear with the boundary values at x=0, M=0, and at x=l_1, $M = \frac{Pl_1 l_2}{L}$.

Let us now take an imaginary cut at a distance x from the left support in the region $l_1 \le x \le L$ to determine the shear force and bending moment in the beam sections to the right of the concentrated load P. The free-body diagram of the beam portion to the left of the cut section with the shear force $V(x)$ and bending moment $M(x)$ is shown in Fig. 3.13 (b). Writing the force equilibrium equation in the y direction, one obtains the shear force to the right of the concentrated load P as

$$V(x) + R_A - P = 0, \qquad l_1 \le x \le L$$

$$V(x) = P - R_A = P - \frac{Pl_2}{L} = \frac{Pl_1}{L}, \tag{3.11}$$

which shows that the shear force is constant in the region $l_1 \le x \le L$. The moment equilibrium equation about the cut section provides

$$M(x) + P(x - l_1) - R_A x = 0, \qquad l_1 \le x \le L$$

$$M(x) = R_A x - P(x - l_1) = \frac{Pl_2}{L} x - P(x - l_1),$$

$$M(x) = \frac{Pl_1(L - x)}{L}. \tag{3.12}$$

Thus, the bending moment in the region $l_1 \le x \le L$ also varies linearly with the boundary values at x=l_1, $M = \frac{Pl_1 l_2}{L}$ and at x=L, M=0.

The values of the shear forces provided by Eqs. (3.9) and (3.11) to the left and to the right of the concentrated load P, respectively, are plotted in Fig. 3.14 (a) as a function of x measured along the length of the beam to obtain the shear force variation over its entire span. The resulting plot is the SF diagram for the present case. On plotting the bending moment values as a function of x provided by Eqs. (3.10) and (3.12), one obtains the bending moment diagram with the maximum value $M = \frac{Pl_1 l_2}{L}$ occurring at x=l_1 as shown in Fig. 3.14 (b).

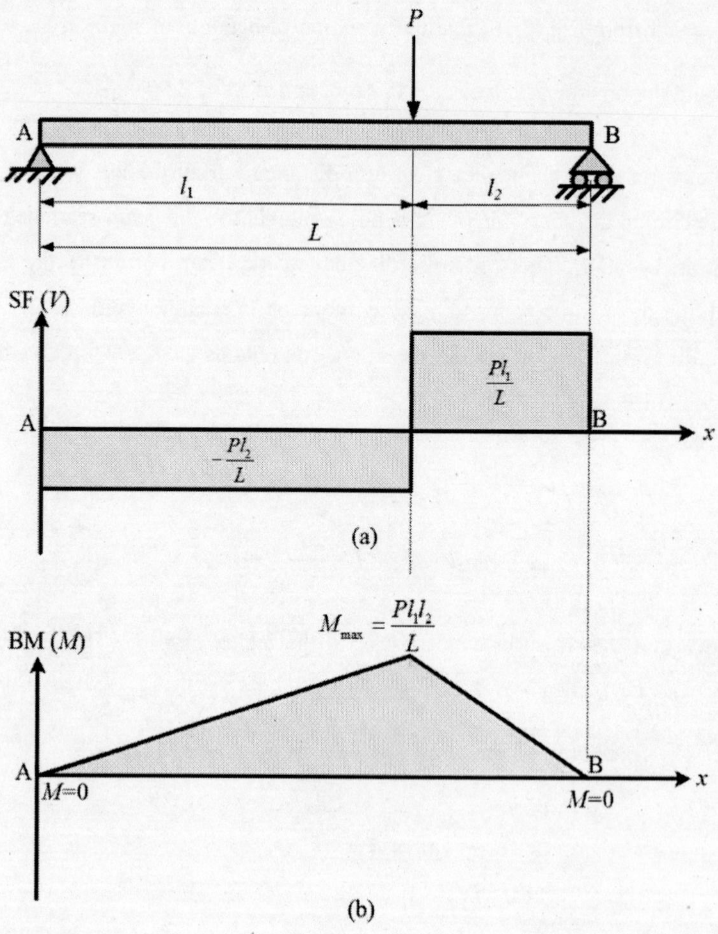

Fig. 3.14 A simply supported beam carrying a concentrated load:

(a) schematic and shear force diagram and (b) bending moment diagram

3.8.2 SF and BM diagrams for cantilever beam carrying a concentrated load

Consider a cantilever beam AB of length L subjected to a concentrated load at its free end B, as shown in Fig. 3.15 (a). The free-body diagram of the beam is drawn in Fig. 3.15 (b). To construct the SF and BM diagram, the first step is to determine the support reactions R_A, H_A, and M_A at point A. Writing the equations of force equilibrium along the axis of the beam *viz.*, the x direction, transverse to its axis *viz.*, in the y direction, and equation of moment balance about point A, the support reactions are obtained as

$$H_A = 0, \quad R_A = P, \quad M_A = -PL. \tag{3.13}$$

The negative sign for the moment reaction M_A indicates that its direction should be reversed to that considered in drawing the free body diagram.

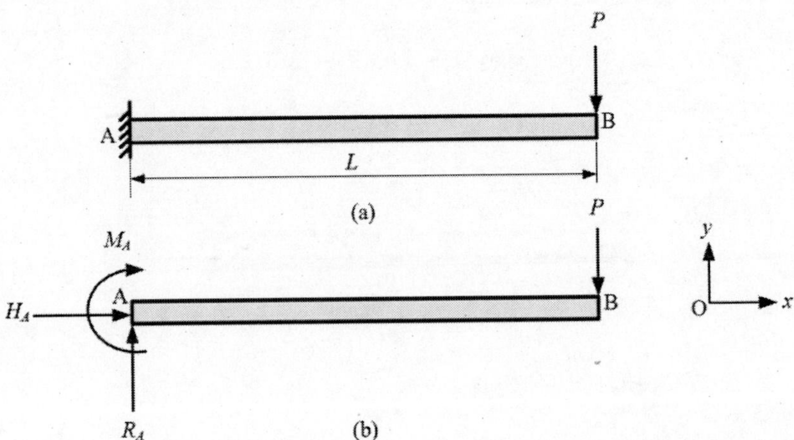

Fig. 3.15 A cantilever beam carrying a concentrated load: (a) schematic and (b) free body diagram

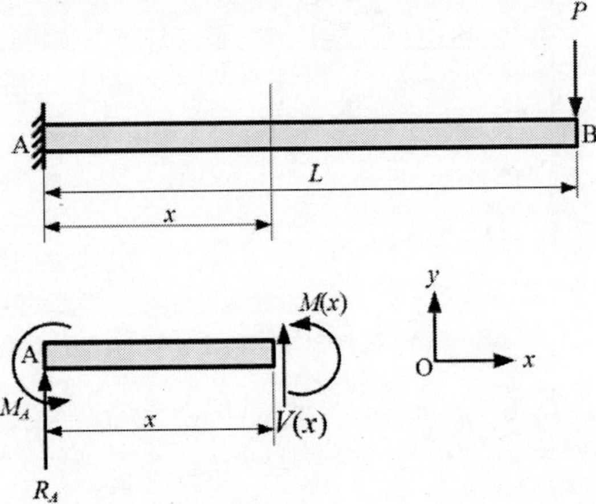

Fig. 3.16 Free body diagram of the beam portion to the left of the cut section.

Now, to obtain the shear force and bending moment as a function of length, an imaginary cut section is passed across the beam cross-section at a distance x from the fixed end A as shown in Fig. 3.16. A free-body diagram of the beam segment left to the cut section is drawn showing the shear force $V(x)$ and bending moment $M(x)$ at the cut section taken in the positive sense. Using force equilibrium equation in the y direction, the shear force function is obtained as

$$V(x) = -P, \tag{3.14}$$

which is constant in the region to the left of the concentrated load P at the free end, *i.e.*, over the entire beam span. The moment equilibrium equation written about the cut section provides the bending moment function as

$$M(x) = Px - PL. \tag{3.15}$$

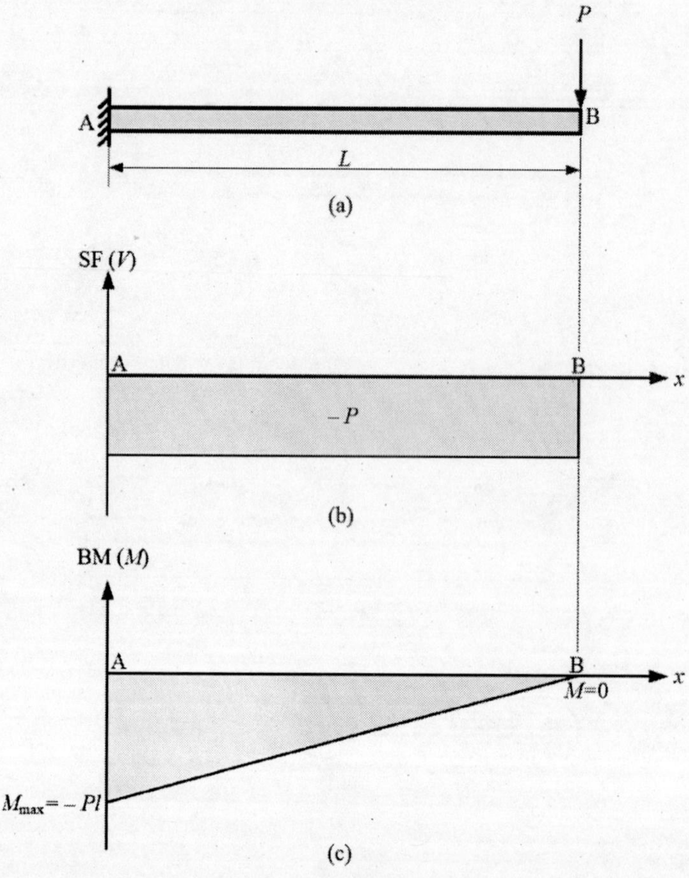

Fig. 3.17 (a) Shear force and (b) bending moment diagrams for cantilever beam carrying a concentrated load at the free end.

According to Eq. (3.15), the bending moment M over the entire span varies linearly from $M = -PL$ at the fixed end A at x=0 to M =0 at the free end B at x=L. The variation of shear force and bending moment given by Eqs. (3.14) and (3.15) are plotted against the beam length taken along the x-axis to obtain the SF and BM diagrams, as shown in Figs. 3.17 (a) and (b), respectively. It is observed that the maximum value of bending moment occurs at the fixed end A, and its value is $M_{max} = -PL$.

3.8.3 SF and BM diagrams for overhanging beam carrying a concentrated load

An overhanging beam is constructed by extending a span of l_2 from the roller support at point B of a simply supported beam of span l_1 as shown in Fig. 3.18 (a). The length of the overhanging beam AC is taken as L subjected to only a concentrated load at point C in the overhang portion. The free-body diagram of the beam showing the support reactions at A and B is shown in Fig. 3.18 (b). Writing the force equilibrium equations in the x and y directions and the moment equilibrium equation (moments evaluated about the point A), the support reactions at points A and B are obtained as

$$H_A = 0, \quad R_A = -\frac{Pl_2}{l_1}, \quad R_B = \frac{PL}{l_1}. \tag{3.16}$$

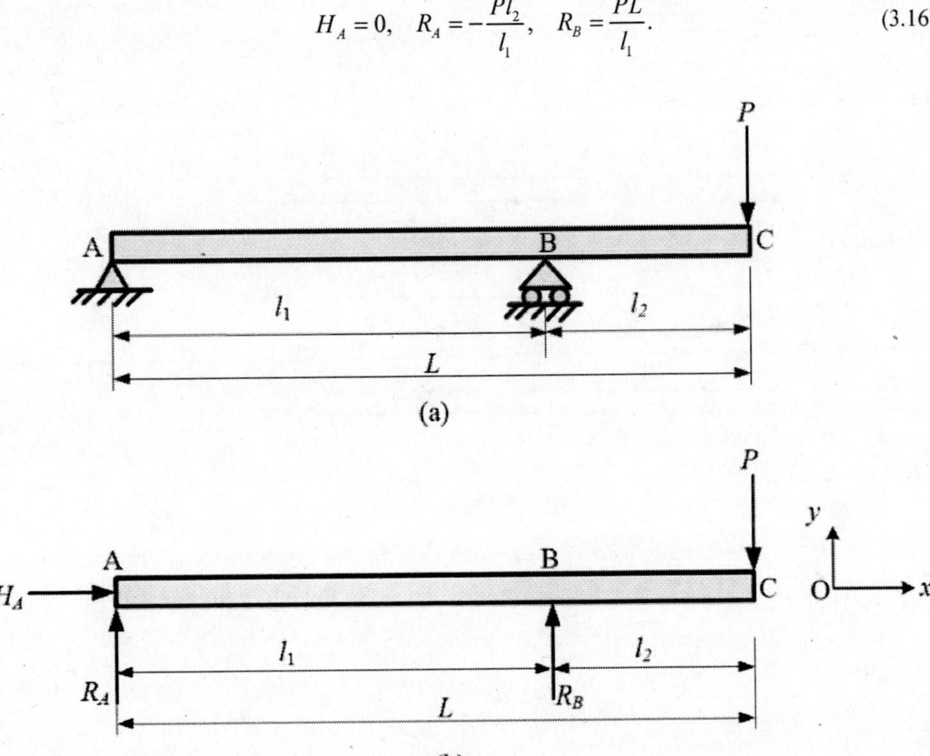

Fig. 3.18 An overhanging beam carrying a concentrated load: (a) schematic and (b) free body diagram

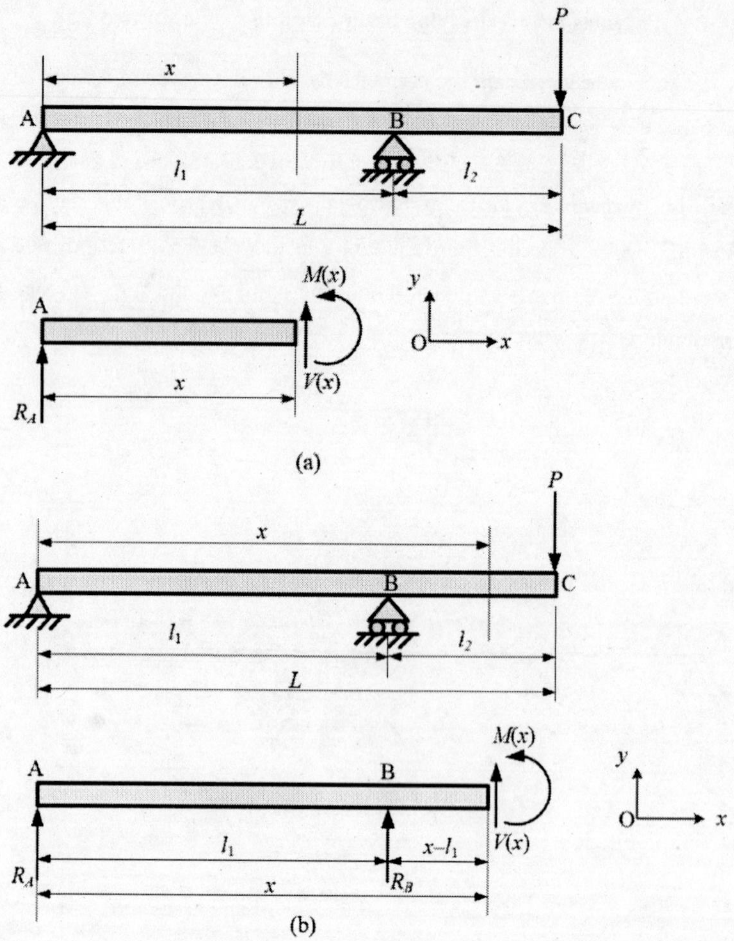

Fig. 3.19 Free body diagram of the beam portion (a) to the left of the cut section taken in between the supports at A and B and (b) to the left of the cut section taken in the overhang portion.

To determine the shear force and bending moment function in the segment AB between the two supports, an imaginary cut section is passed through the beam cross-section in that segment at a distance x from the left end A as shown in Fig. 3.19 (a). The corresponding free-body diagram of the beam portion to the left of the cut section is also shown in Fig. 3.19 (a), revealing the shear force $V(x)$ and bending moment $M(x)$ at the cut section. Using the equations of force equilibrium in the y direction and moment equilibrium equation evaluating moment about the cut section, one obtains the shear force and bending moment function in the region $0 \leq x \leq l_1$ as

$$V(x) = \frac{Pl_2}{l_1}, \qquad 0 \le x \le l_1 \tag{3.17}$$

$$M(x) = -\frac{Pl_2}{l_1}x. \qquad 0 \le x \le l_1 \tag{3.18}$$

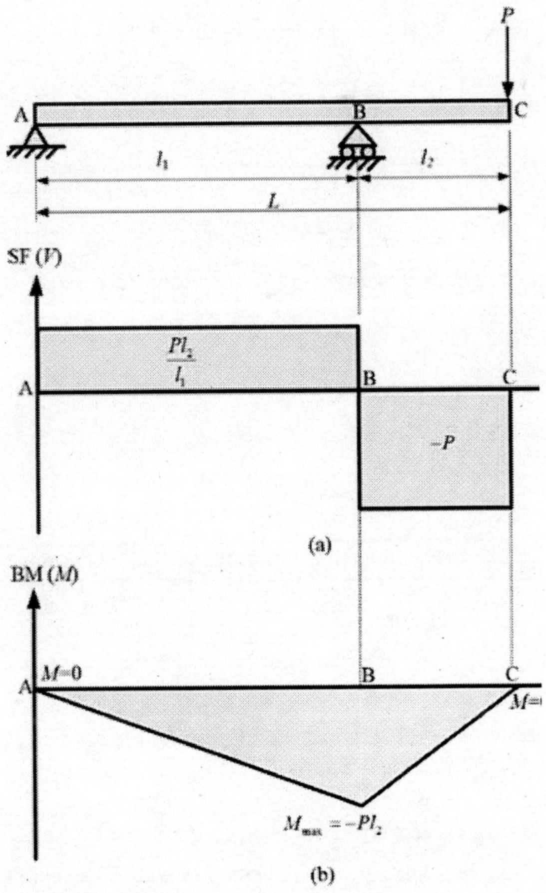

Fig. 3.20 An overhanging beam carrying a concentrated load in the overhang portion: (a) schematic and shear force diagram and (b) bending moment diagram

The shear force and bending moment function in segment BC can be obtained by considering an imaginary cut in that segment at a distance x from the end A, as depicted in Fig. 3.19 (b), along with the free body diagram of the portion left to the cut section. Similarly, writing the force and moment equilibrium equations, the shear force and bending moment functions for the region just to the right of the support at B, *i.e.*, $l_1 \le x \le L$ are obtained as

$$V(x) = -P, \qquad l_1 \le x \le L \tag{3.19}$$

$$M(x) = Px - PL. \qquad l_1 \le x \le L \tag{3.20}$$

Now, from Eqs. (3.17) and (3.19), it is seen that the shear force in the segments AB and BC are constants that change suddenly from $\frac{Pl_2}{l_1}$ at point B in segment AB to $-P$ at point B in segment BC. This variation of shear force along the length of the beam is shown in Fig. 3.20 (a) to obtain the SF diagram for the present case. The bending moment functions given by Eqs. (3.18) and (3.20) show that the bending moment varies linearly from M=0 at x=0 at point A to M= $-Pl_2$ at x=l_1 at point B in the segment AB and from M= $-Pl_2$ at x=l_1 at B to M=0 at x=L at point C in the segment BC. This variation of bending moment over the beam span is plotted as a function of its length to obtain the BM diagram, as shown in Fig. 3.20 (b).

Example 3.1 Draw the shear force and bending moment diagram for the beam shown in the following figure.

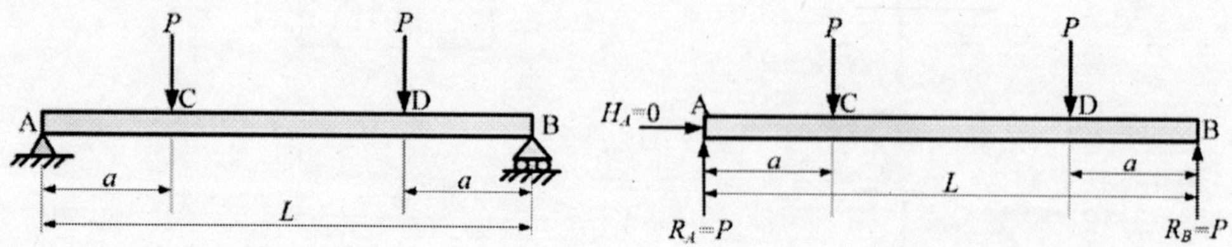

Free body diagram of the beam

Solution

Support reactions: The support reactions are at points A and B are determined using the equations of equilibrium as H_A=0, R_A=R_B=P, which are shown in the free body diagram of the beam.

Shear force and bending moment functions: The shear force and bending moment functions in different segments of the beam are evaluated by taking an imaginary cut in the segment of interest at a distance x from the left end and then drawing the free body diagrams of the portion left to each cut section as follows:

For the segment AC ($0 \le x \le a$):

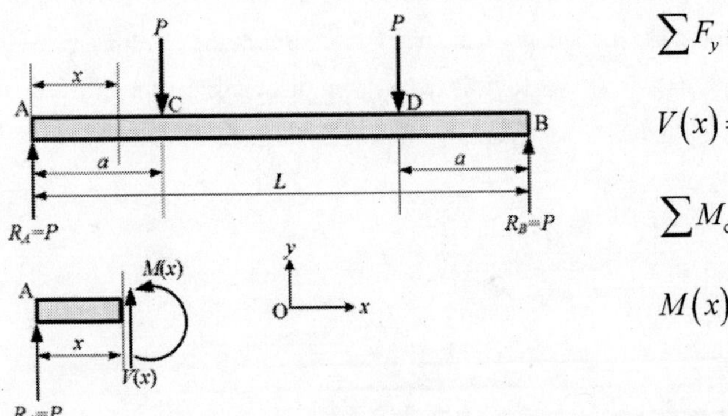

$$\sum F_y = 0,\ V(x) + R_A = 0,$$

$$V(x) = -P. \tag{i}$$

$$\sum M_{\text{cut section}} = 0,\ M(x) - R_A x = 0,$$

$$M(x) = Px. \tag{ii}$$

For the segment CD ($a \le x \le L-a$):

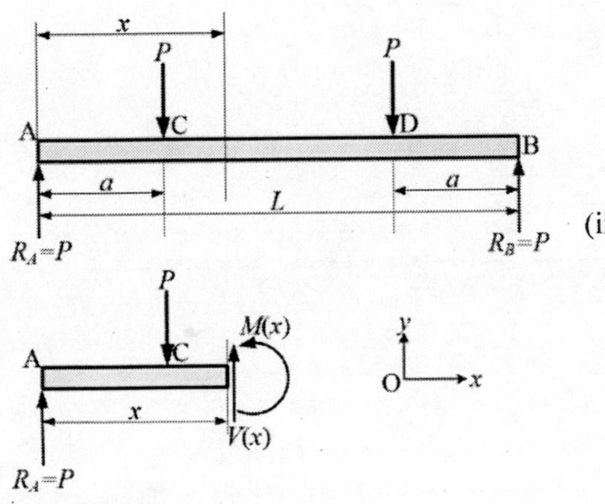

$$\sum F_y = 0,\ V(x) + R_A - P = 0,$$

$$V(x) = 0. \tag{iii}$$

$$\sum M_{\text{cut section}} = 0,$$

$$M(x) + P(x-a) - R_A x = 0,$$

$$M(x) = Pa. \tag{iv}$$

For the segment DB ($L-a \le x \le L$):

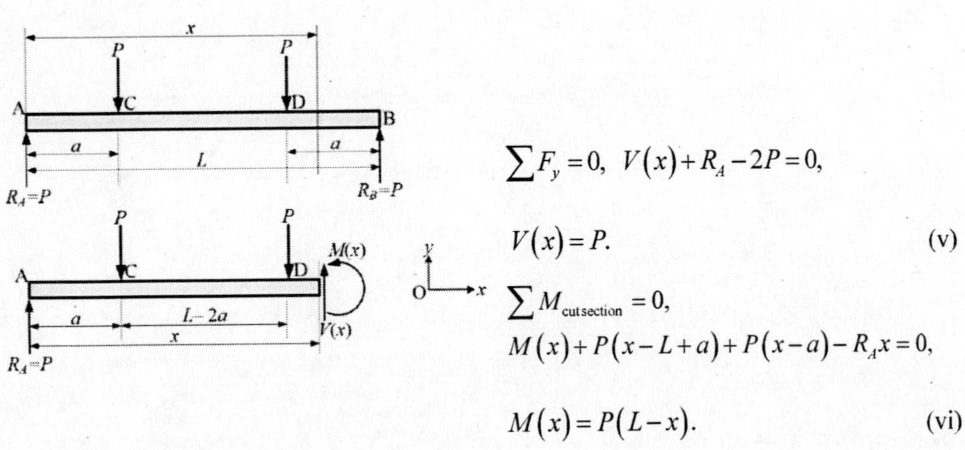

$$\sum F_y = 0,\ V(x) + R_A - 2P = 0,$$

$$V(x) = P. \tag{v}$$

$$\sum M_{\text{cut section}} = 0,$$

$$M(x) + P(x - L + a) + P(x-a) - R_A x = 0,$$

$$M(x) = P(L-x). \tag{vi}$$

S.F. and B.M. diagrams: Using Eqs. (i), (iii), and (v), the shear force variation along the length of the beam is plotted to obtain the shear force diagram. Equations (ii), (iv), and (vi) are used to plot the variation of bending moment along the length of the beam to construct the resulting bending moment diagram, as shown in the following figure. It is to be noted that the shear force is zero in segment CD, and thus, the bending moment is constant in this segment. This verifies Eq. (3.3).

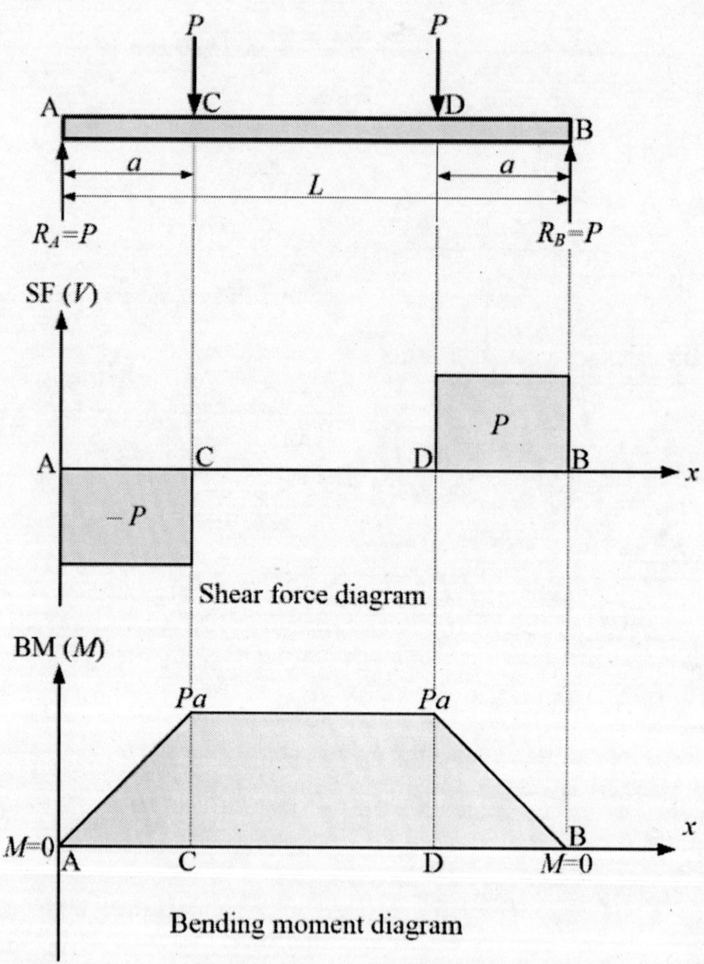

3.9 SF and BM Diagrams for Beams Subjected to Uniformly Distributed Load

In this section, the shear force and bending moment diagrams will be constructed for a beam subjected to uniformly distributed load following the same procedure as discussed in Section 3.8. The beam may be subjected to uniformly distributed load over the entire span or over a certain part. As an example, let us consider a simply supported beam AB subjected to a uniformly distributed load of intensity q over the entire span L, as shown in Fig. 3.21 (a).

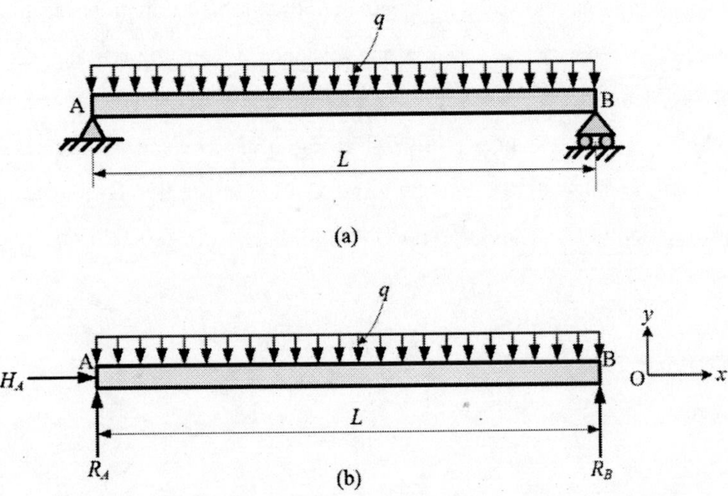

Fig. 3.21 A simply supported beam subjected to uniformly distributed load over the entire span and: (a) schematic and (b) free body diagram

First, it is required to determine the support reactions at points of support at A and B. A free-body diagram of the beam is drawn showing the support reactions H_A and R_A at point A and R_B at point B, as shown in Fig. 3.21 (b). Due to the force equilibrium in the x direction H_A vanishes straightway. The solution of the force equilibrium equation in the y direction and the moment equilibrium equation written taking the moments about point A, the support reactions R_A and R_B are obtained as

$$R_A = R_B = \frac{qL}{2}. \tag{3.21}$$

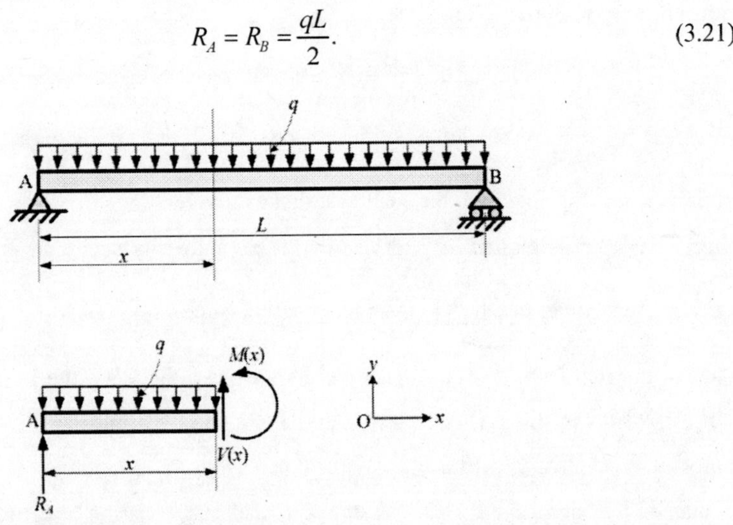

Fig. 3.22 Free body diagram of the cantilever beam portion carrying uniformly distributed load to the left of the cut section.

Now, to formulate the shear force and bending moment functions, an imaginary cut is passed through the beam cross-section at any distance x from the left support. A free-body diagram of the beam segment left to the cut section is drawn containing the uniformly distributed load q over the span x, as shown in Fig. 3.22. The shear force $V(x)$ and bending moment $M(x)$ at the cut section are taken to be positive in the free body diagram. The force equilibrium equation in the y direction provides the shear force function for the entire span of the beam as

$$V(x) - qx + R_A = 0,$$

$$V(x) = qx - \frac{qL}{2}. \tag{3.22}$$

Taking the moments about the cut section, the moment equilibrium equation takes the following form:

$$M(x) + qx\frac{x}{2} - R_A x = 0,$$

$$M(x) = -q\frac{x^2}{2} + \frac{qLx}{2}. \tag{3.23}$$

Equation (3.23) represents the bending moment function at any cross-section considered in the entire span of the beam.

The shear force function given by Eq. (3.22) reveals that the shear force varies linearly with x from $V = -\frac{qL}{2}$ at the left support at x=0 to $V = \frac{qL}{2}$ at the right support at $x= L$. This observation is in line with the load and shear force relationship given by Eq. (3.1). The shear force variation is plotted in Fig. 3.23 (a). It can be easily seen that the maximum magnitude of the shear force, *i.e.*, $|V_{\max}| = \frac{qL}{2}$ occurs at the support points with a change in sign from the left to the right support. The shear force vanishes in between the left and right support. The location of vanishing shear force can be obtained by putting V=0 in Eq. (3.22), which provides x=L/2, *i.e.*, at the mid-span of the beam. The bending moment variation can be obtained by using Eq. (3.23). This shows a quadratic variation of M with x. At x=0, *i.e.*, at the left support, and at x=L, *i.e.*, at the right support, Eq. (3.23) provides M=0. At the mid-span, *i.e.*, at $x=L/2$, Eq. (3.23) provides the value of the bending moment as $M=\frac{qL^2}{8}$. It can be easily verified by equating the first derivative of the bending moment evaluated from Eq. (3.22) to .zero and then conducting a second derivative test that the bending moment occurring at $x=L/2$ is the maximum. It is worth noting that the maximum bending moment occurs at the location where the shear force is zero. This observation is consistent with Eq. (3.3). A bending moment diagram for the present case can be constructed, as shown in Fig. 3.23 (b). It is seen that the distribution of bending moment along the length of the beam is parabolic in nature.

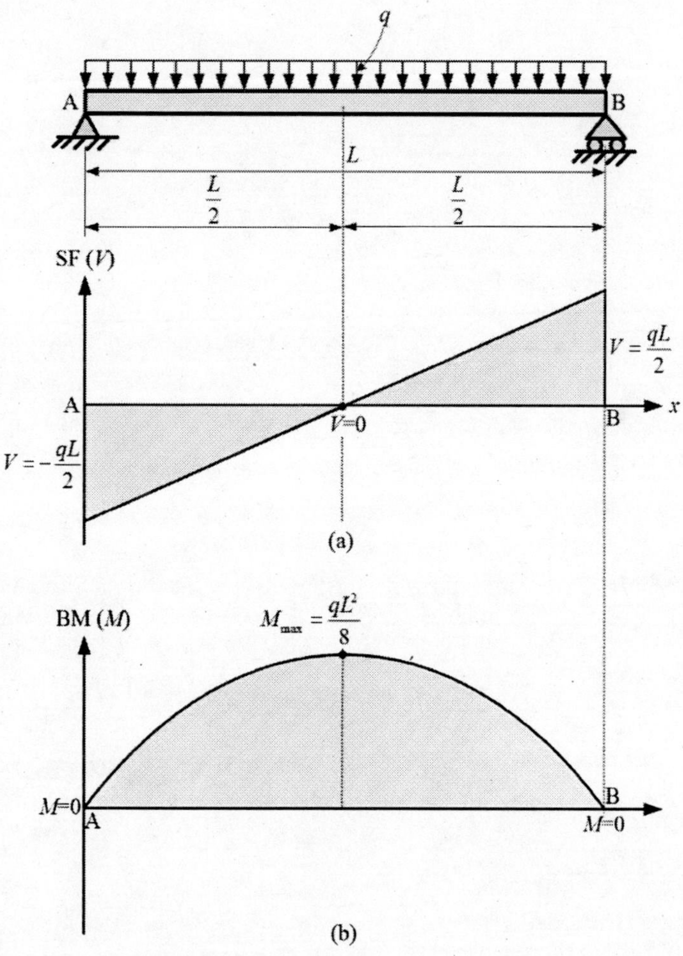

Fig. 3.23 A simply supported beam carrying uniformly distributed load over the entire span: (a) schematic and shear force diagram and (b) bending moment diagram

Example 3.2 Draw the shear force and bending moment diagrams for a cantilever beam subjected to a uniformly distributed load over the entire span. Also, locate the position of the maximum bending moment.

Solution

A cantilever beam fixed at the left end A subjected to a uniformly distributed load of intensity q over the span L is shown along with its free body diagram in the following figure.

Support reactions: The support reactions at point A are determined using the equations of static equilibrium as H_A=0, R_A=qL and $M_A = -\frac{qL^2}{2}$.

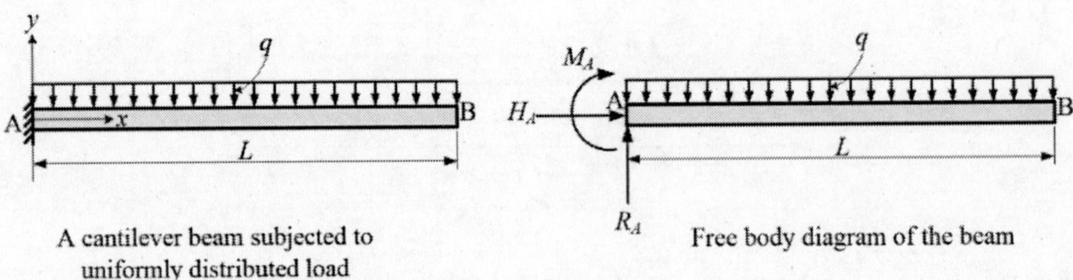

A cantilever beam subjected to uniformly distributed load

Free body diagram of the beam

Shear force and bending moment functions: To obtain the shear force and bending moment functions, let us pass an imaginary cut across the beam cross section at any distance x from the fixed end. A free body diagram of the portion left to the cut section is drawn and the equations of equilibrium are written to arrive at the shear force and bending moment functions as follows:

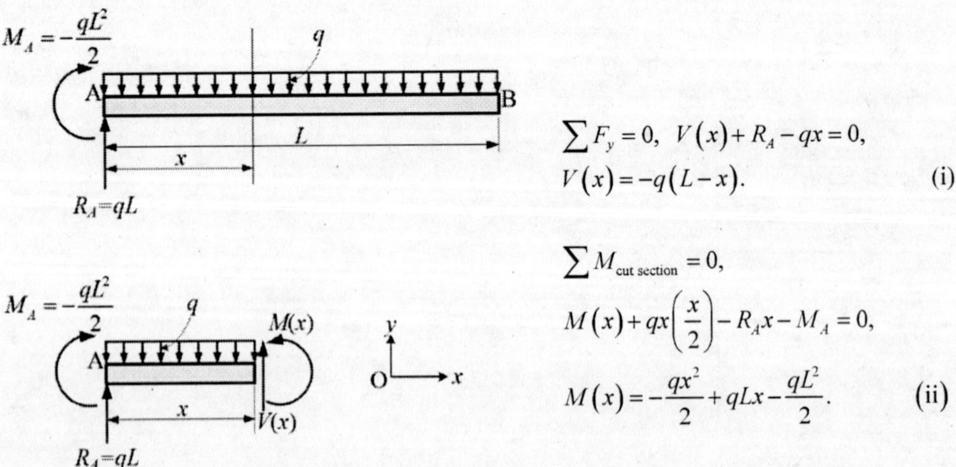

$$\sum F_y = 0,\ V(x) + R_A - qx = 0,$$

$$V(x) = -q(L-x). \tag{i}$$

$$\sum M_{\text{cut section}} = 0,$$

$$M(x) + qx\left(\frac{x}{2}\right) - R_A x - M_A = 0,$$

$$M(x) = -\frac{qx^2}{2} + qLx - \frac{qL^2}{2}. \tag{ii}$$

Now, using Eqs. (i) and (ii), the shear force and bending moments at any location along the length of the beam can be determined. Equation (i) provides a linear variation of shear force with $V=-qL$ at $x=0$ and $V=0$ at $x=L$. The bending moment variation is parabolic according to Eq. (ii) with $M=-\frac{qL^2}{2}$ at $x=0$ and $M=0$ at $x=L$. The shear force and bending moment diagram for the present case is constructed in the following figure.

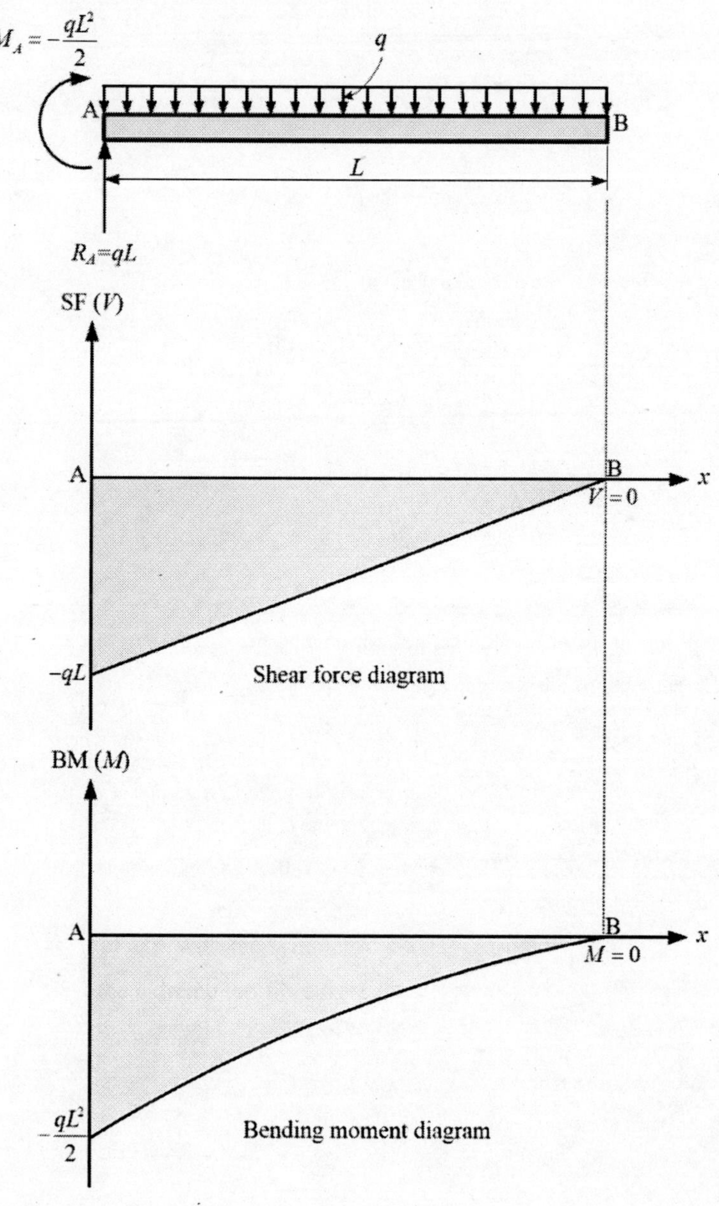

From the bending moment diagram, it is observed that the maximum bending moment occurs at the fixed end A, and its magnitude is $|M_{max}| = \dfrac{qL^2}{2}$.

Example 3.3 Draw the shear force and bending moment diagram for the beam shown in the following figure and locate the position of the maximum bending moment.

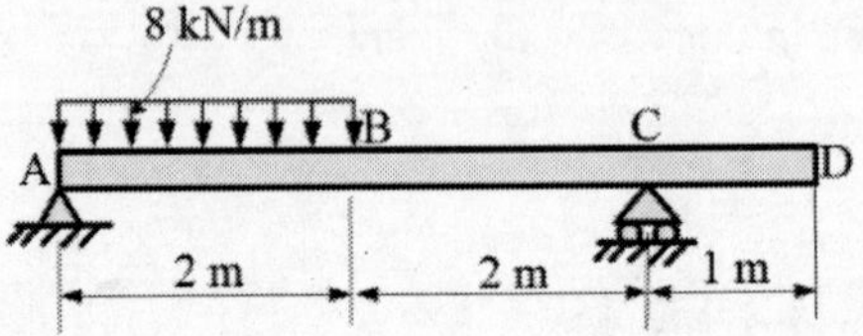

Solution

Support reactions: The support reactions in the given beam at points A and C are evaluated as H_A=0, R_A=12 kN, and R_C=4 kN considering the static equilibrium of the entire beam. The support reactions are shown in the free-body diagram of the beam.

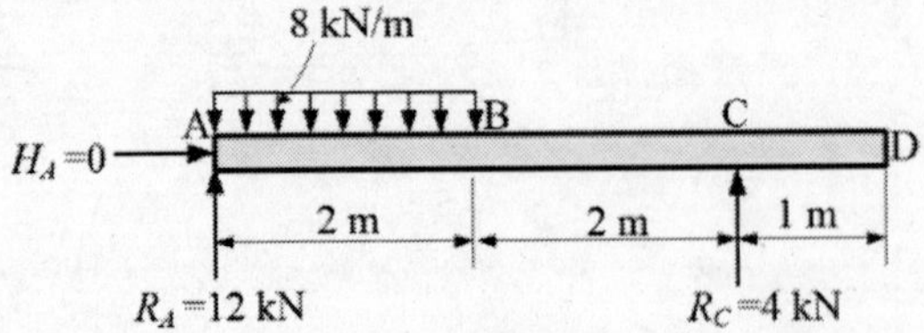

Free body diagram of the beam

Shear force and bending moment functions: The shear force and bending moment functions for the different segments of the beam are obtained considering the equilibrium of the beam portions left to an imaginary cut section considered in each segment.

Segment AB (0≤x≤2):

$$\sum F_y = 0,\ V(x) + 12 - 8x = 0,$$

$$V(x) = 8x - 12. \qquad \text{(i)}$$

$$\sum M_{\text{cut section}} = 0,\ M(x) + 8x\left(\frac{x}{2}\right) - 12x = 0,$$

$$M(x) = -4x^2 + 12x. \qquad \text{(ii)}$$

Segment BC ($2 \le x \le 4$):

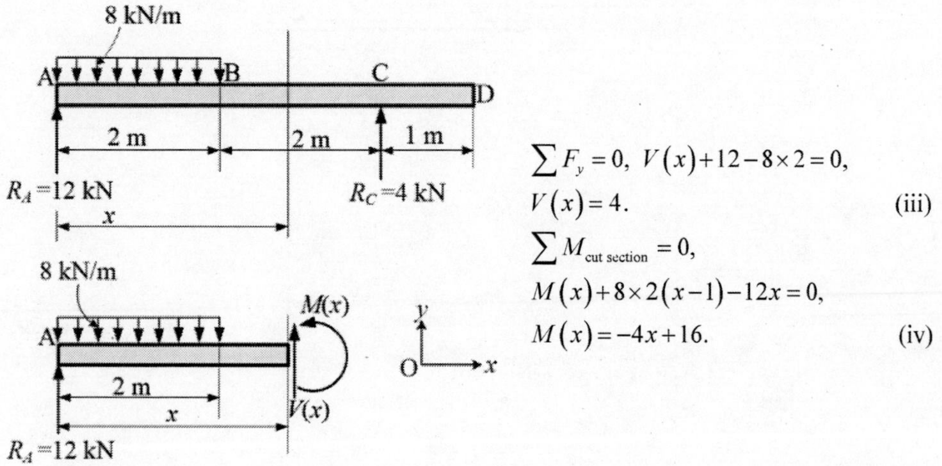

$$\sum F_y = 0,\ V(x) + 12 - 8 \times 2 = 0,$$
$$V(x) = 4. \qquad \text{(iii)}$$
$$\sum M_{\text{cut section}} = 0,$$
$$M(x) + 8 \times 2(x-1) - 12x = 0,$$
$$M(x) = -4x + 16. \qquad \text{(iv)}$$

Segment CD ($4 \le x \le 5$):

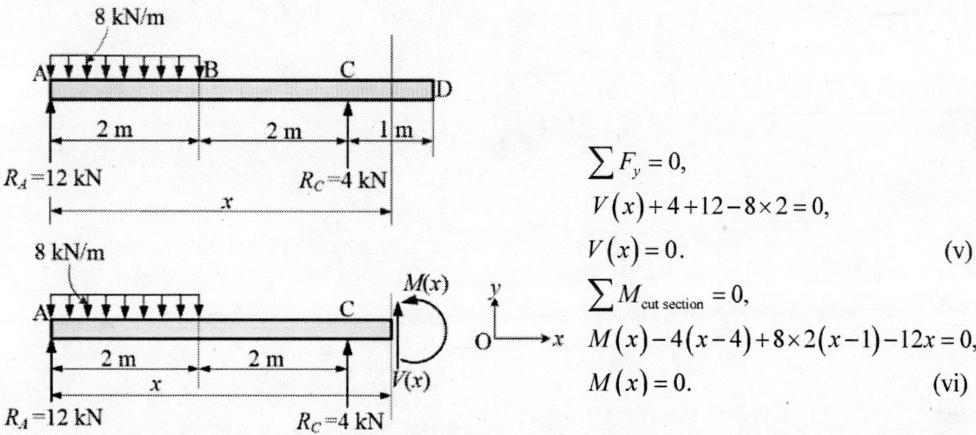

$$\sum F_y = 0,$$
$$V(x) + 4 + 12 - 8 \times 2 = 0,$$
$$V(x) = 0. \qquad \text{(v)}$$
$$\sum M_{\text{cut section}} = 0,$$
$$M(x) - 4(x-4) + 8 \times 2(x-1) - 12x = 0,$$
$$M(x) = 0. \qquad \text{(vi)}$$

Shear force and bending moment diagrams: Using Eqs. (i), (iii), and (v), the shear force diagram is constructed. In segment AB, the shear force varies linearly from $V = -12$ kN at $x=0$ to $V=4$ kN at $x=2$ m. In segment BC, the shear force has a constant value equal to 4 kN and in segment CD, the shear force is zero. The bending moment diagram is constructed using Es. (ii), (iv), and (vi). The bending moment varies in a parabolic manner in the segment AB with $M=0$ at $x=0$, $M=5$ kNm at $x=0.5$ m, and $M=8$ kNm at $x=2$ m. The bending moment varies linearly from point B with $M=8$ kNm to vanish at point C. The bending moment is zero in the segment CD.

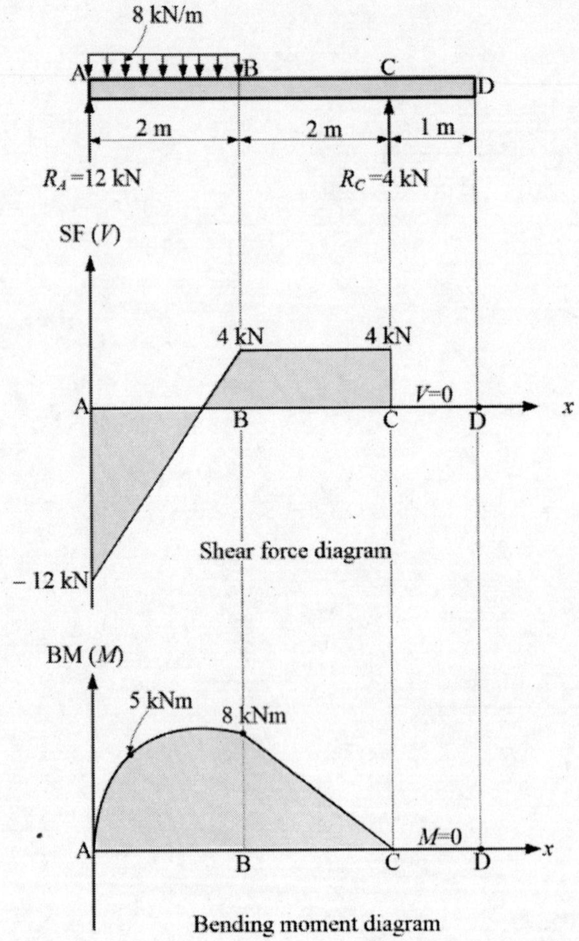

3.10 SF and BM Diagrams for Beams Subjected to Combined Concentrated and Uniformly Distributed Loads

To demonstrate the SF and BM diagrams for beams subjected to combined concentrated and uniformly distributed loads, let us consider the example of an overhanging beam, as shown in Fig. 3.24 (a). The beam is supported at points A and C by a hinge and a roller, respectively. The span between the supports is subjected to a uniformly distributed load of intensity 5 kN/m. At a distance of 2 m from the left support at point B and at the end D of the overhang portion CD, the beam is loaded with concentrated loads 10 kN and 20 kN, respectively. The free-body diagram of the beam is shown in Fig. 3.24 (b).

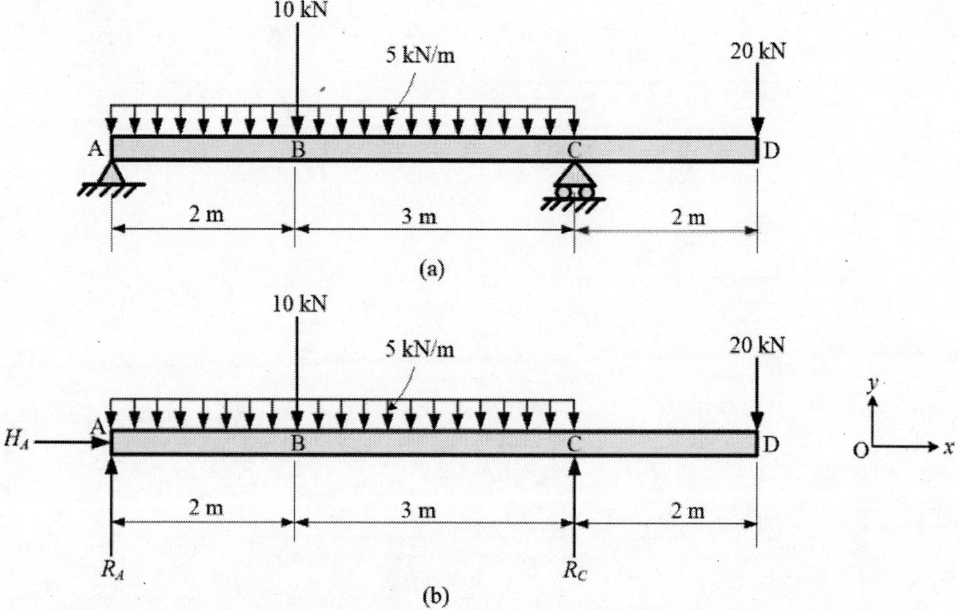

Fig. 3.24 An overhanging beam subjected to simultaneous action of concentrated and uniformly distributed loads: (a) schematic and (b) free body diagram

Using the equations of static equilibrium, the support reactions at points A and C are calculated as H_A=0, R_A=10.5 kN, and R_C =44.5 kN. The shear forces and bending moments in the beam are now calculated by taking imaginary cuts in the segments AB, BC and CD, respectively and then constructing the free body diagrams of the portions left to the cut sections as shown in Figs. 3.25 (a), (b), and (c).

Referring to the free body diagram of Fig. 3.25 (a), the vertical force equilibrium and the moment equilibrium about the cut section provides the shear force and bending moment function in the region AB ($0 \le x \le 2$) as

$$\sum F_y = 0, \quad V(x) - 5x + R_A = 0,$$

$$V(x) = 5x - 10.5, \tag{3.24}$$

$$\sum M = 0, \quad M(x) + 5x\left(\frac{x}{2}\right) - R_A x = 0,$$

$$M(x) = -2.5x^2 + 10.5x. \tag{3.25}$$

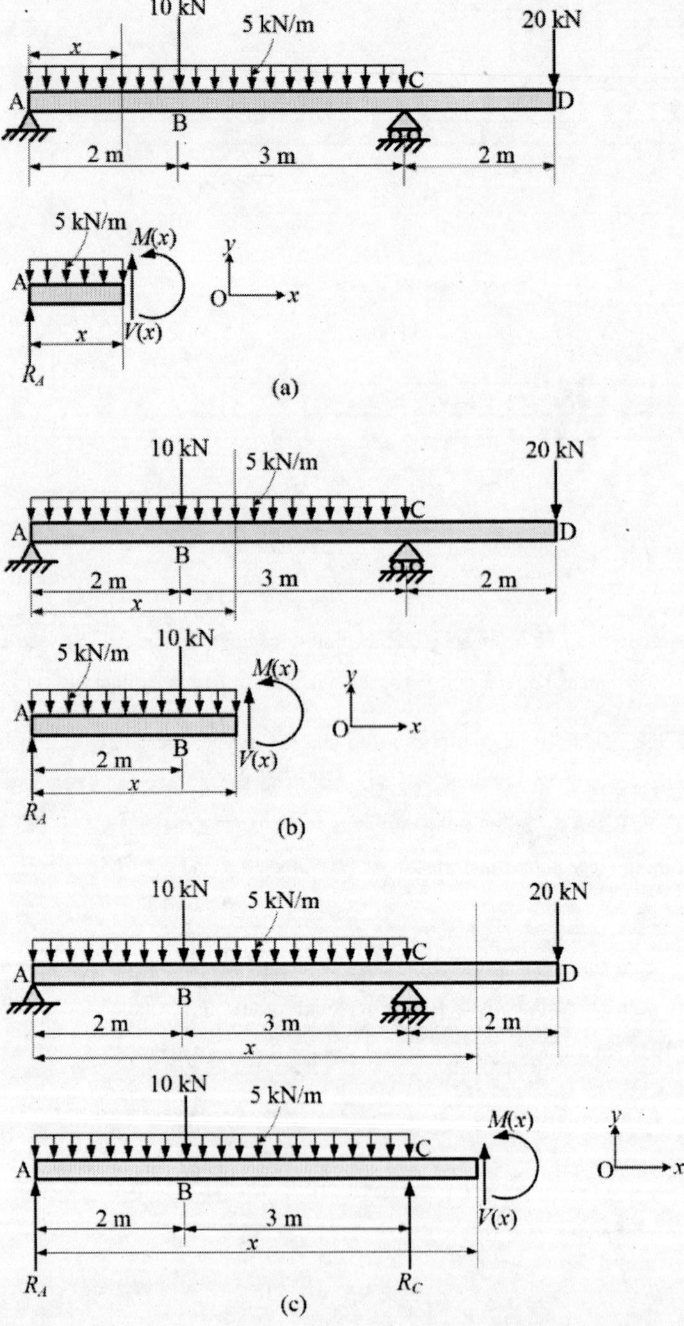

Fig. 3.25 Free body diagrams of the beam portion to the left of the cut section taken in the segments (a) AB, (b) BC and (d) CD.

It is clear from Eq. (3.24) that in the region $0 \le x \le 2$, the shear force varies linearly with x from $V = -10.5$ kN at $x=0$ to $V = -0.5$ kN at $x=2$ m (just to the left of the concentrated load 10 kN). Equation (3.25) shows that the bending moment in the region $0 \le x \le 2$ varies as a quadratic function of x (in a parabolic manner) with the boundary values $M=0$ at $x=0$ and $M=11$ kNm at $x=2$ m.

Similarly, referring to the free body diagrams of Figs. 3.25 (b) and (c), the shear force and bending moment functions in the regions BC ($2 \le x \le 5$) and CD ($5 \le x \le 7$), respectively, are obtained as follows:

In the region BC ($2 \le x \le 5$):

$$\sum F_y = 0, \quad V(x) - 5x - 10 + R_A = 0,$$

$$V(x) = 5x - 0.5, \tag{3.26}$$

$$\sum M = 0, \quad M(x) + 10(x-2) + 5x\left(\frac{x}{2}\right) - R_A x = 0,$$

$$M(x) = -2.5x^2 + 0.5x + 20. \tag{3.27}$$

In the region CD ($5 \le x \le 7$):

$$\sum F_y = 0, \quad V(x) + R_C - 10 - 5\times5 + R_A = 0,$$

$$V(x) = -20, \tag{3.28}$$

$$\sum M = 0, \quad M(x) - R_C(x-5) + 5\times5(x-2.5) + 10(x-2) - R_A x = 0,$$

$$M(x) = 20x - 140. \tag{3.29}$$

In the region BC ($2 \le x \le 5$), the shear force and bending moment variation with x is similar to the region AB ($0 \le x \le 2$). Equation (3.26) provides that the shear force varies from $V=9.5$ kN at $x=2$ m to $V=24.5$ kN at $x=5$ m. The bending moment varies from $M=11$ kNm at $x=2$ m to $M=-40$ kNm at $x=5$ m, according to Eq. (3.27). Further, Eq. (3.28) shows that in the region CD at $x=5$ m to $x=7$ m, the shear force has a constant value equal to -20 kN. According to Eq. (3.29), the bending moment in this region varies linearly with x from $M=-40$ kNm at $x=5$ m to $M=0$ at $x=7$ m. The variations of shear force and bending moment, as discussed above, given by Eqs. (3.24) – (3.29) are plotted in Fig. 3.26 to obtain the shear force and bending moment diagrams. It is observed that the magnitude of the maximum bending moment occurs at point C, which is $|M_{max}| = 40\,\text{kNm}$.

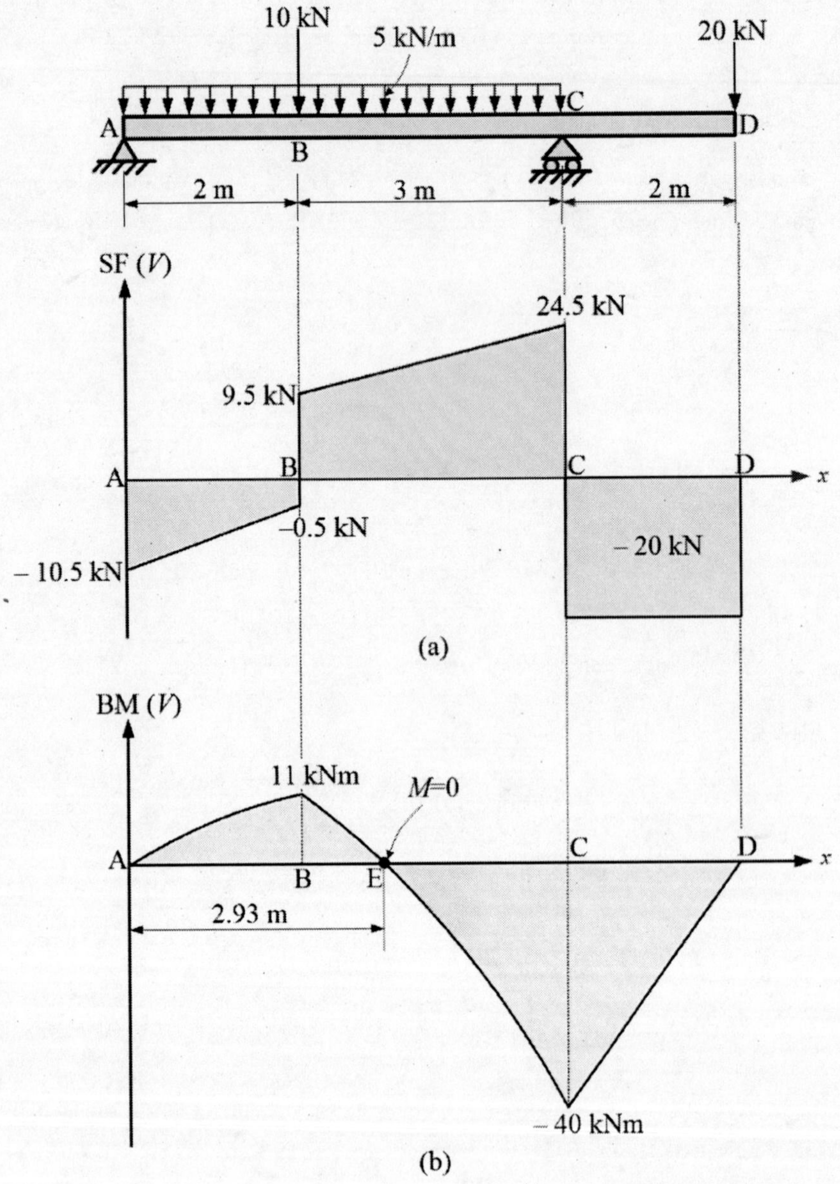

Fig. 3.26 An overhanging beam subjected to combined concentrated and distributed loads:

(a) schematic and shear force and (b) bending moment diagrams

3.11 Points of Contra flexure

From the bending moment diagram for the beam shown in Fig. 3.26, it is evident that the bending moment changes sign from positive to negative between points B and C (BM at B is positive and BM at C is negative) at point E. This point E, where the transition of bending moment from positive to negative takes place, is called the point of contra flexure. At point E, the bending moment instantaneously becomes zero. Point E is also called the point of inflexion. Thus, the point of contraflexure or point of inflexion in a beam can be defined as the point where the bending moment changes sign from positive to negative or vice-versa. In other words, it is the point where the curvature of the beam changes (from sagging to hogging or vice-versa).

The position of the point of contra flexure can be obtained by equating the corresponding bending moment function in the region where it occurs to zero and then solving it for x. For the beam shown in Fig. 3.26, the point of contra flexure can be obtained by equating the bending moment function given by Eq. (3.27) valid in the region BC to zero. Thus,

$$-2.5x^2 + 0.5x + 20 = 0. \tag{3.30}$$

Solving the quadratic Eq. (3.30), one obtains $x = -2.73$, 2.93. The first solution can be ignored as it lies outside the beam region. The second solution can be accepted, which lies in between the points B and C. Thus, the point of contra flexure for the beam must be at a distance of 2.93 m from the left support or 0.93 m from point B.

3.12 S.F. and B.M. Diagrams for Beams Subjected to a Couple or Moment

Consider a simply supported beam subjected to an applied moment M_o at point C at a distance of l_1 from the left support at A and l_2 from that of the right support at B as shown in Fig. 3.27 (a). Drawing the free body diagram of the beam in Fig. 3.27 (b) and using the equations of equilibrium, the support reactions at points A and B are evaluated as

$$H_A = 0, \quad R_A = \frac{M_o}{L}, \quad R_B = -\frac{M_o}{L}. \tag{3.31}$$

Now, in the segment AC, *i.e.* in the region just left to the applied moment M_o ($0 \le x \le l_1$), the shear force and bending moment function can be constructed by taking an imaginary cut in that segment and drawing the free body diagram of the portion to the left of the cut section as shown in Fig. 3.28 (a). The force equilibrium in the y direction provides the shear force function as

$$V(x) = -R_A = -\frac{M_o}{L}, \tag{3.32}$$

which is constant from point A to the just left of point C. Evaluating the moments about the cut section and writing the equation of moment equilibrium, the bending moment function in the segment CB is obtained as

$$M(x) = -\frac{M_o}{L}x, \tag{3.33}$$

which varies linearly with x from M=0 at point A to $M = -\frac{M_o}{L}l_1$ at point C.

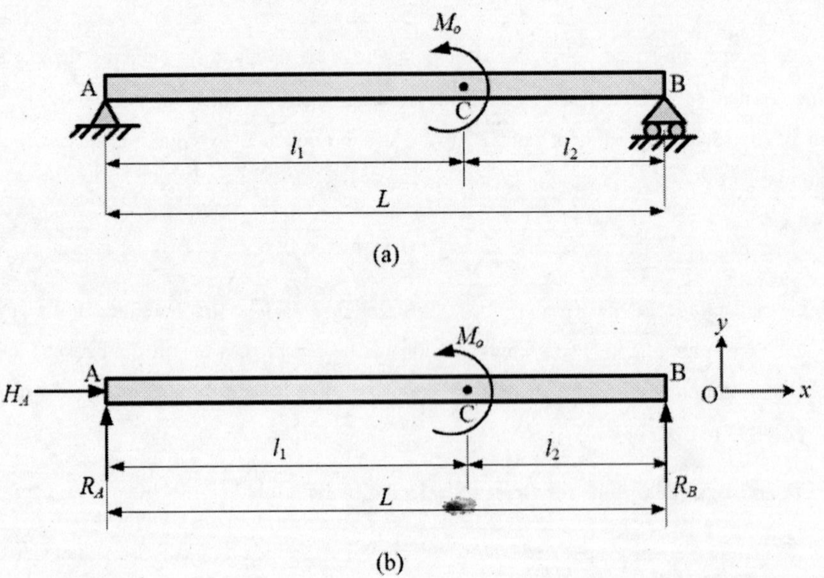

Fig. 3.27 A simply supported beam carrying a concentrated moment: (a) schematic and (b) free body diagram

Proceeding similarly, taking an imaginary cut in the segment CB (refer Fig. 3.28 (b)), the shear force and bending moment functions in the region $l_1 \le x \le L$ are obtained as

$$V(x) = -\frac{M_o}{L}, \tag{3.34}$$

$$M(x) = \frac{M_o}{L}x - M_o. \tag{3.35}$$

It is evident from Eq. (3.34) that the shear force is constant in segment CB. Further comparing it with Eq. (3.32), it reveals no variation of shear force from the left to the right portion of the applied concentrated moment. This verifies the conclusion we made in Case 3 of Section 3.6. Equation (3.35) shows a linear variation of the bending moment as expected from $M = \frac{M_o}{L} l_1$ at $x=l_1$ at point C to $M=0$ at $x=L$ at point B. The shear force and bending moment diagrams for the present beam are shown in Figs. 3.29 (a) and (b). It is to be noted that the applied moment M_o causes a sudden change in the bending moment from $-\frac{M_o}{L} l_1$ to $\frac{M_o}{L} l_1$ at $x=l_1$, *i.e.*, at the point of application of M_o.

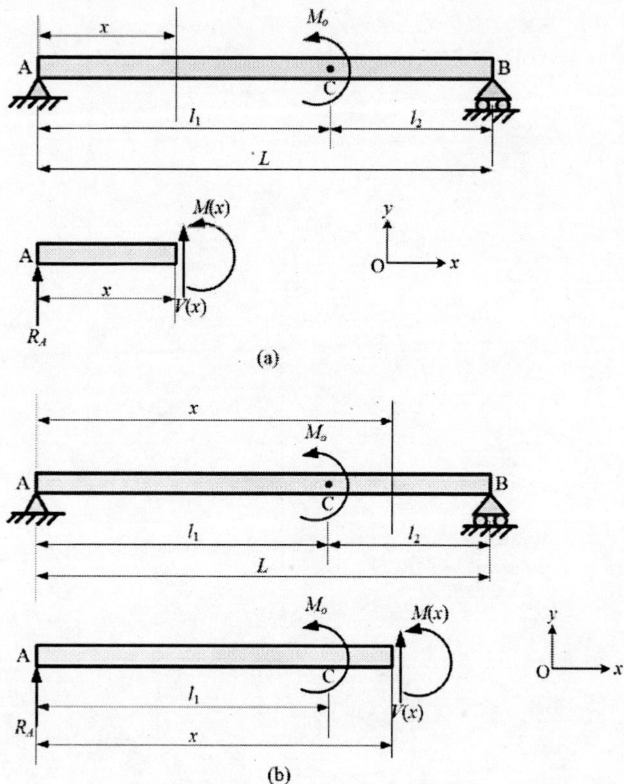

Fig. 3.28 Free body diagrams of the beam portion to the left of the cut section taken in the segments (a) AC and (b) CB.

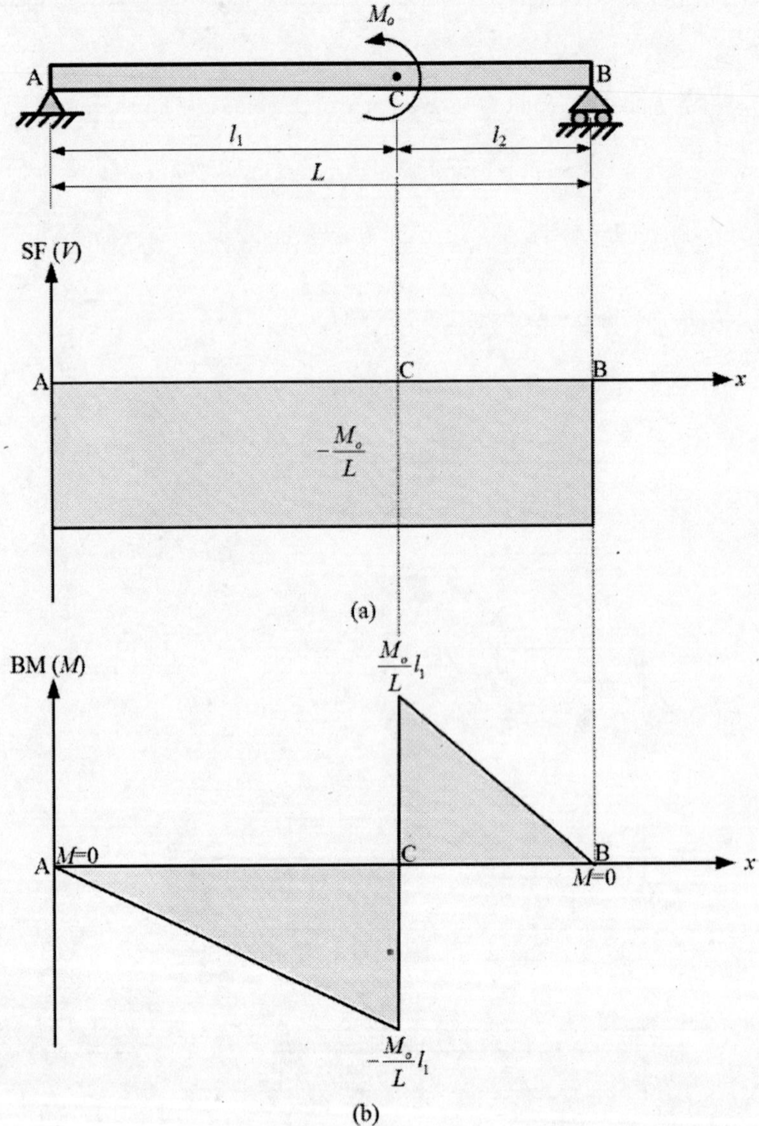

Fig. 3.29 a simply supported beam carrying a concentrated moment:

(a) schematic and shear force diagram and (b) bending moment diagram

3.13 SF and BM Diagrams for Beams Subjected to Gradually Varying Distributed Load

To demonstrate the construction of shear force and bending moment diagrams for beams subjected to gradually varying distributed load, a cantilever beam carrying a triangular distribution of load over the entire span along with its free body diagram is shown in Fig. 3.30. The equilibrium requirement in the x direction automatically provides horizontal reaction H_A at the support as zero.

The force equilibrium equation in the y direction provides the vertical reaction R_A at the fixed support as

$$R_A - \frac{qL}{2} = 0, \quad R_A = \frac{qL}{2}. \tag{3.36}$$

Evaluating the moment about point A and invoking the moment equilibrium condition, the reactive moment MA at the fixed support is obtained as

$$M_A + \frac{qL}{2}\left(\frac{L}{3}\right) = 0, \quad M_A = -\frac{qL^2}{6}. \tag{3.37}$$

The negative sign in Eq. (3.37) indicates that the direction of the reactive moment should be reversed to the one considered while drawing the free-body diagram.

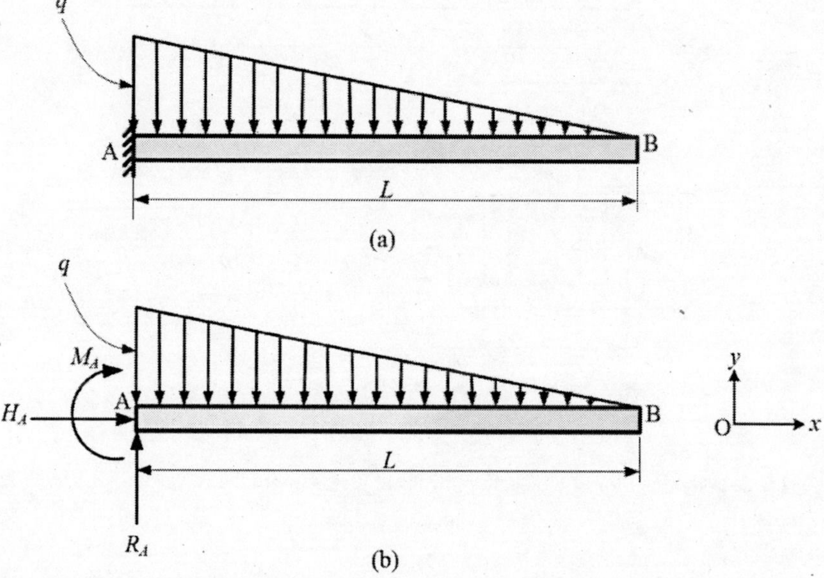

Fig. 3.30 A cantilever beam subjected to a gradually varying distributed load over the entire span: (a) schematic and (b) free body diagram

Now, to reveal the shear force and bending moment in the cross-section of the beam, let us pass an imaginary cut across the beam section at any distance x from the fixed support, as shown in Fig. 3.31. It is considered that the imaginary cut is taken across point D, where the intensity of the distributed load is q_2. The maximum intensity of the triangular distribution of load q is represented by CA. If one draws the free body diagram of the left cut half of the beam portion, it can be thought of as carrying a triangular distribution of load of intensity q_1

superposed over the uniformly distributed load of intensity q_2. From the similarity of the triangles ABC and CDE, one can write

$$\frac{x}{L}=\frac{q_1}{q}, \quad q_1=\frac{q}{L}x. \tag{3.38}$$

Thus, the uniformly distributed load intensity q_2 can be obtained as

$$q_2=q-q_1=q\left(1-\frac{x}{L}\right). \tag{3.39}$$

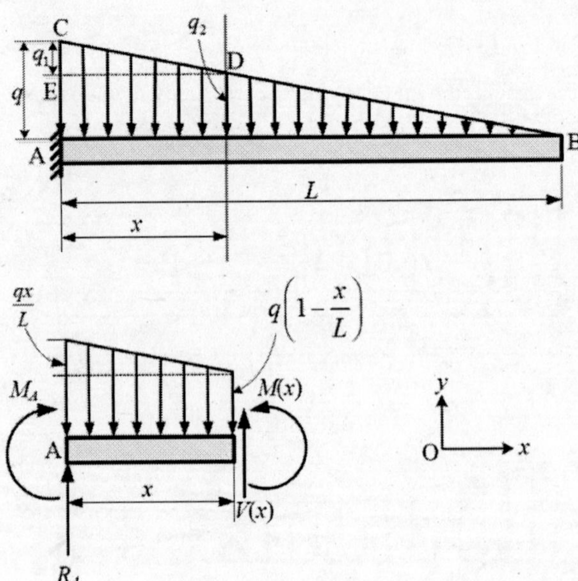

Fig. 3.31 Free body diagram of the beam portion subjected to gradually varying distributed load left to the cut section.

From the free body diagram of the left cut half of the beam portion, using the vertical force equilibrium, the shear force function can be obtained as

$$V(x)+R_A-\frac{1}{2}\left(\frac{qx}{L}\right)x-q\left(1-\frac{x}{L}\right)x=0,$$

$$V(x)=-\frac{qx^2}{2L}+qx-\frac{qL}{2}. \tag{3.40}$$

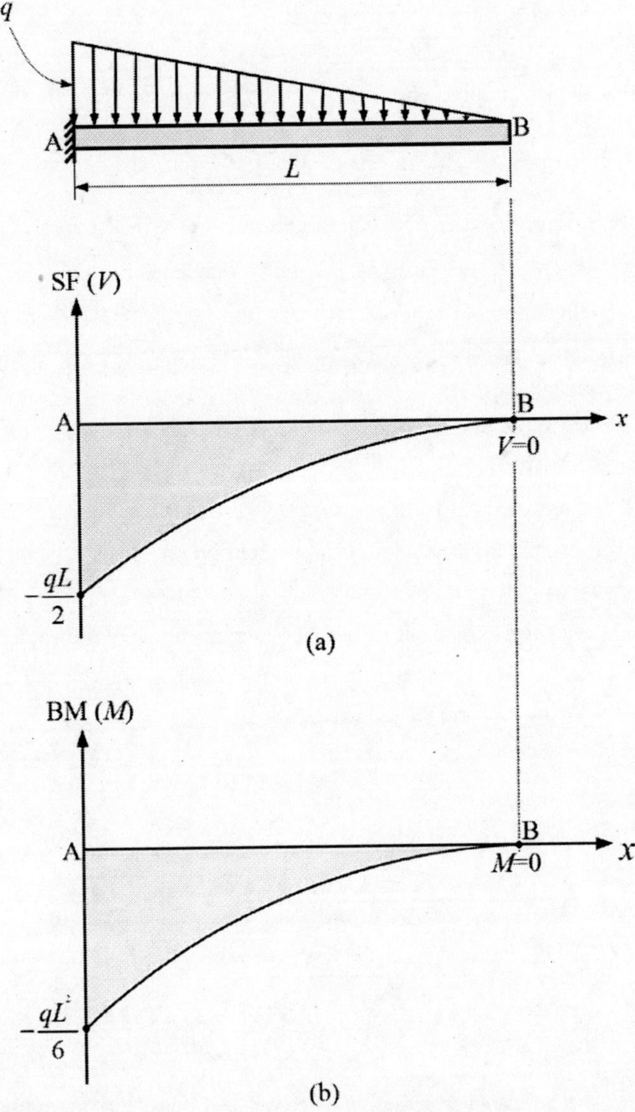

Fig. 3.32 A cantilever beam carrying gradually varying distributed load over the entire span (a) schematic and shear force diagram and (b) bending moment diagram

Considering the moment equilibrium taking the moment about the cut section, the bending moment function can be obtained as

$$M(x)+q\left(1-\frac{x}{L}\right)x\left(\frac{x}{2}\right)+\frac{1}{2}\left(\frac{qx}{L}\right)x\left(\frac{2x}{3}\right)-R_A x-M_A=0,$$

$$M(x)=\frac{qx^3}{6L}-\frac{qx^2}{2}+\frac{qLx}{2}-\frac{qL^2}{6}. \tag{3.41}$$

It is observed that the shear force varies in a parabolic manner, according to Eq. (3.40), from $V=-\frac{qL}{2}$ at the fixed support to vanish at the free end. The corresponding shear force diagram is shown in Fig. 3.32 (a). The bending moment at any distance x along the length of the beam is calculated using Eq. (3.41) and plotted in Fig. 3.32 (b) to obtain the corresponding bending moment diagram. As dictated by Eq. (3.41) and also from the BM diagram, it is clear that the bending moment along the length of the beam varies cubically from $M=-\frac{qL^2}{6}$ at the fixed end to vanish at the free end.

Example 3.4 A 8 m long beam AB is supported at points A and C, as shown in the following figure. The beam carries a triangular distribution of load over the portion AC with the maximum intensity of 40 kN/m and the overhang portion CB is subjected to the uniformly distributed load of intensity 5 kN/m. At point C, a clockwise moment of 60 kNm is applied. Draw the shear force and bending moment diagram. Determine the position of the maximum bending moment and its magnitude. Also, determine the position of the point of contraflexure, if any.

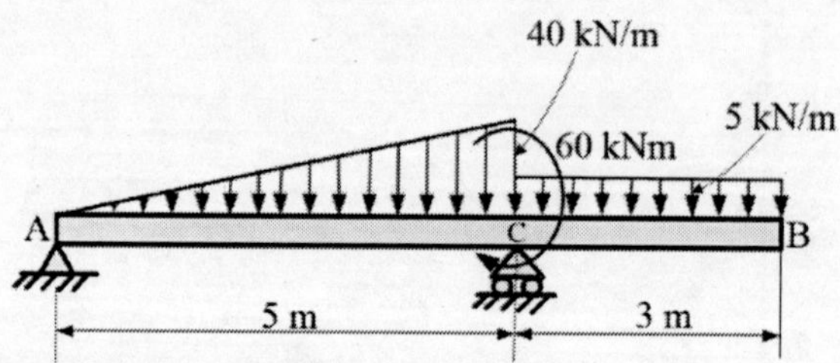

Solution

Support reactions: The horizontal reaction H_A becomes zero instantaneously from the equilibrium condition in the x direction. Taking the moment about point C, the moment equilibrium equation provides

$$-60-5\times3\times1.5+\frac{1}{2}\times5\times40\times\frac{5}{3}-R_A\times5=0, \quad R_A=16.83\text{ kN}.$$

The force equilibrium in the y direction provides

$$R_A+R_B=5\times3+\frac{1}{2}\times5\times40=115, \quad R_B=115-R_A=98.17\text{kN}.$$

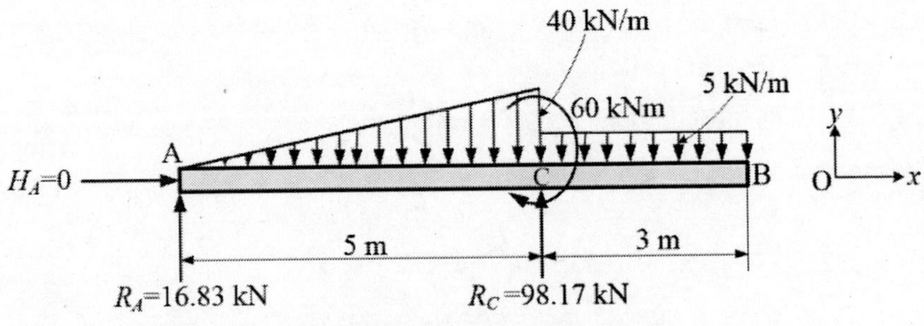

Free body diagram of the beam

Shear force and bending moment functions: The shear force and bending moment functions for different segments of the beam separated by different loads are formulated as follows:

Segment AC (0≤x≤5):

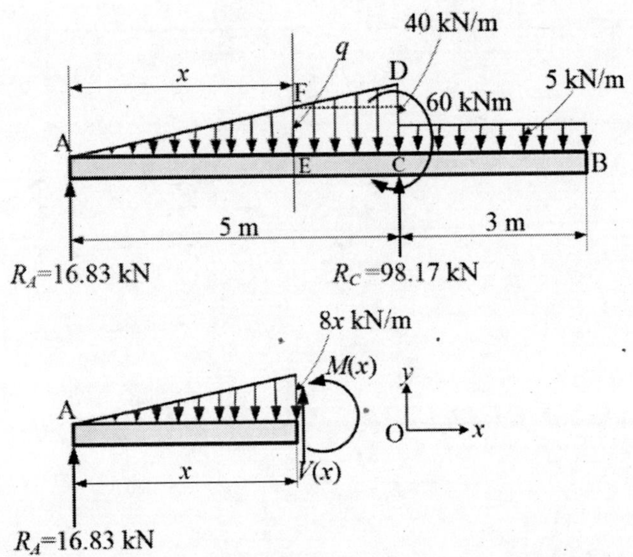

An imaginary cut is taken at any distance x from the left end between points A and C. The left cut portion of the beam of length x carrying the triangular load distribution is isolated from the rest of the beam portion, and a free-body diagram is constructed. Let the intensity of the distributed load at the cut section be q. Now, from the similarity of the triangles ACD and AEF,

$$\frac{q}{x} = \frac{40}{5}, \quad q = 8x \text{ kN/m}$$

The force equilibrium in the y direction provides the shear force function as

$$V(x)+R_A-\frac{1}{2}(8x)x=0, \quad V(x)=4x^2-16.83. \tag{i}$$

Writing the moment equilibrium equation taking the moment about the cut section, the bending moment function is obtained as

$$M(x)+\frac{1}{2}(8x)x\left(\frac{x}{3}\right)-R_Ax=0, \quad M(x)=-\frac{4}{3}x^3+16.83x. \tag{ii}$$

Segment CB ($5 \le x \le 8$):

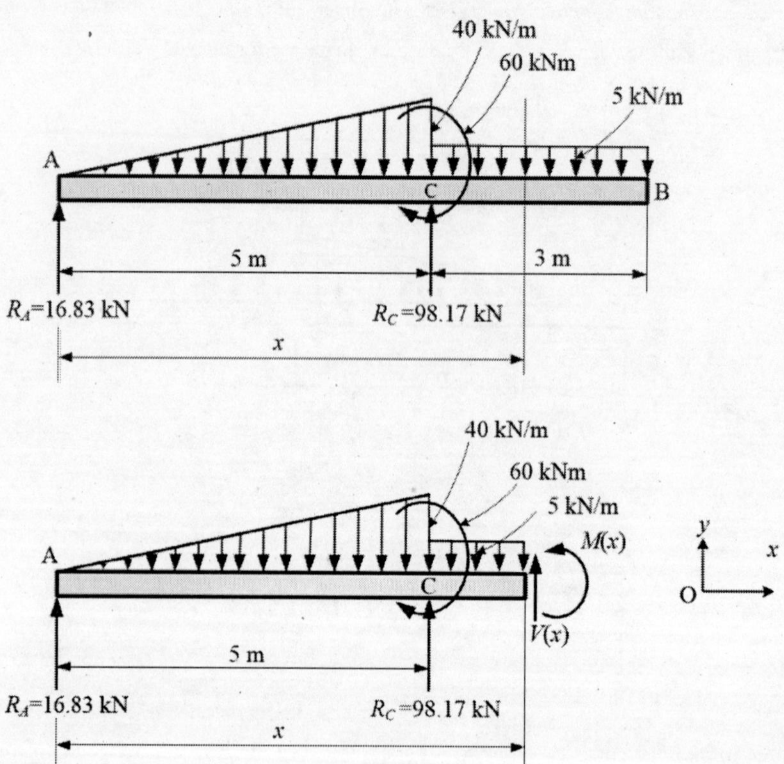

Taking an imaginary cut in between points C and B at a distance of x from the left end, the left cut portion of the beam is isolated from the rest of the beam portion, and a free-body diagram is drawn. The force equilibrium equation in the y direction provides the shear force function as

$$V(x)+R_A+R_C-5(x-5)+\frac{1}{2}\times5\times40=0, \quad V(x)=5x-40. \tag{iii}$$

The moment equilibrium equation is written taking the moment about the cut section to obtain the bending moment function as

$$M(x)+5(x-5)\left(\frac{x-5}{2}\right)+\frac{1}{2}\times 40\times 5\left(\frac{5}{3}+x-5\right)-60-R_A x-R_C(x-5)=0,$$

$$M(x)=-\frac{5}{2}(x-5)^2-100\left(x-\frac{10}{3}\right)+60+16.83x+98.17(x-5). \qquad \text{(iv)}$$

Shear force and bending moment diagrams: The shear force diagram is constructed evaluating the shear forces at the boundary points as well as certain intermediate points using Eqs. (i) and (iii) in the respective segments. It is observed that the shear force distribution is parabolic from $V=-16.83$ kN at point A to $V=83.17$ kN just to the left of point C, vanishing in between at a distance of 2.05 m from the left end. The shear force becomes –15 kN just to the right of point C and then varies linearly to zero at point B. The bending moments at different locations along the length of the beam are evaluated using Eqs. (ii) and (iv) in the respective segments and plotted to obtain the bending moment diagram. It is observed that the bending moment varies cubically from A to C. Due to the applied moment at point C, there is jump in the value of the bending moment from –82.52 kNm just to the left of point C to –22.52 kNm just to the right of point C. From point C to B bending moment varies in a parabolic manner. The bending moment at points A and B vanishes.

Position of the maximum bending moment and its magnitude: For the maximum or minimum, from Eq. (ii)

$$\frac{dM(x)}{dx}=0,\quad -\frac{4}{3}\times 3x^2+16.83=0,$$
$$x=2.05 \text{ (considering only the positive root)}$$

Thus, the maximum or minimum occurs at a distance of 2.05 from the left end. A second derivative test ($\frac{d^2M}{dx^2}<0$) shows that the value of the bending moment corresponding to x=2.05 m is actually the maximum one. This is also the location where the shear force vanishes. The magnitude of the maximum bending moment is obtained by substituting x=2.05 in Eq. (ii) as M_{max}=23.01 kNm.

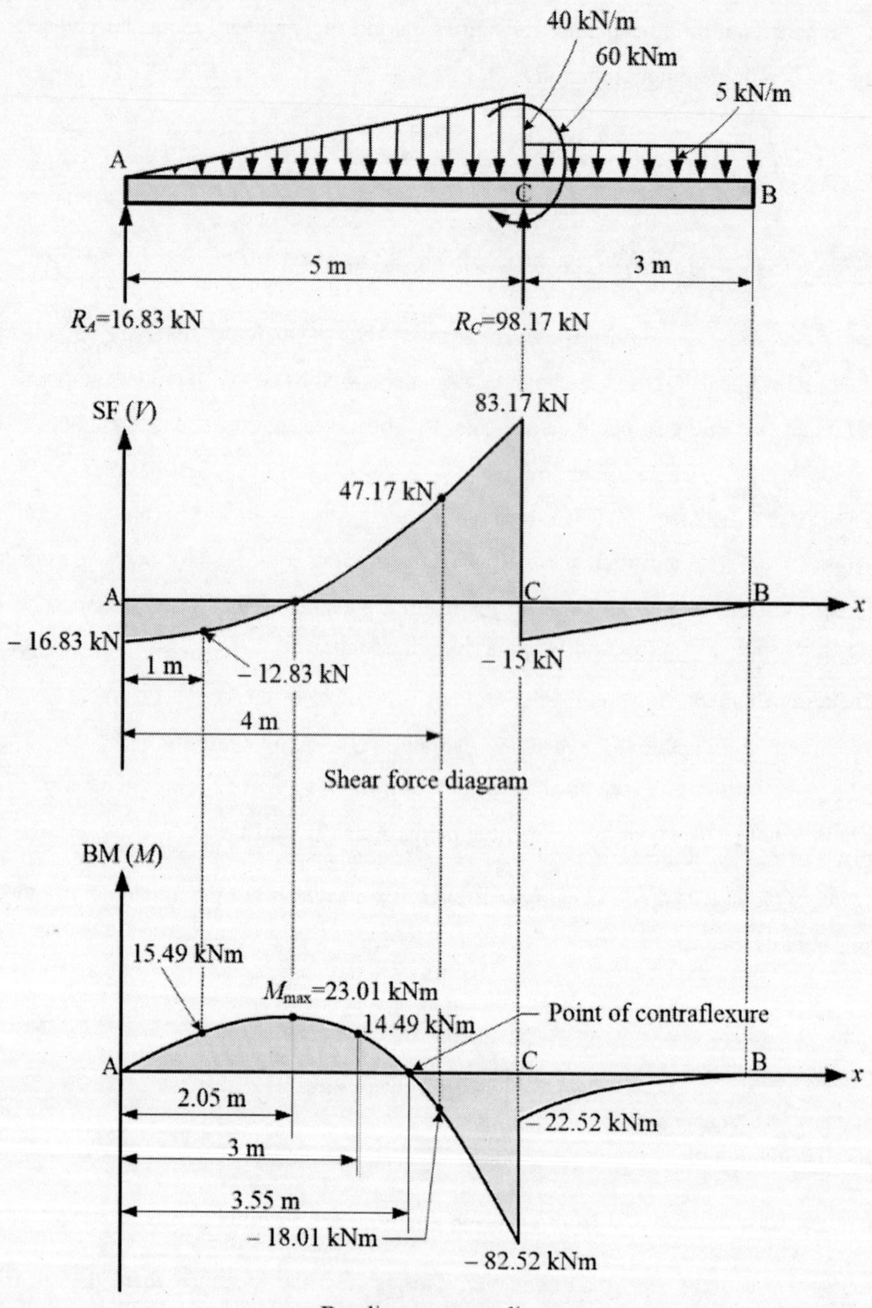

Point of contraflexure: It is observed that the bending moment changes sign from positive to negative at a certain point between points A and C and it becomes zero instantaneously at that point. This point is the point of contraflexure for the given beam. To locate the point of contraflexure, the bending moment given by Eq. (ii) is equated to zero. This provides x=3.55 m. Thus, the point of contraflexure is located at a distance of 3.55 m from the left end.

3.14 Summary

In this unit, the concept of internal forces induced in the beam cross-section, *i.e.*, shear force and bending moment due to the externally applied loads, are introduced. A detailed discussion on the construction of shear force and bending moment diagrams for various beams carrying different types of transverse loads is presented. From the discussions presented in this unit, the method for constructing the SF and BM diagrams can be summarized as follows:

a) First, determine the support reactions.
b) The beam is then divided into different segments separated by loads. An imaginary cut is taken in each segment from the left end at a distance of x, and draw the free body diagram of either the left or right portion of the beam.
c) Write the equations of equilibrium (only two equations of equilibrium are available as the horizontal force equilibrium has no relevance) to construct the shear force and bending moment functions for each segment.
d) Use the shear force and bending moment functions to evaluate the shear force and bending moment at any location along the length of the beam. Preferably, the corresponding values at the end points, load application points, and at certain conveniently chosen intermediate locations are obtained.
e) Using the shear force and bending moment values at different locations as in (d), the shear force and bending moment diagrams are constructed plotting the shear force/bending moment in the ordinate (y-axis) against any location x along the length of the beam in abscissa (x-axis).

It is worth noting that the maximum bending moment occurs at the point where shear force vanishes. If the shear force over a certain span of the beam is zero, then the bending moment over that span is constant or uniform. Further, if the bending moment changes sign from positive to negative or vice-versa (curvature changes from sagging to hogging or vice-versa) at any location between the two ends of a beam vanishing bending moment instantaneously, then that location is called the point of contraflexure. A beam can have more than one point of contraflexure.

Know More

Exercises

Multiple Choice Questions

3.1 If the SF diagram for a beam is parallel to abscissa forming rectangles from one portion to the other portion, then the beam is acted upon by a

(a) point load (b) concentrated moment

(c) uniformly distributed load (d) Uniformly varying load

3.2 If the bending moment distribution is parabolic over the certain span of a beam, then that span of the beam is acted upon by a

(a) point load (b) concentrated moment

(c) uniformly distributed load (d) Uniformly varying load

3.3 Shear force and bending moment are related by

(a) $\frac{dV}{dx} = M$ (b) $\frac{dM}{dx} = -V$

(c) $M = Vx$ (d) $\frac{d^2M}{dx^2} = V$

3.4 A portion of the beam is carrying a uniformly distributed load of intensity q (q being positive directed upwards), then the relationship between load q and the shear force V is given by

(a) $\frac{dV}{dx} = q$ (b) $\frac{dq}{dx} = V$

(c) $\frac{dq}{dx} = -V$ (d) $\frac{dV}{dx} = -q$

3.5 The shear force diagram of the beam shown in the following figure is

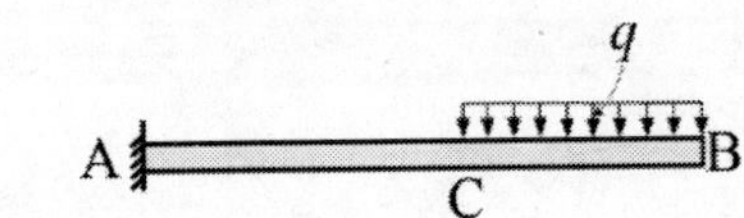

(a)

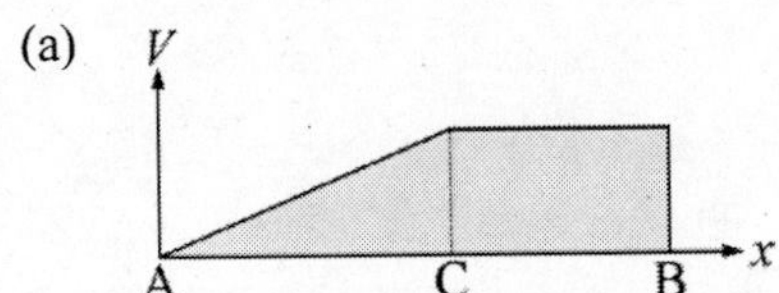

(b)

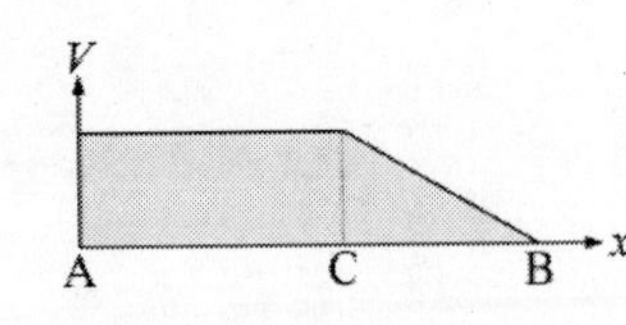

(c)

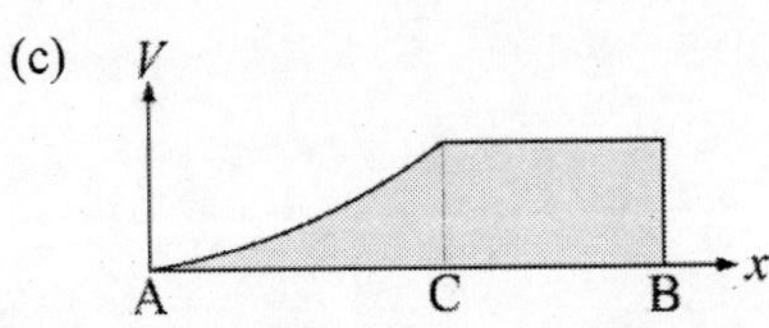

(d)

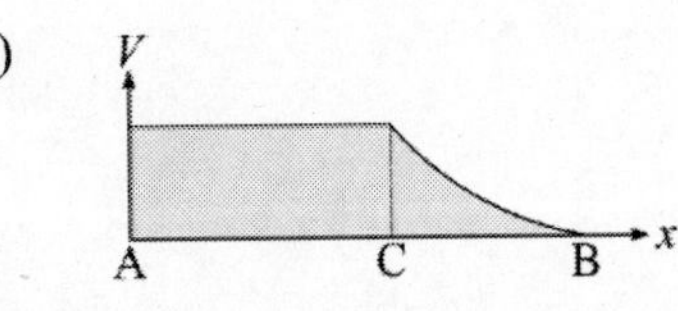

3.6 A simply supported beam of length 6 m is subjected to a uniformly distributed load of intensity 48 kN/m over its entire span. The magnitude of the maximum bending moment is

(a) 216 kNm (b) 144 kNm

(c) 432 kNm. (d) 864 kNm

3.7 In Q. 3.6, the maximum bending moment occurs at

(a) 2 m from the left support (b) 2 m from the left support

(c) 1.5 m from the left support (d) at the mid-span

3.8 A uniformly distributed load q is acting over the entire span of a cantilever beam of length 4 m. If the shear force at the mid-span of the beam is 10 kN, the value of q is

(a) zero (b) 2.5 kNm

(c) 5 kNm (d) 7.5 kNm

3.9 A simply supported beam is loaded, as shown in the figure. The absolute magnitude of shear force just to the right of point C is

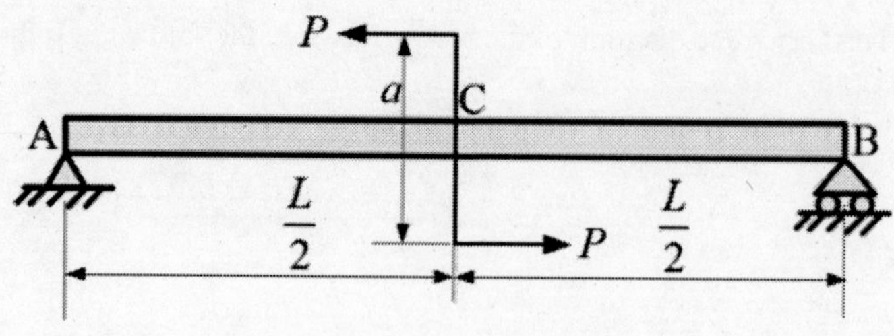

(a) P (b) $2P$

(c) $\frac{P}{L}$ (d) $\frac{Pa}{L}$

3.10 At the point of contraflexure

(a) the shear force is zero (b) the bending moment is zero

(c) both shear force and bending moment are zero (d) bending moment becomes the maximum

Answers of Multiple Choice Questions

3.1 (a), 3.2 (c), 3.3 (b), 3.4 (d), 3.5 (b), 3.6 (a), 3.7 (d), 3.8 (c), 3.9 (d), 3.10 (b).

Short and Long Answer Type Questions

Category I

3.1 What are shear force and bending moment?

3.2 Why is it important to evaluate the shear force and bending moment at a beam cross-section?

3.3 What are shear force and bending moment diagrams and their physical significance?

3.4 When the shear force at all cross sections over a certain portion of a beam is zero, what happens to the bending moment over that portion?

3.5 If the uniformly distributed load over a certain span of a beam is absent, then what information does it provide for the shear force variation over that span?

3.6 The bending moment diagram for a beam is shown in the following figure. Draw the corresponding diagram of the beam along with its loading.

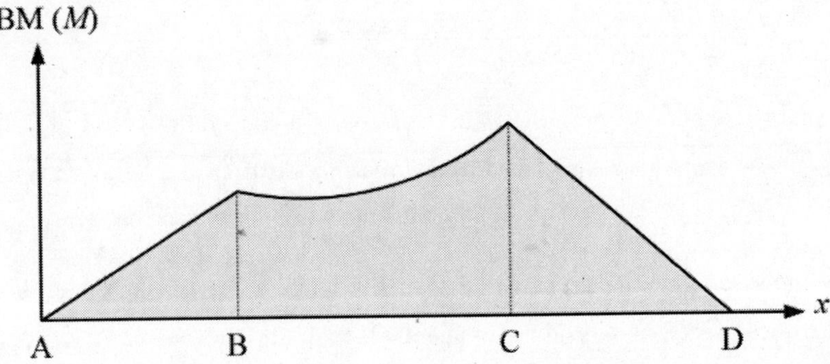

Category II

3.7 Derive the relationship between the bending moment, shearing force, and intensity of loading of a laterally loaded beam.

3.8 What is the point of contraflexure? Explain the occurrence of a point of contraflexure in a beam with an example.

3.9 Does it so happen that over a certain portion of a beam, both the shear force and bending moment are zero at all cross sections? Explain with an example.

Numerical Problems

3.10 Draw the shear force and bending moment diagram for the beam loaded, as shown in the following figure. Also, find the position of the maximum shear force and bending moment and their corresponding magnitudes.

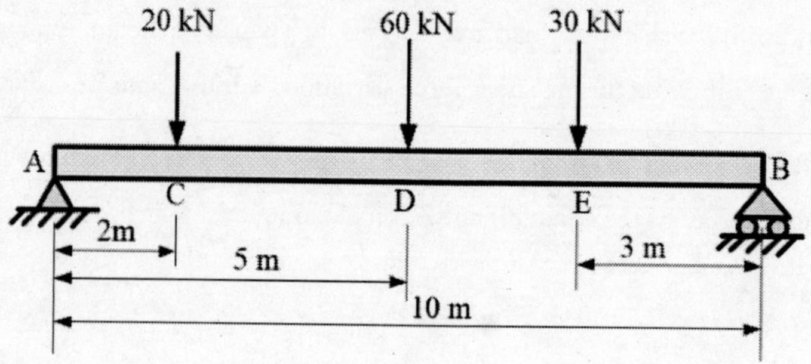

3.11 A simply supported beam of length 6 m carries a concentrated load of 120 kN at the mid-span. If the same load is replaced by a uniformly distributed load to act over the entire span, then what is the value of the maximum bending moment? (**Ans.** 90 kNm)

3.12 A simply supported beam carries a load P through a bracket, as shown in the figure. Draw the shear force and bending moment diagram for the beam. Also, determine the position of the maximum bending moment and its magnitude.

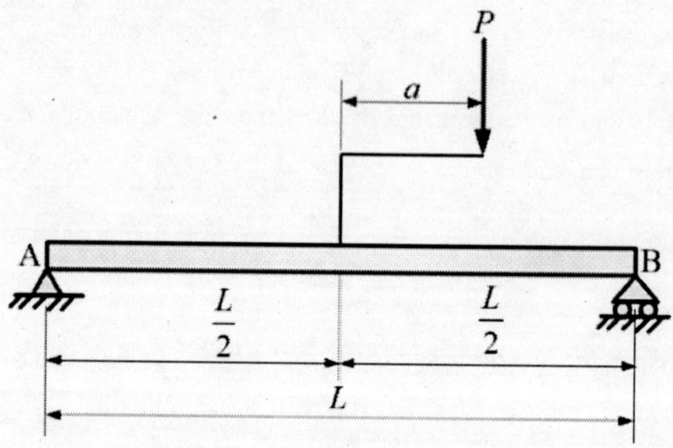

3.13 Consider the loadings on the aircraft wing, as shown in the following figure. The wing is fixed to the fuselage at point A. Draw the shear force and bending moment diagram for the wing. Determine the position of the maximum bending moment and its magnitude.

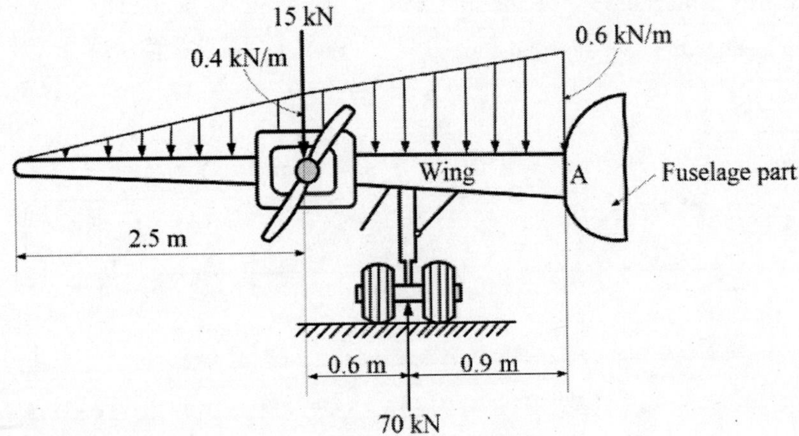

3.14 Draw the shear force and bending moment diagrams for the beams shown in the following figure indicating salient features such as nature, maximum values, and points of contraflexure if any.

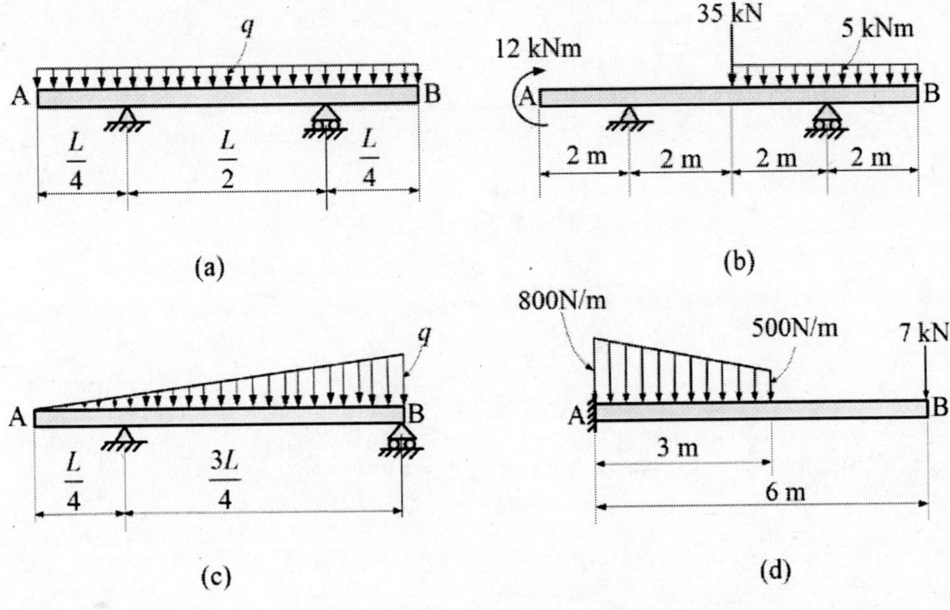

3.15 Shear force diagrams for beams are shown in the following figure. Draw the diagram of the beam along with its loading and corresponding bending moment diagram.

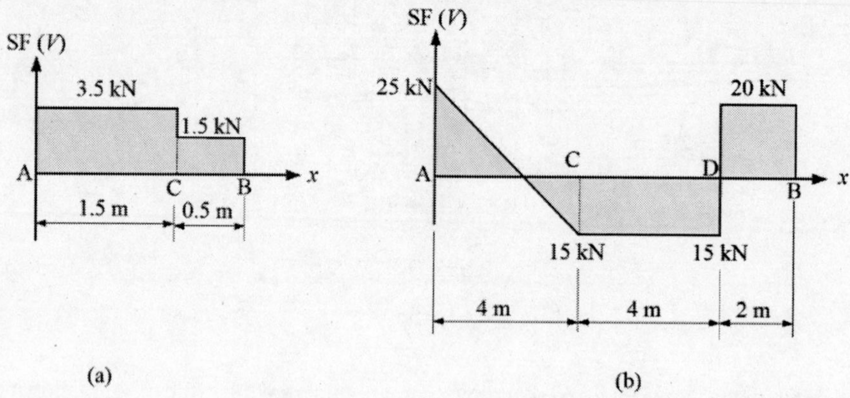

Unit 4

Bending Stresses

UNIT SPECIFICS

The following topics are covered in this unit:

- Pure and non-uniform bending;
- Geometrical properties of a beam cross-section;
- Theory of pure bending- derivation of the flexure formula;
- Evaluation of section modulus for simple and composite beam sections;
- Design of simple beam sections.

RATIONALE

The generation of internal forces, *viz.*, shear force and bending moment due to transversely applied loads on a beam and their evaluation is discussed in Unit 3. Knowing the magnitudes of these internal forces, one can determine the associated stresses induced at a given beam cross-section. As in general, the axial length of a beam is much longer than its cross-sectional dimensions, the stress associated with the bending moment, *i.e.*, bending or flexure stress dominates the beam design. It is therefore, in this unit it is devoted to analyze the bending or flexure stress beam treating the beam under pure bending.

PRE-REQUISITIES

Engineering Mechanics;

Bending moment diagram.

UNIT OUTCOMES

After completing this unit, students will be able to

U4-O1: understand the concept of bending or flexure stress induced in beam cross-section.

U4-O2: derive the bending or flexural equation.

U4-O3: evaluate the bending stress in determinate beams with different cross-sections subjected to different kinds of loading.

U4-O4: design beam of simple cross-sections.

Course Outcomes	Expected Mapping with Course Outcomes - CE (1- Weak Correlation; 2- Medium correlation; 3- Strong Correlation)			
	CO-1	CO-2	CO-3	CO-4
U3-O1	3	-	-	-
U3-O2	3	-	-	-
U3-O3	3	-	-	3
U3-O4	3	-	-	3

Course Outcomes	Expected Mapping with Course Outcomes - ME (1- Weak Correlation; 2- Medium correlation; 3- Strong Correlation)	
	CO-1	CO-2
U3-O1	3	-
U3-O2	3	3
U3-O3	3	-
U3-O4	3	3

4.1 Introduction

In Unit 3, it has been discussed how the internal forces at the beam cross-section are induced in the form of shear force and bending moment due to externally applied transverse loads on a beam. The variation of these internal forces along the length of the beam was also discussed. Knowing the shear force and bending moment at the beam cross-section at any location along the length of the beam, one can evaluate the associated stresses at that location. The loads acting on a beam cause it to deform such that a class of straight lines in the form of a curve, which is called bending or flexing of beam. This unit is devoted to the analysis of normal stresses induced in the beam cross-section due to pure bending. These normal stresses are called bending stress or flexural stress. A formula for bending or flexural stress for pure bending will be developed relating to the bending moment, the second moment of the area of cross-section and amount of curvature produced due to bending based on certain simplifying assumptions. The developed flexural stress formulation due to pure bending can reasonably be used to determine the bending stresses in non-uniform bending also when the effect of shear force is negligible.

4.2 Pure and Non-Uniform Bending

Pure bending refers to the bending load that causes uniform bending moment over the entire span or over a part of span of a beam without inducing any shear force. For example, one may refer to the shear force and bending moment diagrams of the simply supported beam loaded symmetrically with two concentrated loads of equal magnitudes *P* in Example Problem 3.1. It is evident from the shear force and bending moment diagrams of the beam that the shear force is zero and bending moment is constant over the central span (CD) of the beam; this span undergoes pure bending. On the other hand, in the extreme left and right portions (AC and DB) of the beam, the bending moment is not constant and is accompanied by shear forces. Thus, the portions AC and DB undergo non-uniform bending.

4.3 Geometrical Properties of a Beam Cross-section

The objective of this unit is to evaluate the bending stresses at a given cross-section of the beam associated with the bending moment. One shall appreciate later that the computation of bending stresses requires the knowledge of certain geometrical properties of the cross-section. The students might have studied in detail about such cross-sectional properties in a course on engineering mechanics. However, for the sake of continuity, these properties are briefly reviewed in this section before proceeding to the analysis of bending stresses in beams at a given cross-section.

4.3.1 First moment of area, centroidal axes and centroid

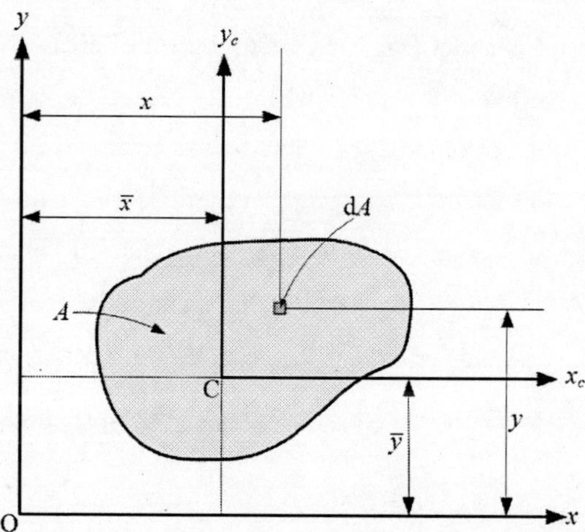

Fig. 4.1 A general cross-section of a beam to illustrate first and second moments of area.

Consider an arbitrary cross-section of area A as shown in Fig. 4.1 in x-y plane. An infinitesimally small element of area dA is considered on the cross-section at a location (x, y). If one takes the moment of the small area dA about x and y axes and integrates them over the total area A, then the integral quantities $\int_A y\mathrm{d}A$ and $\int_A x\mathrm{d}A$ are called as the first moment of area A about x and y axis, respectively. If one takes a set of axes x_c-y_c parallel to the original x-y axes at distances of $\bar{y}$and $\bar{x}$, respectively, the first moment of area A of the cross-section with respect to x_c and y_c can be written as

$$(FM)_{x_c} = \int_A (y - \bar{y})\,\mathrm{d}A = \int_A y\mathrm{d}A - \bar{y}\int_A \mathrm{d}A = \int_A y\mathrm{d}A - \bar{y}A, \tag{4.1}$$

$$(FM)_{y_c} = \int_A (x - \bar{x})\,\mathrm{d}A = \int_A x\mathrm{d}A - \bar{x}\int_A \mathrm{d}A = \int_A x\mathrm{d}A - \bar{x}A, \tag{4.2}$$

where $(FM)_{x_c}$ and $(FM)_{y_c}$ are used to represent the first moment of area of the cross-section with respect to the new set of axes x_c and y_c, respectively. Equations. (4.1) and (4.2) indicate that $(FM)_{x_c}$ and $(FM)_{y_c}$ vanish if

$$\int_A y\mathrm{d}A = \bar{y}A, \tag{4.3}$$

$$\int_A x\mathrm{d}A = \bar{x}A. \tag{4.4}$$

These set of axes x_c and y_c about which the first moment of area of the cross-section vanish are known as centroidal axes. The point where the centroidal axes intersect is called the centroid of the cross-section. Suppose the entire area is concentrated at the centroid, then the first moment of area about x- and y-axis is given by right hand sides of Eqs. (4.3) and (4.4). Thus, centroid of a cross-section can be defined as a point at which the entire area can be assumed to be concentrated to calculate the first moment of the area. In general, the centroid of a cross-section may lie inside or outside the section area. The distances $\bar{x}$ and $\bar{y}$provide the coordinate of the centroid $(\bar{x}, \bar{y})$, which can be obtained from Eqs. (4.3) and (4.4) as

$$\bar{x} = \frac{\int_A x\mathrm{d}A}{A}, \tag{4.5}$$

$$\bar{y} = \frac{\int_A y\mathrm{d}A}{A}. \tag{4.6}$$

4.3.2 Second moment of area or moment of inertia of cross-section

For an arbitrary cross-sectional area A as shown in Fig. 4.1, if one takes the moment of the first moment of the elemental area dA with respect to x and y axes and integrate them over the area A, then the values of the integral obtained are called as the second moment of area of the cross-section. Second moments of area about x and y axes are denoted by I_{xx} and I_{yy} in this unit. Thus,

$$I_{xx} = \int_A y^2 \mathrm{d}A, \tag{4.7}$$

$$I_{yy} = \int_A x^2 \mathrm{d}A. \tag{4.8}$$

The second moment of area of a cross-section is always positive. It is also termed as the moment of inertia of the cross-section. It provides a measure of resistance to bending about an axis. Often one comes across situations where the second moment of area of a cross-section needs to be determined about different axes. For this purpose, there are two useful theorems of second moment of area, *viz*., the parallel axes theorem and the perpendicular axes theorem, which are described next.

4.3.2.1 The parallel axis theorem of second moment of area

The parallel axes theorem relates the second moment of area of a cross-section about any axes in the plane of the area to the second moment of area evaluated with respect to a set of parallel centroidal axes. By knowing the second moment of area of a cross-section about its centroidal axes, one can easily evaluate the second moment of area about a set of non-centroidal axes parallel to the centroidal axes using the parallel axes theorem and vice-versa.

Referring to Fig. 4.1, the second moment of area of the arbitrary cross-section about the centroidal x_c axis is given by

$$I_{x_c x_c} = \int_A (y - \bar{y})^2 \mathrm{d}A. \tag{4.9}$$

Taking $y - \bar{y} = y'$, Eq. (4.9) can be expressed as

$$I_{x_c x_c} = \int_A y'^2 \mathrm{d}A. \tag{4.10}$$

The second moment of area of the cross-section about the non-centroidal x-axis parallel to the centroidal axis x_c is given by Eq. (4.7), which can be rewritten in the following form:

$$I_{xx} = \int_A \{\bar{y} + (y - \bar{y})\}^2 \mathrm{d}A = \int_A (\bar{y} + y')^2 \mathrm{d}A,$$

$$= \int_A \bar{y}^2 \mathrm{d}A + \int_A 2\bar{y}y' \mathrm{d}A + \int_A y'^2 \mathrm{d}A,$$

$$I_{xx} = \bar{y}^2 \int_A \mathrm{d}A + 2\bar{y} \int_A y' \mathrm{d}A + \int_A y'^2 \mathrm{d}A. \tag{4.11}$$

In Eq. (4.11), the first term is the square of the y coordinate of the centroid multiplied by the total area A, the second term vanishes as $\int_A y' \mathrm{d}A$ is the first moment of the area about the centroidal axis which is zero and the third term represents the second moment of the area about the centroidal axis x_c given by Eq. (4.10). Thus, Eq. (4.11) reduces to

$$I_{xx} = I_{x_c x_c} + A\bar{y}^2. \tag{4.12}$$

Equation (4.12) is the parallel axis theorem for the set of parallel centroidal and non-centroidal x-axis. Similarly, one can derive an equation of parallel axis theorem for the set of parallel centroidal and non-centroidal y axes and is given by

$$I_{yy} = I_{y_c y_c} + A\bar{x}^2. \tag{4.13}$$

The parallel axes theorem given by Eqs. (4.12) and (4.13) are quite useful in solving the problem of bending stresses in beam, which is the main focus of the present unit.

4.3.2.2 The perpendicular axis theorem of second moment of area: the polar moment of inertia

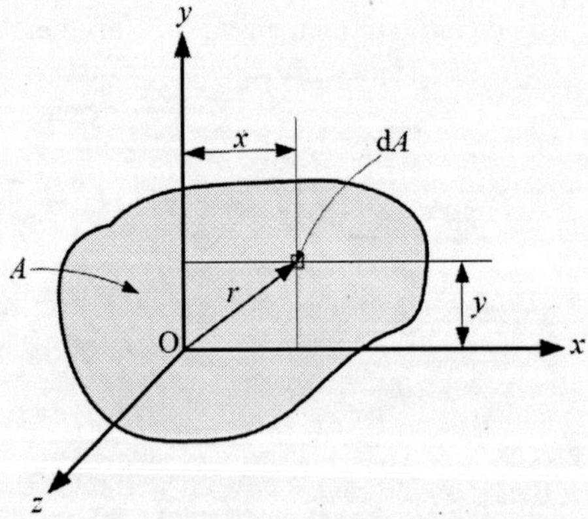

Fig. 4.2 A general cross-section of a member to illustrate polar moment of inertia.

The perpendicular axis theorem provides the second moment of area or moment of inertia of a cross-section about an axis perpendicular to the plane of the cross-section. This is also called the polar moment of inertia. In order to evaluate the polar moment of inertia, let us consider an arbitrary area A in xy-plane as shown in Fig. 4.2. The z-axis is the axis perpendicular to the plane of the area pointing outwards. If one considers a small element of area dA at a radial position of r from the z-axis, then the moment of inertia of the elemental area about the z-axis perpendicular to the xy-plane is given by

$$dI_{zz} = r^2 dA. \tag{4.14}$$

The integration of Eq. (4.14) over the area A of the cross-section provides the moment of inertia of the entire area about the z axis, which is the polar moment of inertia or the second moment of area about the perpendicular axis given by

$$I_{zz} = I_p = \int_A r^2 dA. \tag{4.15}$$

One can see from Fig. 4.2 that $r^2=x^2+y^2$. Thus, the polar moment of inertia of the arbitrary cross-section can be expressed as

$$I_p = \int_A \left(x^2+y^2\right) dA = \int_A x^2 dA + \int_A y^2 dA = I_{yy} + I_{xx}. \tag{4.16}$$

Equation (4.16) states that the polar moment of inertia of a cross-sectional area is equal to the algebraic sum of the moments of inertia of the area about two mutually perpendicular axes in the plane of the area.

It is worth noting that the polar moment of inertia is an important property of the cross-section to be evaluated for a member subjected to a twisting moment or torsion. The polar moment of inertia provides a measure of resistance to twist about an axis perpendicular to the plane of the cross-section. The concept described here will serve as the background knowledge while evaluating the torsional shear stress in circular bars in Unit 7.

4.4 Theory of Pure Bending: The Flexure Formula

In this section, the theory of pure bending is developed for prismatic beam. The formulations for bending normal stress induced in the beam cross-section relating to the bending moment and sectional properties such as second moment of area are obtained considering certain simplified assumptions. It is, therefore, the theory introduced here is often termed as the theory of simple bending.

4.4.1 Assumptions in the theory of pure bending

Following assumptions are employed in developing a theory of pure bending:

a) The beam is straight in its unstressed state, *i.e.*, its curvature is zero. In other words, the radius of the curvature of the beam is infinite.

b) The beam is made up of homogeneous and isotropic material with identical Young's modulus of elasticity in tension and compression.

c) The cross-section of the beam is at least symmetric about the vertical *y*-axis, *e.g.*, a beam with trapezoidal cross-section as depicted in Fig. 4.3.

d) The resultant of applied loads lies in the plane containing the vertical axis of symmetry of all cross-sections; this plane is called the plane of symmetry. At any location in the beam, the loading is uniform across the width direction, *i.e.*, it is not a function of *z*. In fact, the loading is not a function of *x* and *y* also. However, in most of the cases, theory of plane bending is applied even for the cases where bending moment changes along longitudinal direction, i.e., loading is a function of *x*. In Fig. 4.3, the applied moments *M* at the end sections of the beam are shown to act on the plane of symmetry. The bending occurs in the plane of symmetry (and in all planes parallel to it). Hence, the plane of symmetry is also called the plane of bending.

e) The plane sections remain plane and perpendicular to the centroidal axis of the beam before and after bending.

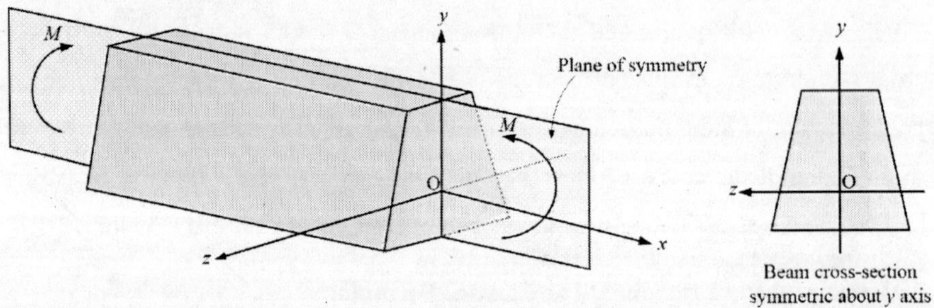

Fig. 4.3 A beam with trapezoidal cross-section loaded with equal moments at the ends

4.4.2 Longitudinal normal strain induced in the beam

Let us consider a straight unstressed beam as shown in Fig. 4.4 (a). Now, the beam is considered to be subjected to equal moments *M* at each end. The loaded beam is shown in Fig. 4.4 (b). The applied equal moments at each end induce a constant or uniform positive bending moment equal to *M* over the entire beam span with no shear force (pure bending) and causes the beam to bend. The bending moment distribution in the beam is shown in Fig. 4.4 (c) and the bent configuration of a portion of the beam between Sections 1-1 and 2-2 is depicted in Fig. 4.4 (d). When the beam bends, all its longitudinal lines take up the form of concentric circular arcs whose centre is situated at O. The point O is termed as the centre of curvature of the beam. Due to the bending deformation caused by a positive bending moment *M*, the longitudinal lines on the upper part of the bent beam undergoes contraction and the longitudinal lines on its lower part undergoes extension. Thus, the upper part of the beam is in compression and its lower part is in tension. In between a layer exists which is neither subjected to contraction nor extension; its length remains the same as in the unstressed configuration. This layer is called as the neutral surface of the beam. In Fig. 4.4, the neutral surface of the beam is represented by the dashed line in its undeformed configuration and by the corresponding dashed arc in the deformed configuration. The intersection of any cross-sectional plane with the neutral surface is called as the neutral axis of the beam cross-section. For example, the z-axis is the neutral axis of the typical cross-section shown in Fig. 4.4 (d). The distance measured from the centre of curvature O to the neutral surface of the beam is called the radius of curvature R of the beam.

For the analysis of the beam, two parallel imaginary cuts PQ and RS across the cross-sections are taken in the unstressed beam, which are separated by an infinitesimal distance dx. Attention is focussed on the small element PQRS. After bending, the originally parallel cut sections PQ and RS rotate with respect to each other, which are represented by P′Q′ and R′S′. The rotation about the neutral axis P′Q′ and R′S′ subtend a small angle dθ at the centre of curvature as shown in Fig. 4.4 (d). The sections P′Q′ and R′S′ remain plane and perpendicular to the neutral surface in the bent configuration of the beam. The element P′Q′R′S′ is isolated from the rest of the beam parts and is shown exaggeratedly in Fig. 4.4 (e). Thė parallel cut sections PQ and RS intersect the neutral surface at points C and D, which are represented by C′ and D′ on the neutral surface in the bent configuration. Thus, the lengths of CD and C′D′ are the same, which is dx. If a line element EF is considered at a distance y from the neutral surface, after bending, the line element contracts to E′F′. As the radius of curvature of the arc C′D′ is R, the radius of curvature of the arc E′F′ will be $(R–y)$. The length of the line element EF after bending is equal to the arc length E′F′, *i.e.*,

$$E'F' = (R - y)\mathrm{d}\theta = R\mathrm{d}\theta - y\mathrm{d}\theta = \mathrm{d}x - \frac{y}{R}\mathrm{d}x. \tag{4.17}$$

The original length of the arc $E'F'$ is given by the line element EF=dx. Hence, the longitudinal strain induced in the line element EF due to bending is obtained by

$$\varepsilon_{xx} = \frac{E'F' - EF}{EF} = \frac{dx - \frac{y}{R}dx - dx}{dx} = -\frac{y}{R}. \tag{4.18}$$

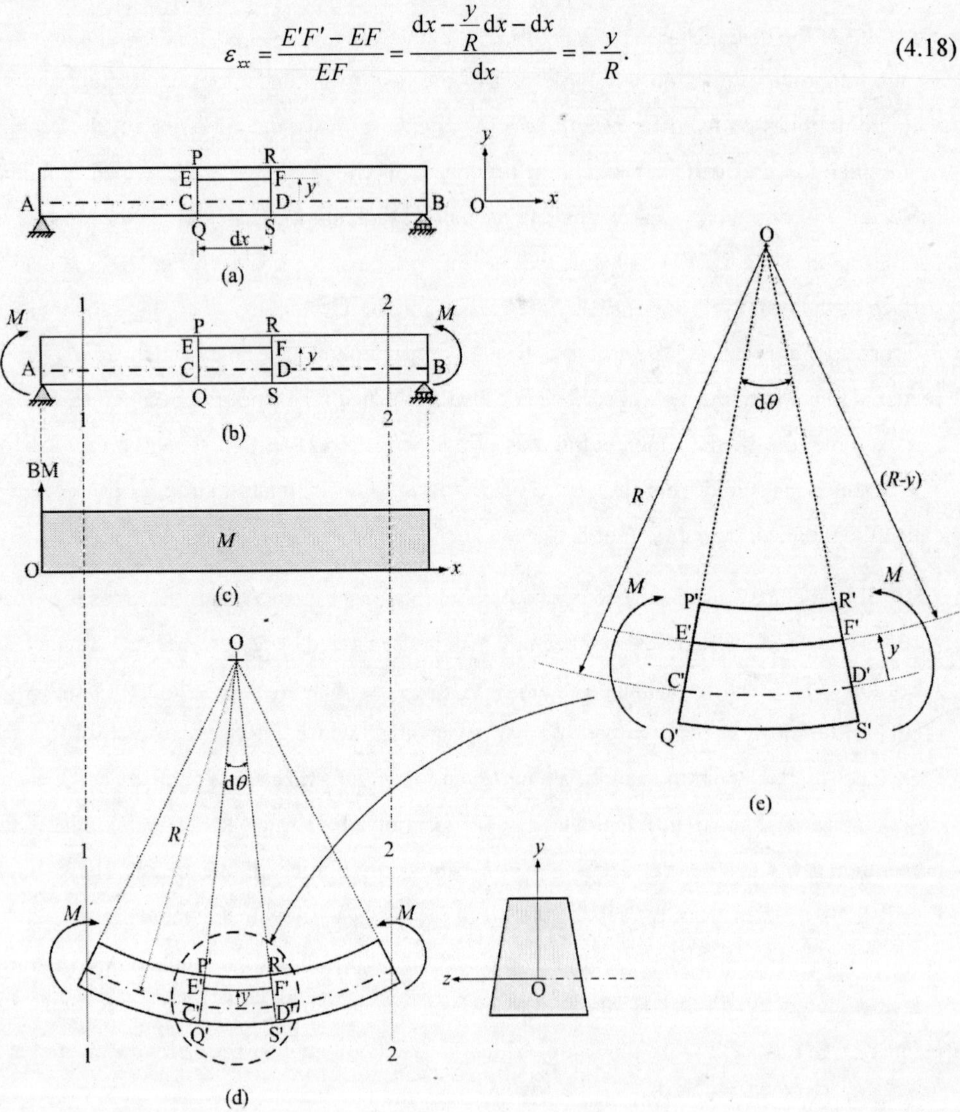

Fig. 4.4 A beam subjected to pure bending: (a) unstressed beam, (b) beam loaded with equal moments at the ends, (c) bending moment diagram, (c) deformed configuration of a portion of the beam subjected to pure bending and (e) free body diagram of the deformed element P′Q′R′S′.

4.4.3 Normal stress induced in the beam cross-section

Assume that under the action of bending moment, the deformation behaviour of the beam is purely elastic and linear. The stresses induced in the beam cross-section can be determined from the uniaxial stress-strain curve of the material up to linear elastic limit. Once the longitudinal strains of the lines located at any distance y from the neutral surface of the beam is known from Eq. (4.18), the normal stress induced in the beam cross-section can be obtained using Hooke's law as

$$\sigma_{xx} = E\varepsilon_{xx} = -E\frac{y}{R}, \tag{4.19}$$

where E is the Young's modulus of elasticity of the beam material. In Eq. (4.19), the normal stress is denoted by σ_{xx} as the longitudinal stress acting on the beam cross-section is directed along x-axis. The normal stress induced in the beam cross-section varies linearly, being zero at the neutral surface.

4.4.4 Determination of the position of neutral axis on the beam cross-section

The determination of the position of neutral axis is crucial in order to obtain the bending stress distribution on the cross-section of the beam. The position of the neutral axis can be obtained by writing the equation of static equilibrium of force in the x direction. Let us consider an element of area $\mathrm{d}A$ on the beam cross-section at a distance y from the neutral axis as shown in Fig. 4.5. The normal stress acting on the element is given by Eq. (4.19). Thus, the elemental force acting on the element is

$$\mathrm{d}F_x = \sigma_{xx}\mathrm{d}A = -E\frac{y}{R}\mathrm{d}A. \tag{4.20}$$

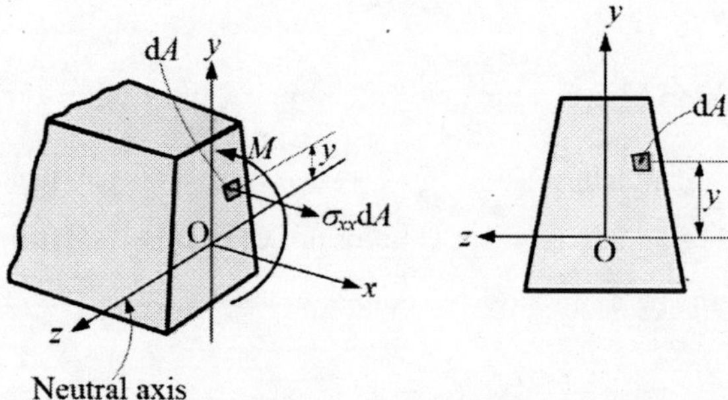

Fig. 4.5 Elemental force acting on a small area dA considered on the beam cross-section at a distance y from the neutral axis.

The net force acting on the entire area A of the cross-section of the beam is obtained by integrating Eq. (4.20) over the area A. Thus,

$$F_x = \int_A \mathrm{d}F_x = \int_A -E\frac{y}{R}\mathrm{d}A. \tag{4.21}$$

The static equilibrium of force in the x direction requires the vanishing of the net force acting on the cross-section of area A. Thus,

$$\int -E\frac{y}{R}\mathrm{d}A = 0. \tag{4.22}$$

As E and R are nonzero constants over a cross-section, Eq. (4.22) can be written as

$$\int y\mathrm{d}A = 0. \tag{4.23}$$

Use of Eq. (4.3) in Eq. (4.23) provides

$$A\bar{y} = 0. \tag{4.24}$$

As A cannot be zero, the only condition to satisfy (4.24) is $\bar{y} = 0$, which indicates that the first moment of the area of the beam cross-section evaluated with respect to the neutral axis vanishes. Thus, the neutral axis, *viz.*, the z-axis in Fig. 4.5 must be located at the centroid of the cross-section. In other words, y=0 indicates a neutral axis or neutral surface. The strains and stresses at the neutral axis or neutral surface are zero as evident from Eqs. (4.18) and (4.19), respectively.

4.4.5 The relationship between the bending moment and radius of curvature

In order to obtain the relationship between the bending moment M and the radius of curvature R of the beam, the moment equilibrium equations is considered. Referring to Fig. 4.5, the elemental moment of the force acting on the element of area A about the neutral axis is given by

$$\mathrm{d}M = -\sigma_{xx} y\mathrm{d}A, \tag{4.25}$$

where the negative sign indicates that the elemental moment dM is acting in a direction opposite to the positive bending moment M. For equilibrium, the integral of Eq. (4.25) over the entire cross-sectional area A must be equal to the bending moment M. Thus,

$$M = -\int_A \sigma_{xx} y \mathrm{d}A. \tag{4.26}$$

Substituting the value of σ_{xx} from Eq. (4.19) in Eq. (4.26), one obtains

$$M = \int_A \frac{Ey}{R} y \mathrm{d}A,$$

$$M = \frac{E}{R} \int_A y^2 \mathrm{d}A. \tag{4.27}$$

In Eq. (4.27), the integral term represents the second of the area of cross-section about the neutral axis, denoted by I. Thus, Eq. (4.27) can be expressed as

$$M = \frac{E}{R} I,$$

$$\frac{M}{I} = \frac{E}{R}. \tag{4.28}$$

Equation (4.28) provides the relationship between the bending moment M and the radius of curvature R of the beam.

4.4.6 The Bending or Flexural Equation

Denoting the normal stress σ_{xx} induced in the beam cross-section due to pure bending by f, which is usually used to represent bending or flexural stress, Eq. (4.19) can be rewritten as

$$-\frac{f}{y} = \frac{E}{R}. \tag{4.29}$$

Combining Eqs. (4.28) and (4.29), one obtains

$$\frac{M}{I} = -\frac{f}{y} = \frac{E}{R}, \tag{4.30}$$

where M is the bending moment, f the bending stress, I the second moment of the area of beam cross-section about the neutral axis, y the distance from the neutral axis, E the Young's modulus of elasticity of the beam material and R is the radius of curvature of the beam. Equation (4.30) is well-known as the bending or flexural equation, which can be used for the design of beams based on strength as well as stiffness.

Know More

4.4.7 Determination of bending stresses

Knowing the bending moment M induced at the given beam cross-section and the sectional property I, one can obtain the distribution of the bending stress as a linear function of the distance from the neutral axis y. From Eq. (4.30),

$$f = -\frac{My}{I}, \tag{4.31}$$

where the bending moment M at the given section is either specified or one can evaluate at the desired location along the length of the beam for the given loading situation. It is to be noted that the distance y measured above the neutral axis is positive and that below it is negative. It is seen from Eq. (4.31) that for a positive bending moment M, the fibres above the neutral axis are subjected to compressive bending stress. The maximum compressive bending stress is induced at the fibre located at the farthest distance from the neutral axis, *i.e.*, at the top fibre. The fibres below the neutral axis are subjected to tensile bending stress with the maximum value at the bottom fibre. If the bending moment M at the beam cross-section is negative, the fibres above the neutral axis are subjected to tensile bending stress with the maximum value at the top fibre. On the other hand, the fibres below the neutral axis are subjected to compressive bending stress with the maximum value at the bottom fibre. The typical distribution of bending stress in a beam cross-section with only a vertical axis of symmetry due to positive and negative bending moments are shown in Fig. 4.6. If the cross-section of the beam is symmetric about both vertical and horizontal axes (y and z), *e.g*, a rectangular section, then the magnitudes of the maximum tensile and compressive bending stresses at the extreme fibres are the same. This is because the distance of the extreme fibres at the extreme top and bottom fibres from the neutral axis is the same for such cross-sections.

A general procedure for determining bending stresses at a point in a beam cross-section is as follows:

a) Evaluate the bending moment M at the desired section of the beam.

b) Locate the neutral axis of the cross-section. This is same as locating the centroidal axis.
c) Determine the second moment of area of the cross-section about neutral axis.
d) Locate the y coordinate of the point on the given cross-section, *i.e.*, the distance from neutral axis.
e) Use Eq. (4.31) to evaluate the bending stress f.

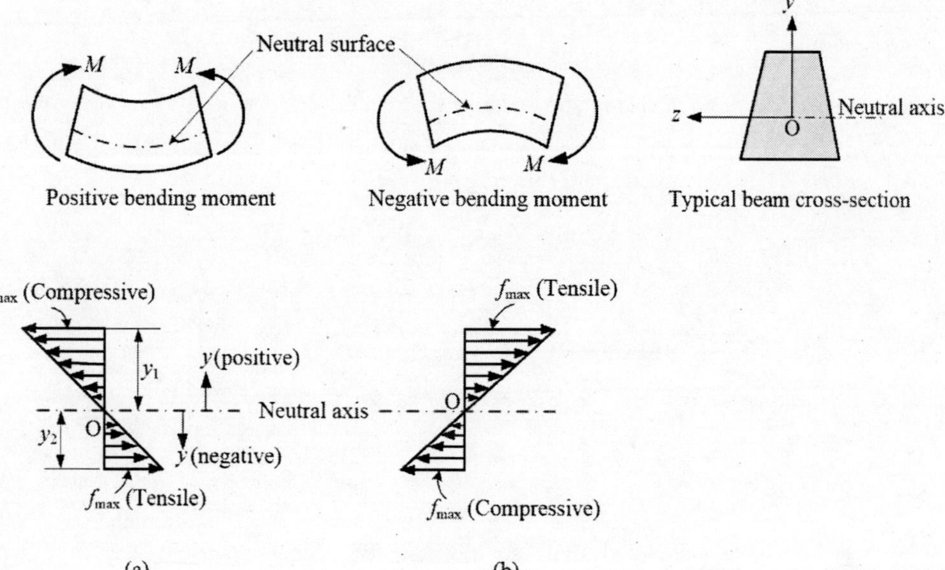

Fig. 4.6 Bending stress distribution in a typical beam cross-section subjected to (a) positive bending moment, (b) negative bending moment.

4.4.8 Limitations of bending equation

The bending or flexural equation developed in this unit is valid for the case of pure bending of a prismatic beam under certain simplified assumptions as stated in Subsection 4.4.1. Further, the theory is applicable for beam of homogeneous material subjected to small linearly elastic deformation. If a beam is subjected to non-uniform bending, it associates shear force in the beam cross-section along with the bending moment. In the presence of associated shear force, the beam cross-section is prone to out of plane distortion or warping. The warping of beam cross-section due to shear deformation invalidates certain assumptions that are considered in developing the present bending theory. For example, due to warping, the plane sections in the originally straight unstressed beam is no longer remain plane after bending. However, it has been established through detailed investigation that the bending stresses evaluated from the bending or flexural equation are not significantly different even in the presence of shear forces for the beams with a much greater length to depth ratio. The bending equation provides a reasonably accurate solution for bending stresses in the regions slightly away from the supports and the points of concentrated loads according to St. Venant's principle. At the points of supports and concentrated loads, localized stresses are induced which are much larger in magnitude than the stresses evaluated from the equation of pure bending.

Example 4.1 The beam loaded as shown in the figure has a rectangular cross-section of width b= 60 mm and depth h= 90 mm. Determine the maximum bending stress induced in the beam and its location.

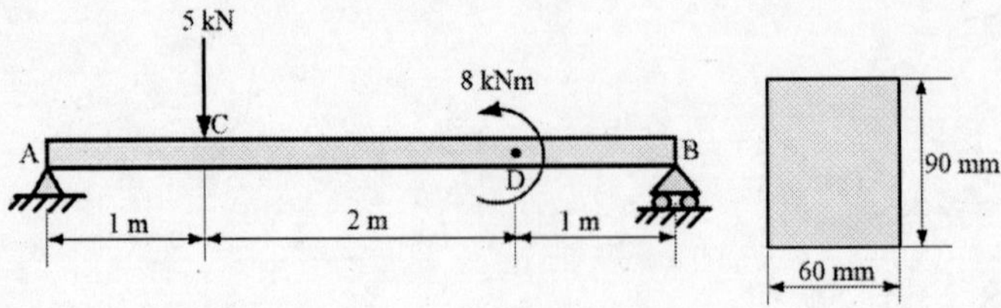

Solution

Using the equations of static equilibrium, the support reactions at A and B are obtained as

$$R_A = 5.75\text{kN}, \quad R_B = -0.75\text{kN}$$

Now, the bending moment (BM) variation over the beam span is obtained following the procedure presented in Unit 3 and is shown in the following figure.

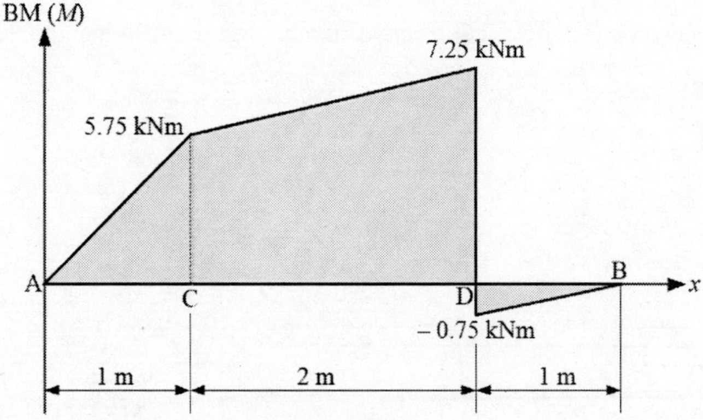

Bending moment diagram

It is clear from the BM diagram of the beam that the maximum bending moment occurs at a location just to the left of point D, which is at a distance of 3 m from the left support. The magnitude of maximum bending moment is M_{max}=7.25 kNm=7.25×10^6 Nmm. For the given rectangular beam cross-section, the extreme fibres are located at a distance of y_{max}=45 mm. The second moment of area of the section is obtained as

$$I = \frac{bh^3}{12} = \frac{60 \times 90^3}{12} = 36.45 \times 10^5 \text{ mm}^4.$$

Now, using the bending equation, the magnitude of the maximum bending stress induced in the beam is evaluated as

$$f_{max} = \frac{M_{max} y_{max}}{I} = \frac{7.25 \times 10^6 \times 45}{36.45 \times 10^5} = 89.51 \text{MPa}.$$

As the maximum bending moment acting at the section is positive, the nature of the maximum bending stress at the extreme top fibre is compressive and that at the extreme bottom fibre is tensile.

The maximum bending stress in the beam is located at a section where the bending moment is the maximum, *i.e.*, at the section which is located just to the left of point D at a distance of 3 m from the left support in the beam.

Example 4.2 The simply supported beam shown in the figure is loaded with two concentrated (point) loads each of magnitude P at a distance of 2 m from each support. Consider that the cross-section of the beam is a trapezoidal section with dimensions shown in the figure. If the maximum bending stress in the beam is limited to 90 MPa, find the maximum magnitude of P.

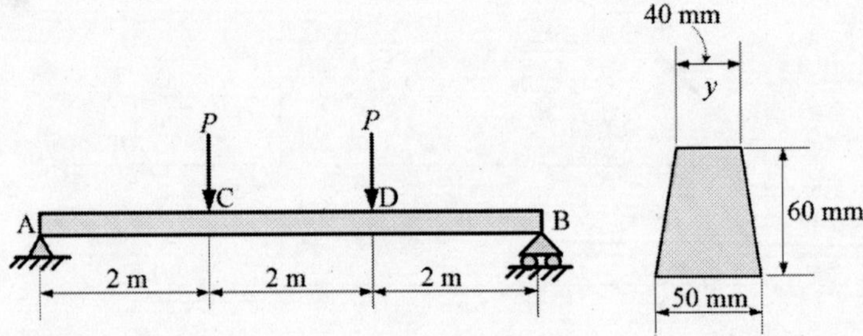

Solution

First, the bending moment diagram for the beam is constructed and is shown in the figure. The maximum bending moment (M_{max}) induced in the beam is equal to $2P$ Nm and occurs at any section in the segment CD. Next, the neutral axis of the beam section is located, which is the centroidal axis of the section. The z-coordinate of the centroidal axis lies on the y-axis of symmetry. Let the y coordinate of the centroid from the bottom fibre of the section is y_2. Dividing the trapezoidal section into two triangular areas and one rectangular area, the coordinate y_2 is obtained as

$$y_2 = \frac{2\left(\frac{1}{2}\times 5\times 60\times \frac{60}{3}\right)+40\times 60\times 30}{2\left(\frac{1}{2}\times 5\times 60\right)+40\times 60} = 28.89\,\text{mm}.$$

One can also directly use the following formula to obtain y_1 (see the figure for the meaning of a, b and h):

$$y_2 = \frac{(b+2a)h}{3(a+b)} = \frac{(50+2\times 40)60}{3(40+50)} = 28.89\,\text{mm}.$$

Thus, the neutral axis is located at a distance of y_2= 28.89 mm from the extreme bottom fibre. The intersection of the neutral axis with the symmetric y-axis, *i.e.*, point O is the centroid of the section. The distance of the extreme top fibre from the neutral axis is y_1=60–28.89=31.11 mm.

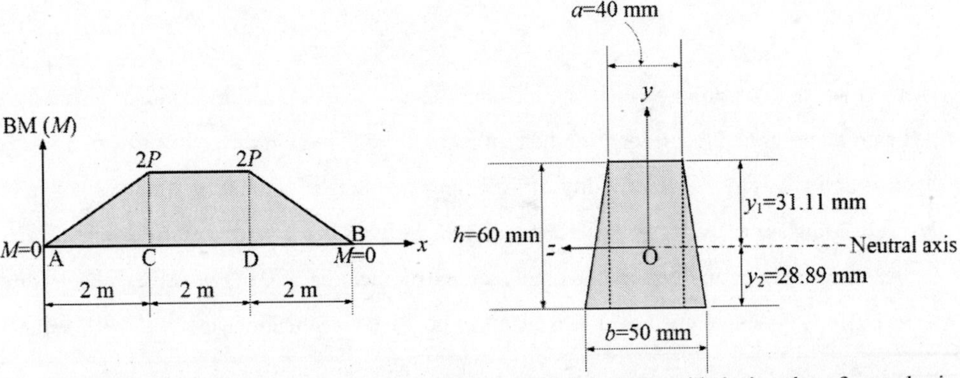

Bending moment diagram

Cross-section of the beam with the location of neutral axis

Using the parallel axis theorem, the second moment of area of the section about the neutral axis is obtained as

$$I=\frac{h^3\left(a^2+4ab+b^2\right)}{36(a+b)}=\frac{60^3\left(40^2+4\times 40\times 50+50^2\right)}{36(40+50)}=80.67\times 10^4\ \text{mm}^4.$$

The maximum bending stress in the beam is induced at any section in the segment CD for the given loading situation. The maximum compressive bending stress occurs at the extreme top fibre and the maximum tensile bending stress occurs at the extreme bottom fibre. In the present case, the magnitude of the maximum bending stress is the maximum compressive bending stress as the top fibre of the section is located at the farthest distance from the neutral axis and it is given by

$$\left|f_{\max}\right|=\frac{M_{\max}y_2}{I}.$$

It is given that the limiting value of the maximum bending stress is 150 MPa. Thus, equating the right hand side of the above equation to the limiting value of the maximum bending stress, one obtains the maximum magnitude of P as

$$50=\frac{2P\times 10^3\times 31.11}{80.67\times 10^4},$$

$$P=1.94\ \text{kN}.$$

4.5 The Flexural Rigidity

From the bending equation (Eq. (4.13)), one can write

$$\frac{1}{R}=\frac{M}{EI}, \tag{4.32}$$

where $1/R$ is the curvature of the beam. The product of the Young's modulus of elasticity of the beam material and the second moment of area of cross-section of the beam, *i.e.*, EI in Eq. (4.32) is called as the flexural rigidity of the beam and is measured in the SI unit of Nm^2. The flexural rigidity of a beam is always a positive quantity. Therefore, the sign for curvature of the beam depends on the direction of the bending moment M. If M is positive, the curvature of the beam is concave upwards and is taken as positive. On the other hand, if M is negative, the curvature of the beam is convex upwards and is taken as negative.

The flexural rigidity of a beam provides the measure of stiffness of the beam that signifies the resistance offered by the member against bending. It is seen from Eq. (4.32) that the curvature of the beam is inversely related to the flexural rigidity. The higher the value of flexural rigidity, the smaller is the curvature of the beam. For a given curvature, bending stress is not proportional to flexural rigidity, rather it is proportional to Young's modulus. For a given bending moment, bending stress is inversely proportional to I.

4.6 The Section Modulus

The absolute magnitude of maximum bending stresses at the extreme top and bottom fibres of any beam cross-section can be expressed from Eq. (4.31) as

$$f_{\max}=\frac{My_{\max}}{I}=\frac{M}{Z}, \tag{4.33}$$

where y_{max} denotes the distance of the extreme top or bottom fibre of the section from the neutral axis and

$$Z=\frac{I}{y_{\max}}. \tag{4.34}$$

The quantity Z in Eq. (4.34) which is the ratio of the second moment of area to the distance of the extreme fibre from the neutral axis of a section is known as the section modulus. The section modulus of a cross-section is expressed in the unit of length to the third power, *e.g.*, m^3, mm^3. As I and y_{max} are the beam's cross-sectional properties, the section modulus Z is also a cross-sectional property of the beam. Expressing the maximum bending stress in terms of section modulus is advantageous as it combines the relevant cross-sectional properties of the beam into a single quantity, which is very convenient to be used by the designers for the design of beam cross-sections. In calculating the section modulus, the distances of the top and bottom fibres from the neutral axis are always taken as positive quantities.

The maximum bending moment that can be carried by a beam cross-section of a particular shape for any given maximum bending stress is expressed from Eq. (4.33) as

$$M = Zf_{max}. \tag{4.35}$$

Equation (4.35) states that the higher is the value of section modulus Z for cross-section of a particular shape, the higher is the bending moment carrying capacity of the beam for a given maximum bending stress.

For cross-sections with both axes of symmetry, y_{max} is same for both top and bottom fibre. Thus, taking $y_{max}=y$, one can define only one value of section modulus from Eq. (4.34). The corresponding maximum bending stresses at the top and bottom fibre of the cross-section subjected to positive bending moment M are given by

$$f_{max1} = -\frac{My}{I} = -\frac{M}{Z}, \qquad f_{max2} = \frac{My}{I} = \frac{M}{Z}, \tag{4.36}$$

where f_{max1}, f_{max2} represent the maximum bending stresses at the extreme top and bottom fibres, respectively. Knowing that the bending stress is zero at the neutral axis and it varies linear along y-direction, bending stress can be calculated at any point.

For a beam cross-section with only a vertical axis of symmetry only, if y_1 is the distance of the top fibre and y_2 is the distance of the bottom fibre, respectively from the neutral axis as shown in Fig. 4.6 (a), then one has to define two values of section moduli corresponding to the maximum compressive and tensile bending stresses as

$$Z_1 = \frac{I}{y_1}, \qquad Z_2 = \frac{I}{y_2}. \tag{4.37}$$

Accordingly, the maximum bending stresses at the extreme top and bottom fibres of the cross-section subjected to positive bending moment M are given by

$$f_{max1} = -\frac{M}{Z_1}, \qquad f_{max2} = \frac{M}{Z_2}. \tag{4.38}$$

As a conservative approach, the lower value of the section modulus can be taken for calculating the critical stress.

4.7 Section Modulus of Various Beam Cross-sections

In this section, the section moduli of various beam cross-sections are derived. This will serve as the ready references for students as well as practicing engineers for design of typical beam cross-sections. First, the simplest form of cross-sections, *e.g.*, the rectangular and circular (both solid and hollow) are considered. Next, it is extended for the composite beam cross-sections of practical importance, *e.g.*, I-section and T-section.

4.7.1 Rectangular section

Let us consider a solid rectangular section of width b and height h as shown in Fig. 4.7 (a). The second moment of area of cross-section about the neutral axis is

$$I = \frac{bh^3}{12}. \tag{4.39}$$

For rectangular cross-section, $y_{max}=h/2$. Substituting I and y_{max} in Eq. (4.34), the section modulus is obtained as

$$Z = \frac{bh^2}{6}. \tag{4.40}$$

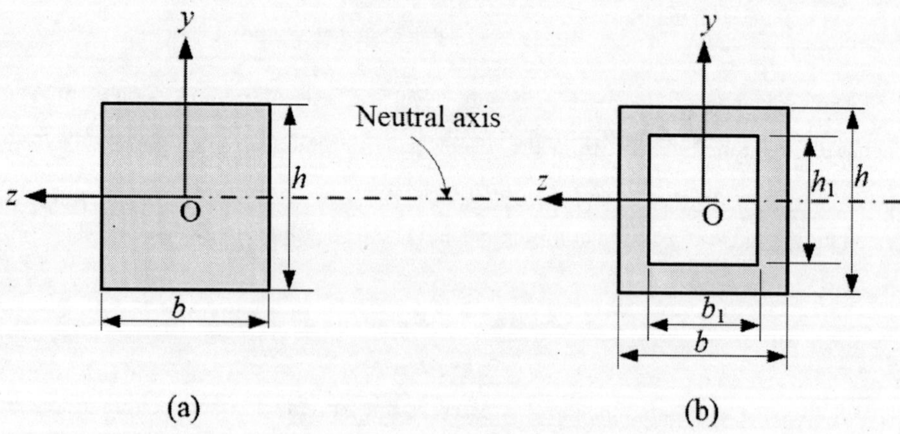

Fig. 4.7 Rectangular section: (a) solid and (b) hollow

If one considers a hollow rectangular section with dimensions shown in Fig. 4.7 (b), the second moment of the area of cross-section about the neutral axis is given by

$$I = \frac{bh^3}{12} - \frac{b_1h_1^3}{12}. \tag{4.41}$$

Using Eq. (4.34), the section modulus of the hollow rectangular section can be obtained as

$$Z = \frac{bh^2}{6} - \frac{b_1h_1^3}{6h}. \tag{4.42}$$

4.7.2 Circular section

Let us consider a solid circular cross-section of a beam with diameter d as shown in Fig. 4.8 (a). The second moment of area of the cross-section about the neutral axis is given by

$$I = \frac{\pi d^4}{64}. \tag{4.43}$$

For the solid circular section $y_{max}=d/2$. Thus, from Eq. (4.34) the section modulus is determined as

$$Z = \frac{\pi d^3}{32}. \tag{4.44}$$

Considering a hollow circular section with inner diameter d_1 and outer diameter d_2 as shown in Fig. 4.8 (b), the second moment of the area about the neutral axis can be expressed as

$$I = \frac{\pi}{64}\left(d_2^4 - d_1^4\right). \tag{4.45}$$

Here, $y_{max}=d_2/2$. Substituting the value of y_{max} and Eq. (4.45) in Eq. (4.34), the section modulus for a hollow circular section is obtained as

$$Z = \frac{\pi}{32d_2}\left(d_2^4 - d_1^4\right). \tag{4.46}$$

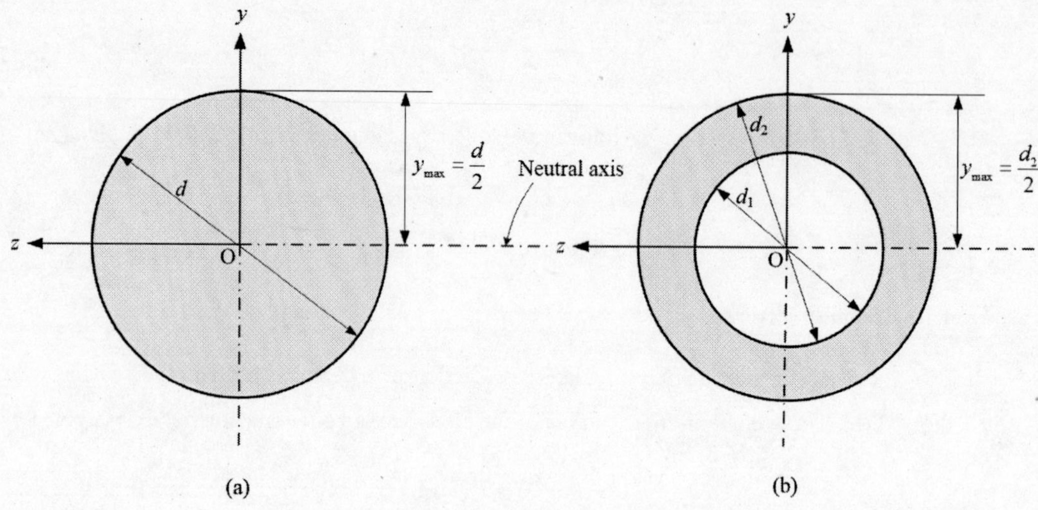

Fig. 4.8 Circular section: (a) Solid and (b) hollow

4.7.3 I-section

An I-section with various dimensions is shown in Fig. 4.9. As the section is symmetric about both horizontal and vertical axes, the horizontal axis of symmetry, *i.e.*, z-axis is the neutral axis for the section. Referring to Fig. 4.9, the second moment of area of the I-section about the neutral axis can be evaluated by subtracting the second moment of the area $(b-t)\times h_1$ from the second moment of the area of the entire rectangular section of dimension $b\times h$ and is obtained as

$$I = \frac{bh^3}{12} - \frac{(b-t)h_1^3}{12} = \frac{1}{12}\left(bh^3 - bh_1^3 + th_1^3\right). \tag{4.47}$$

The location of the extreme top and bottom fibres of the cross-section is at a distance of $y_{max}=h/2$. Thus, the section modulus from Eq. (4.34) can be evaluated as

$$Z = \frac{1}{6h}\left(bh^3 - bh_1^3 + th_1^3\right). \tag{4.48}$$

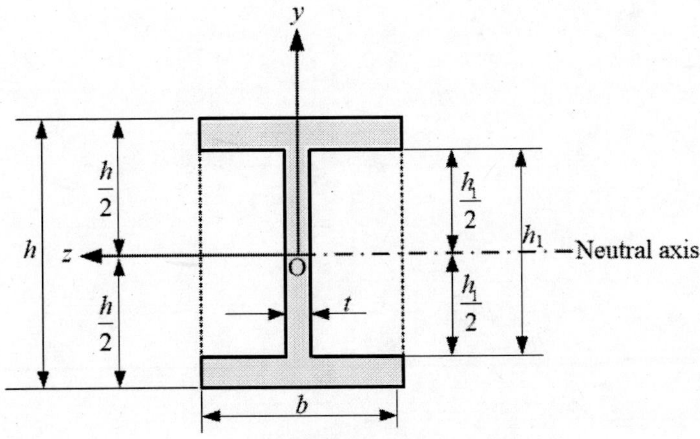

Fig. 4.9 An I-section

4.7.4 T-section

A T-section with different dimensions is shown in Fig. 4.10. The T-section is a composite area connected by two rectangular areas of $h \times t_1$ and $b \times t_2$, respectively. Using the procedures presented in Subsection 4.3.1, the y coordinate of the centroid is evaluated as y_2 from the bottom fibre of the section as shown in Fig. 4.10. Thus, the centroidal z axis is located, which is the neutral axis of the section. Once y_2 is known, the distance of the top fibre from the neutral axis, *i.e.*, y_1, can be easily evaluated. The z coordinate of the centroid is obvious due to vertical axis of symmetry.

Using the parallel axis theorem presented in Subsection 4.3.2, the second moments of the areas of the two rectangular areas of the T-section about the neutral axis are evaluated first and then the quantities are algebraically added to obtain the second moment of the area of the entire section about the neutral axis. Thus, one obtains the second moment of the area of the T-section about the neutral axis as

$$I = \frac{t_1 h^3}{12} + ht_1 \left\{ \frac{bt_2 (h+b)}{2(ht_1 + bt_2)} \right\}^2 + \frac{bt_2^{\ 3}}{12} + bt_2 \left\{ \frac{ht_1 (h+t_2)}{2(ht_1 + bt_2)} \right\}^2 ,$$

$$I = \frac{1}{12}\left(t_1 h^3 + bt_2^{\ 3}\right) + \frac{bht_1 t_2}{4(ht_1 + bt_2)^2} \left\{ bt_2 (h+b)^2 + ht_1 (h+t_2)^2 \right\}. \tag{4.49}$$

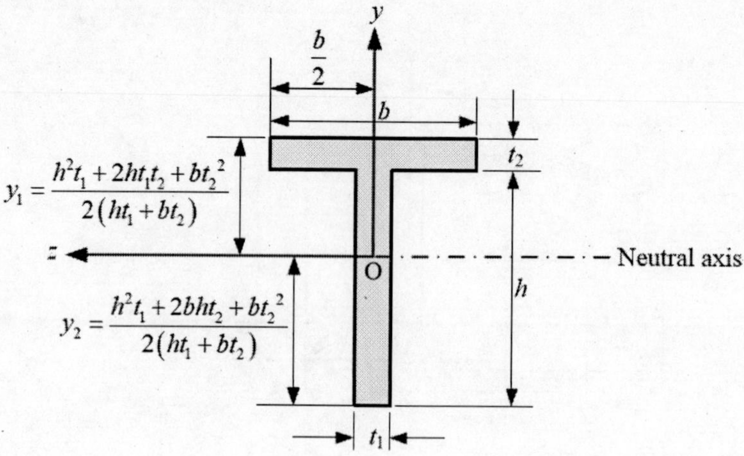

Fig. 4.10 A T-section

For the present cross-section, one has to evaluate two values of section moduli to determine the maximum bending stresses at the top and bottom fibres. Using Eq. (4.37), the section moduli are obtained as

$$Z_1 = \left[\frac{1}{6}\left(t_1h^3 + bt_2^3\right) + \frac{bht_1t_2}{2\left(ht_1 + bt_2\right)^2}\left\{bt_2\left(h+b\right)^2 + ht_1\left(h+t_2\right)^2\right\}\right]\frac{\left(ht_1 + bt_2\right)}{h^2t_1 + 2ht_1t_2 + bt_2^2}, \quad (4.50)$$

$$Z_2 = \left[\frac{1}{6}\left(t_1h^3 + bt_2^3\right) + \frac{bht_1t_2}{2\left(ht_1 + bt_2\right)^2}\left\{bt_2\left(h+b\right)^2 + ht_1\left(h+t_2\right)^2\right\}\right]\frac{\left(ht_1 + bt_2\right)}{h^2t_1 + 2bht_2 + bt_2^2}.$$

(4.51)

In a similar manner, the section moduli for other beam cross-sections such as angle or L-section, channel sections etc. can be evaluated.

Example 4.3 A channel section for a steel beam with dimensions is shown in the figure. Calculate the section moduli of the beam. If the beam is to support a uniformly distributed load of q N/m, over a simply supported span of 3 m, find the value of q, if the allowable stress for steel is 160 MPa.

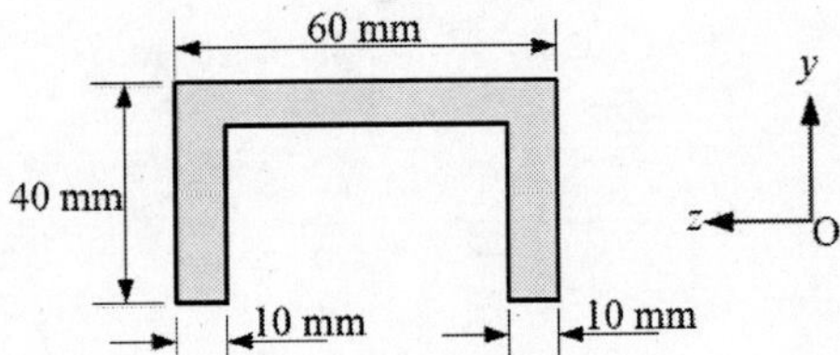

Solution

The neutral axis of the section is located by evaluating the y coordinate of the centroid from the extreme bottom fibres which is obtained as

$$y_2 = \frac{(40\times10)\times20+(40\times10)(30+5)+40\times10\times20}{3(40\times10)} = 25\,\text{mm}.$$

The z coordinate of the centroid lies on the vertical axis of symmetry. The neutral axis thus is located at a distance of y_1=15 mm from the extreme top fibre and y_2=25 mm from the extreme bottom fibres as depicted in the following figure.

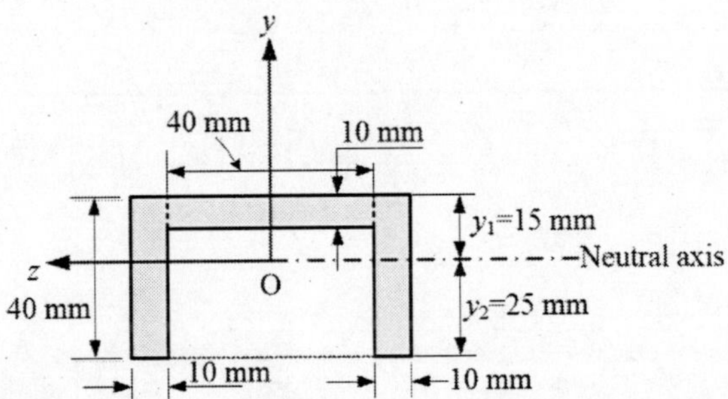

The second moment of area of the section (I) about neutral axis can be obtained by evaluating the second moment of area of the each of the three rectangular area firming the channel section about the neutral axis using the parallel axis theorem and then adding them algebraically. Thus, one obtains

$$I = 2\left\{\frac{10\times40^3}{12}+(40\times10)(20-15)^2\right\}+\frac{40\times10^3}{12}+(40\times10)(15-5)^2 = 1.7\times10^5\ \text{mm}^4.$$

As the section is not symmetric about the horizontal axis, the extreme top and bottom fibres are subjected to different magnitudes of maximum bending stresses. Thus, two values of the section moduli are evaluated as

$$Z_1 = \frac{I}{y_1} = \frac{1.7\times10^5}{15} = 1.13\times10^4\ \text{mm}^3,$$

$$Z_2 = \frac{I}{y_2} = \frac{1.7\times10^5}{25} = 6.8\times10^3\ \text{mm}^3.$$

If the beam is to support a uniformly distributed load of q N/m, over a simply supported span of 3 m, the maximum bending moment occurs at the mid span and its value is

$$M_{\max} = \frac{qL^2}{8} = \frac{q\times3^2}{8} = \frac{9q}{8}\ \text{Nm}.$$

The allowable bending stress for steel beam is 160 MPa. Now, as the magnitude of maximum bending stress for the given section occurs at the extreme bottom fibres, we get

$$\left(f_{\max}\right)_{allowable} = \frac{M_{\max}}{Z_2},$$

$$160\times10^6 = \frac{\frac{9q}{8}}{6.8\times10^3\times10^{-9}},$$

$$q = 967\ \text{N/m}.$$

Thus, the desired value of the uniformly distributed load should not exceed 967 N/m.

4.8 The Economical Beam Sections

In order to illustrate the beam of economical sections, it is important to understand the distribution of bending stresses in a beam cross-section. As an example, let us consider a rectangular beam section of width 200 mm and height 300 mm as shown in Fig. 4.11 (a). Now, if the beam is subjected to a positive bending moment, the bending stress in the section distributes linearly according to the bending equation as depicted in Fig. 4.11 (b). The material at the mid region of the rectangular beam section is stressed less in comparison to top and bottom fibre. This means that the material at the mid region is not fully utilized in carrying the bending moment. Consequently, some materials from the mid region of the rectangular section can be removed and allow the materials to concentrate away from the neutral axis. It is obvious that in order to get an integrated area of connected sections, one cannot remove material fully from the mid-section. Thus, a mere possibility is that to arrive at an I-section of the same cross-sectional area as the original rectangular section as shown in Fig. 4.11 (c). By doing so the contribution of the second moment of area of the section is increased, which provides more resistance to bending. This aspect can easily be seen from the present example. The second moment of area of the rectangular section is evaluated as

$$I = \frac{bh^3}{12} = \frac{200 \times 300^3}{12} = 4.5 \times 10^8 \text{ mm}^4.$$

The second moment of area of the corresponding I-section of same cross-sectional area as that of the rectangular section can be evaluated using Eq. (4.47) and is obtained as

$$I = \frac{1}{12}\left(200 \times 500^3 - 200 \times 400^3 + 10 \times 400^3\right) = 10.70 \times 10^8 \text{ mm}^4.$$

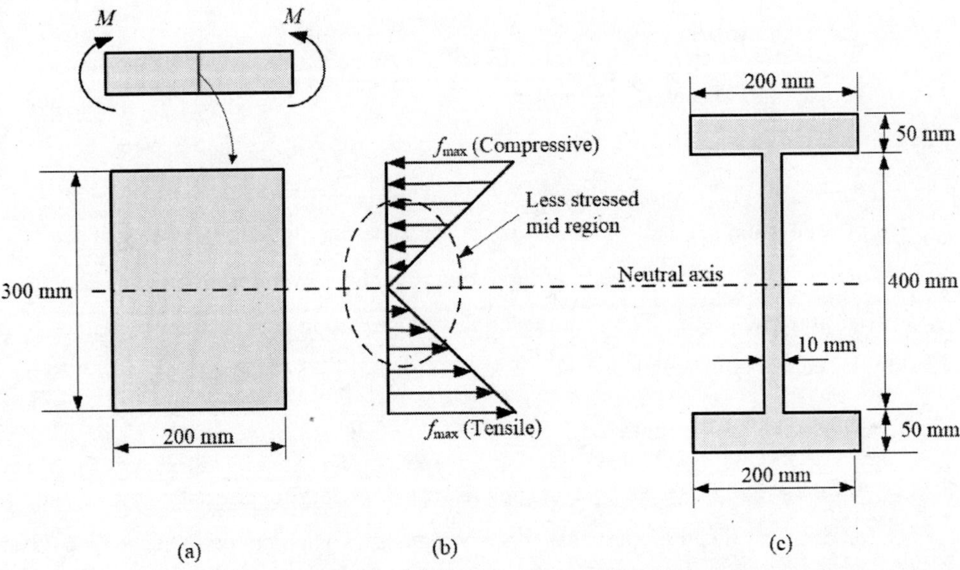

Fig. 4.11 (a) A rectangular beam section, (b) representative bending stress distribution and (c) I-section modified from the rectangular section.

It is seen that the modified I-section of the beam which was obtained by removing material from the mid region of the rectangular section and concentrating the material away from the neutral axis has the higher value of the second moment of the area as compared to that of the corresponding rectangular area. In the present case, it is more than two times than that of its rectangular counterpart. Thus, it follows from the bending equation that the maximum bending stress induced in the beam of I-section is much lesser as compared to that induced in the corresponding beam of rectangular cross-section for the same value of bending moment. This signifies that the beam with I-section is capable of carrying more bending moment. Thus, the I-section is more efficient so far as the bending moment carrying capacity is concerned. Such sections are also termed as the economical beam section. The economical I-section finds a wide range of applications, for instance, beams used to support bridge deck and the cos-section of rails used in railway lines.

Know More

4.9 Design of simple beam sections

The design of simple beam sections is considered here from the standpoints of strength and stiffness. The design task is to determine or select a suitable shape and size of the beam cross-sections such that the maximum bending stresses induced in the beam do not exceed the allowable stress of the material. At the same time, the designer should also keep the deflection of the beam to a narrow limit and thus the curvature of the beam should not exceed an allowable limit. The bending or flexural equation can be used to design beam sections based on both strength and stiffness.

4.9.1 Design based on strength

While designing a beam section for resisting bending, one usually begins with the evaluation of the sectional property called section modulus as described in Section 4.6. Using Eq. (4.35), one can evaluate the desired section modulus Z by dividing the maximum bending moment by the allowable bending stress of the given material, i.e.,

$$Z = \frac{M_{\max}}{f_{\text{allowable}}}. \tag{4.52}$$

The allowable stress for a material is based on the material properties such as yield stress and a suitably selected factor of safety for the desired application. It is worth noting that for a beam with cross-sections symmetric about both vertical and horizontal axis, the allowable bending stress is the same in tension and compression. In this case, one can directly use Eq. (4.52) to evaluate Z. Once the value of Z is known, the suitable size or dimensions of the given cross-section can be obtained by using Eq. (4.34) ensuring that the induced bending stress is not exceeded the allowable limit.

If the beam section is symmetric about only vertical axis, the maximum bending stresses are different in tension and compression and accordingly two values of section moduli are defined. In this case, one has to obtain the size of a given section satisfying both the criterions. This means that the designed dimensions must keep the maximum bending stresses in tension and compression within the allowable limit.

4.9.2 Design based on stiffness

For the design of beams based on stiffness, an allowable condition is usually imposed on the deflection requirement. The deflection of a beam is governed by the geometric parameter called curvature, which can be evaluated from the bending equation as given by Eq. (4.32). Thus, the design of beam cross-sections using bending equation involves specifying the limit of the curvature. First, for the given loading situation, the maximum bending moment induced in the beam is estimated and then it is substituted in Eq. (4.32) along with the flexural rigidity of the beam in terms of the cross-sectional dimensions of the beam and equated it to the specified curvature. This provides the required size or dimension of the given cross-section. It is important to note that if for a beam, both the strength and curvature requirement is specified, the size of the beam section should be such that satisfies both the criteria.

One has to obtain the dimensions of a given beam section to meet the requirements of strength or stiffness or both. The beams are made with a wide variety of cross-sections to suit a number of specific applications. In many instances, one will find handbooks/manuals where the standardized dimensions and properties such as weight, cross-sectional area, second moment of area and section modulus of many kinds of beam cross-sections are listed. For example, the American Institute of Steel Construction (AISC) publishes manuals providing standardized shapes and sizes of structural steel beams. Once the section modulus is evaluated based on the allowable bending stress and maximum bending moment, one may also consider to select a suitable shape and size of the beam cross-section from the available handbooks/manuals to meet the design requirements.

Example 4.4 Consider a vertical post height of 3 m. The post is to be designed for supporting a lateral load P =20 kN at its top end as depicted in the figure. If the post is proposed to construct with a hollow steel circular cross-section, determine the minimum required outer diameter d_2 of the steel tube if its ratio of the outer diameter to the wall thickness is 10 and the allowable bending stress in the steel is 150 MPa?

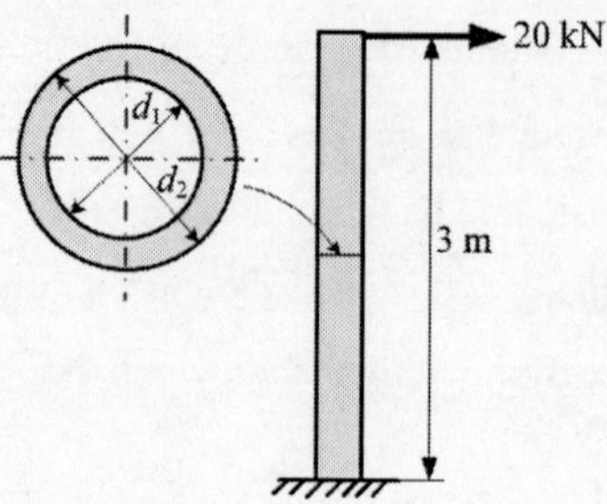

Solution

The post can be considered as a cantilever with load P=20 kN at its free top end and the bottom fixed to the ground. The span of the cantilever is h=3 m. Thus, the maximum bending moment occurs at the bottom of the post and is given by

$$M_{max} = Ph = 20 \times 3 = 60 \text{kNm}$$

To determine the section modulus Z_2 for the hollow circular post, one should first determine the second moment of area I of the cross-section about the neutral axis. The wall thickness of the hollow circular post is $d_2/10=0.1d_2$. Thus, the inner diameter of the post is $d_1=0.8d_2$. The second moment of area of the hollow circular section is calculated as

$$I = \frac{\pi}{64}\left(d_2^4 - d_1^4\right) = \frac{\pi}{64}\left\{d_2^4 - \left(0.8d_2\right)^4\right\} = 0.02897\, d_2^4.$$

The section modulus Z_2 is evaluated as

$$Z_2 = \frac{I}{\frac{d_2}{2}} = \frac{0.02897\, d_2^4}{\frac{d_2}{2}} = 0.05794 d_2^3.$$

Now,

$$Z_2 = \frac{M_{max}}{f_{allowable}},$$

$$0.05794 d_2^3 = \frac{60 \times 10^6}{150},$$

$$d_2 = 190.41 \text{mm}.$$

Thus the required outer diameter is 190.41 mm.

4.10 Summary

In this unit, the theory of simple bending is discussed. The bending or flexural equation is derived based on certain simplified assumptions for pure bending. It is seen that the bending normal stress over the cross-section of a beam varies linearly with distance from the neutral axis or neutral surface. A neutral axis is one which is stress free and remains undeformed after bending. Further, the bending equation shows that the bending stress is directly proportional to the bending moment M and the second moment of the area of cross-section I. The developed pure bending theory can reasonably be used to calculate bending stress in beams subjected to non-uniform bending as well. The terms flexural rigidity and section modulus are also discussed. The flexural rigidity of a beam provides some measure of stiffness of the beam. The section modulus for different cross-sections is determined, which may serve as the ready reference in designing beam cross-sections. At the end, the general guidelines for the design of simple beam sections are discussed based on the strength and stiffness approach.

Know More

Exercises

Multiple Choice Questions

4.1 Consider two beams one with a square cross-section and other with a circular cross-section subjected to equal bending moment. If the side of the square section is a and r is the radius of the circular section, then the ratio of the section modulus of the circular section to the section modulus of square section is

(a) $\frac{3}{2}$ (b) $\frac{3}{2\sqrt{\pi}}$

(c) $\dfrac{2}{3\sqrt{\pi}}$

(d) $\dfrac{2}{3}$

4.2 In Q. 4.1,

(a) the square beam is stronger than the circular beam in carrying the bending moment.

(b) the circular beam is stronger than the square beam in carrying the bending moment.

(c) Both the beams are equally strong in carrying bending moment

(d) The relative strength of the beams depend on the nature of loading.

4.3 A high-strength steel tape of thickness 0.4 mm is bent around a cylindrical drum of diameter 1 m as shown in the figure. If Young's modulus of elasticity of steel is 200 GPa, the maximum bending stress induced in the tape is

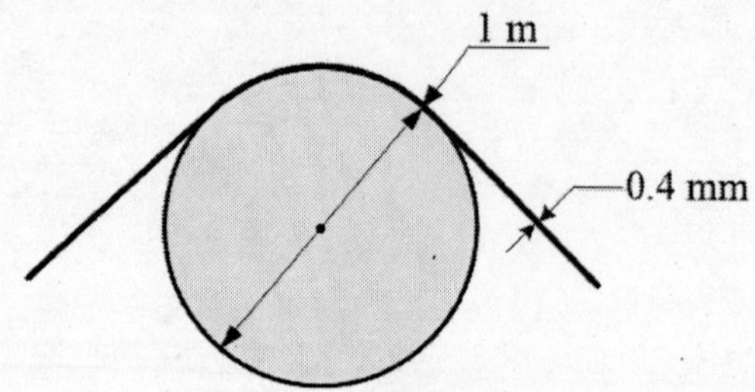

(a) 160 MPa

(b) 120 MPa

(c) 100 MPa

(d) 80 MPa

4.4 A simply supported beam of rectangular cross-section has a width of 100 mm and height 50 mm. If the beam were to be of height 100 mm and width 50 mm, then the beam would be

(a) strengthened 2 times

(b) weakened 2 times

(c) weakened 4 times

(d) strengthened 4 times

4.5 A simply supported beam is subjected to a uniformly distributed load of 3 kN/m over its entire span of 5 m. If the cross-section of the beam is an I-section as shown in the figure, the maximum bending stress induced in the beam is

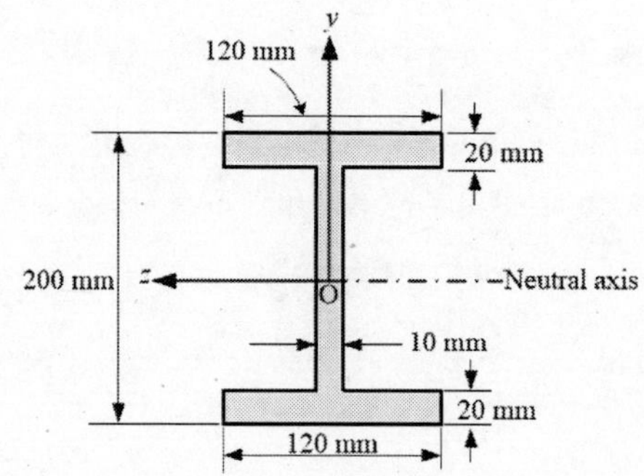

(a) 11.72 MPa (b) 22.08 MPa

(c) 23.44 MPa (d) 24 MPa

4.6 A pipe of outer diameter 60 mm and inner diameter 30 mm is subjected to a point load of 1 kN at the centre while simply supported at its ends. The section modulus of the pipe is

(a) 19.88×10^3 mm^3 (b) 21.20×10^3 mm^3

(c) 2.65×10^3 mm^3 (d) 19.88×10^3 mm^4

4.7 If the span of the pipe is 3 m in Q. 4.6, then the maximum bending stress induced in the pipe is

(a) 79.62 MPa (b) 75.45 MPa

(c) 39.81 MPa (d) 37.73 MPa

4.8 A cantilever steel beam of length 2 m with a rectangular cross-section has a width 40 mm and a depth 60 mm. The beam is subjected to a point load of 180 N at the free end. If the Young's modulus of elasticity of steel is 200 GPa, the flexural rigidity of the beam is

(a) 14.4×10^7 Nmm^2 (b) 14.4×10^9 Nmm^2

(c) 14.4×10^{10} Nmm^2 (d) 3.6 Nmm^2

4.9 In Q. 4.8, the maximum bending stress induced in the beam is

(a) 33.75 MPa (b) 22.5 MPa

(c) 20 MPa (d) 15 MPa

4.10 In Q. 4.8, if the beam cross-section is made to be of a circular cross-section of the same area as that of the rectangular cross-section, what would be the maximum bending stress induced in the beam?

(a) 15 MPa (b) 21.71 MPa

(c) 24.42 MPa (d) 43.41 MPa

Answers of Multiple Choice Questions

4.1 (b), 4.2 (a), 4.3 (d), 4.4 (a), 4.5 (b), 4.6 (a), 4.7 (d), 4.8 (c), 4.9 (d), 4.10 (b).

Short and Long Answer Type Questions

Category I

4.1 What do you mean by pure bending?

4.2 What is the physical significance of the second moment of area of a cross-section?

4.3 What is polar moment of inertia?

4.4 State the assumptions of pure bending theory.

4.5 Consider a beam subjected to pure bending. Draw the Mohr's circle of stress for any generic point on the surface of the beam.

4.6 What is flexural rigidity? How does it influence bending stress?

4.7. What is section modulus? How does it influence bending stress?

4.8 Consider the following two configurations of a rectangular cross-section of a beam. In which case, the resistance to bending is more? Justify your answer.

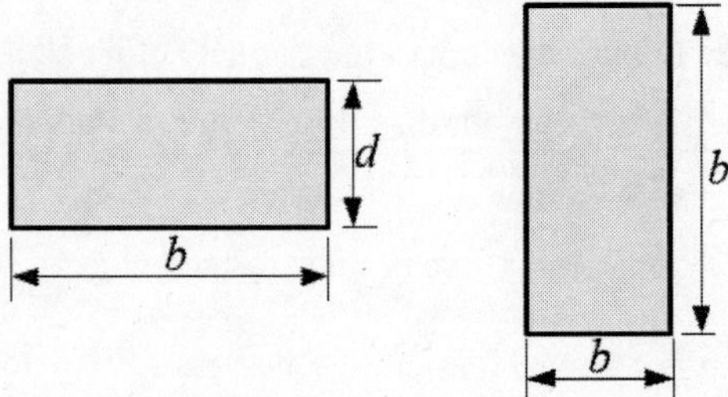

Category II

4.9 Derive the flexural equation. Discuss the application of the flexural equation in the design of beam.

4.10 Why are I-sections preferred in engineering applications when it has to carry bending load? Elaborate your answer.

Numerical Problems

4.11 A beam of triangular cross-section is subjected to pure bending. Derive an expression of second moment of area of the cross-section about its neural axis parallel to its base. The length of the base is b and the height of the triangle is h. Also, obtain the expressions for section moduli. If this beam subjected a pure bending moment such that base side is subjected to tension and opposite vertex to compression, find out the ratio of the magnitudes of maximum tensile and maximum compressive stresses.

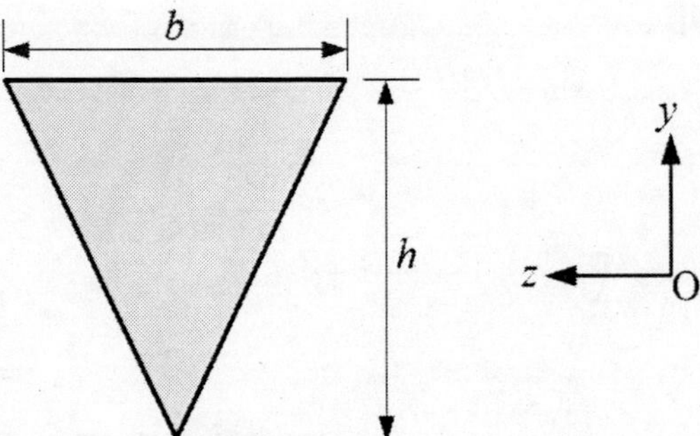

4.12 A steel belt of 0.1 mm thickness and 10 mm width passes on a pulley of 200 mm diameter and 10 mm width. Find out the maximum bending stress on the belt. Take Young's modulus of steel as 210 GPa. What will the impact on the maximum bending stress, if the width of the belt is reduced to 5 mm? What will be the impact on the bending moment coming on the belt? (Ans. $|\sigma|_{max} = 104.95\,\text{MPa}$.)

4.13 A beam is subjected to pure bending in the *xy* plane of bending, such that its top surface becomes convex with radius of curvature as 30 m. Due to Poisson's effect, the top surface will look concave in *yz* plane. Find out the anticlastic curvature of the top surface in *yz* plane, if the Poisson's ratio of the material of the beam is 0.3 and width is 40 mm.

If the width of the beam is 80 mm, find out the flatness (difference in the elevations of the highest and lowest point) in *y-z* plane. (**Ans.** anticlastic curvature=0.01 m^{-1}, flatness=8 μm)

4.14 Consider the loaded beam shown in the following figure. The beam has a rectangular cross-section with width 50 mm and depth 100 mm. If the maximum bending stress in the beam is limited to 60 MPa, then determine the load *P* in kN. If the beam cross-section is replaced by an I-section of the same area with the flange dimension of 50 mm × 10 mm and the web dimension of 10 mm × 400 mm, then what is the value of the maximum bending stress induced in the beam for the same load *P*? Also, calculate the percentage increase in the load carrying capacity of the I-section as compared to the corresponding rectangular section. (**Ans.** *P*=1.25 kN, $(f_{max})_{I\text{-section}}$=11 MPa, % increase in load carrying capacity=81.67%).

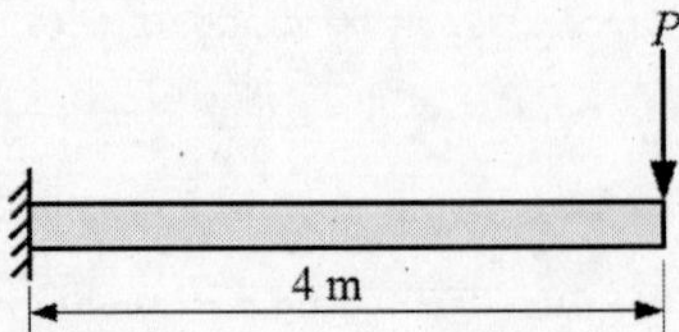

4.15 A simply supported beam of span 5 m is subjected to a uniformly distributed load of 6 kN/m. The cross-section of the beam with the dimensions is shown in the following figure. Determine the ratio of the maximum compressive to the maximum tensile bending stress induced in the beam. (Ans. 1:2)

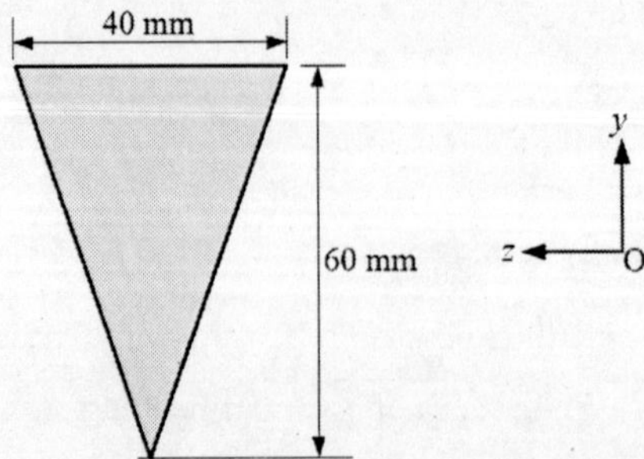

4.16 Consider a beam of rectangular cross-section with width of 60 mm cantilevered to carry a uniformly distributed load of 2 kN/m over the entire span of 3 m. Determine the required depth of the cross-section such that the maximum bending stress induced in the beam does not exceed 40 MPa. (**Ans.** 150 mm)

4.17 A Simply supported beam AB of span 3 m supports a uniformly distributed load of intensity $q = 5$ kN/m spread over the entire span and a concentrated load $P = 1$ kN placed at a distance of 1 m from the right support at B. The beam cross-section is constructed as rectangular with width $b = 80$ mm and depth $h = 160$ mm. Determine the maximum tensile and compressive stresses developed in the beam due to bending. (**Ans.** 17.96 MPa, –17.96 MPa)

4.18 Consider a skateboard (a=60 cm) carrying a 60 kg person at the middle crossing a simply supported plank of length L=1.7 m as shown in the figure below. Determine the position at which the bending moment is the maximum and its magnitude. Evaluate the maximum bending stress if the cross section of the plank is rectangular with 14 cm width and depth of 2 cm. In the figure, x is the position of the skateboard from the left end of the plank at any instant of time. Assume that $x+(a/2)>L/2$. (**Ans.** 0.7 m from the left support at A, M_{max}=169.65 Nm, 18.18 MPa)

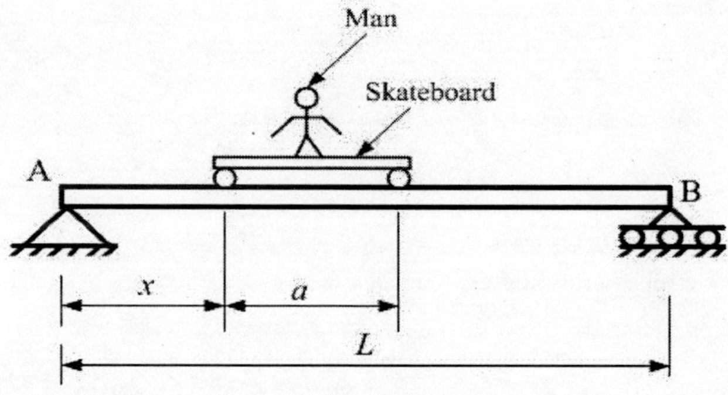

Unit 5

Shear Stresses in Beams

UNIT SPECIFICS

In this unit, the expression of shear stress variation on a beam's cross-section subjected to bending has been derived. Different types of cross-sections that are mostly used in practical settings have been considered, such as rectangular, circular, triangular, I and T angle sections.

RATIONALE

Drawing shear and moment diagrams in Unit 3 taught that shear force and bending moment act along the beam's length when a beam is subjected to a transverse load. The previous unit (Unit 4) covered the relationship between bending moments and normal stresses. However, when beams get shorter and thicker, the transverse shear stress becomes dominant in beam design. In this unit, the dependence of shear stress on the shear force is studied.

PRE-REQUISITES

Bending moment and shear force diagrams (Unit 3)

Theory of simple bending (Unit 4)

UNIT OUTCOMES

After completing this unit, students will be able to

U5-O1: Derive the general expression of shear stress due to shear force acting on a beam's cross-section

U5-O2: Identify the location on the cross-section where the shear stress is maximum for different types of cross-section

Course Outcomes	Expected Mapping with Course Outcomes - CE (1- Weak Correlation; 2- Medium correlation; 3- Strong Correlation)			
	CO-1	CO-2	CO-3	CO-4
U5-O1	-	3	3	1
U5-O2	-	2	3	1

Course Outcomes	Expected Mapping with Course Outcomes - ME (1- Weak Correlation; 2- Medium correlation; 3- Strong Correlation)	
	CO-1	CO-2
U5-O1	3	-
U5-O2	3	-

5.1 Introduction

In general, a deflecting beam is subjected to both bending moment M and shear force V acting on the cross-section. The normal stresses σ_{xx} in beams subjected to the transverse load can be found in the flexural formula. The distribution of shear stress τ on the cross-section for a prescribed shear force V will be discussed in this unit. The discussion will be limited to the elastic analysis.

5.2 Shear stress distribution in beams

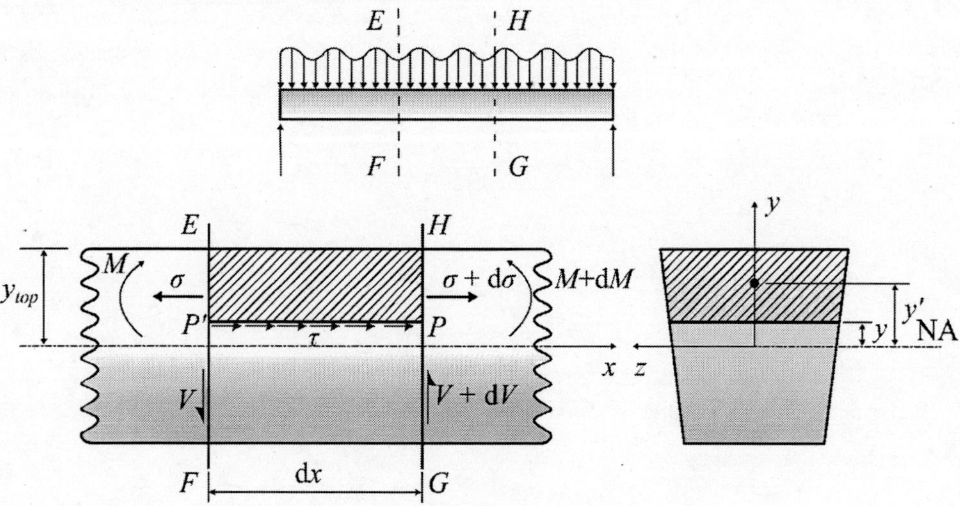

Fig. 5.1 Shear stress in a beam

The shear stress τ in a beam subjected to non-uniform bending can be obtained by considering a differential length $\mathrm{d}x$ along the longitudinal axis of the beam. Fig. 5.1 shows a beam subjected to transverse loading. The beam is cut at two locations using two cutting planes, *EF* and *GH,* which are separated by a distance $\mathrm{d}x$. A portion of the beam enclosing the two cutting plane is shown in the expanded view just below the figure of the beam. At section *EF*, let the bending moment and shear force be *M* and *V*, respectively. Likewise, in section *GH*, let the bending moment and shear force be $M+\mathrm{d}M$ and $V+\mathrm{d}V$, respectively. Let the normal stresses be σ and $\sigma+\mathrm{d}\sigma$ in the sections *EP'* and *HP,* respectively. The force equilibrium equation along the *x*-axis is used to find out the shear stress τ at the *P'P* boundary of the element *P'EHP*. The boundary *P'P* is located at a distance *y* from the neutral axis.

The axial force on the section EP' due to the normal stress σ given by

$$F_{EP'} = -\int_{y}^{y_{top}} \sigma \, \mathrm{d}A, \tag{5.1}$$

y_{top} is the distance of the top surface from the neutral axis. The negative sign in equation (5.1) indicates that the force is along the negative x-axis. The normal stress σ due to bending is related to bending moment M by

$$\sigma = -\frac{My}{I_{zz}} \tag{5.2}$$

Substituting Eq. (5.2) in Eq. (5.1):

$$F_{EP'} = \int_{y}^{y_{top}} \frac{My}{I_{zz}} \mathrm{d}A. \tag{5.3}$$

Similarly, the axial force on the section HP due to the normal stresses will be

$$F_{HP} = \int_{y}^{y_{top}} \frac{-(M + \mathrm{d}M)y}{I_{zz}} \mathrm{d}A. \tag{5.4}$$

The shear stress acts on the x-z plane containing the $P'P$ fiber. The axial force due to the shear stress τ is given by

$$F_{P'P} = -\tau t \mathrm{d}x, \tag{5.5}$$

Note that a positive shear stress is producing a force in the negative x-direction on the boundary $P'P$. The net force along the x-axis should be zero for the static equilibrium. Therefore,

$$F_{HP} + F_{EP'} + F_{P'P} = 0 \text{ or}$$

$$\int_{y}^{y_{top}} \frac{-(M + \mathrm{d}M)y}{I_{zz}} \mathrm{d}A + \int_{y}^{y_{top}} \frac{My}{I_{zz}} \mathrm{d}A - \tau t \mathrm{d}x = 0 \tag{5.6}$$

The shear stress at location y from the neutral axis is given by

$$-\tau = \frac{1}{I_{zz} t} \int_{y}^{y_{top}} \frac{\mathrm{d}M}{\mathrm{d}x} \mathrm{d}A \tag{5.7}$$

The shear force V is related to the bending moment by

$$V = -\frac{\mathrm{d}M}{\mathrm{d}x} \tag{5.8}$$

Combining Eq. (5.7) and (5.8),

$$\tau = \frac{V}{I_{zz}t}\int_{y}^{y_{top}} y\mathrm{d}A \tag{5.9}$$

The quantity $\int_{y}^{y_{top}} t\mathrm{d}A$ is the first moment of the hatched portion, i.e., the area above the location y from the neutral axis. It can be represented by $A\bar{y}$, where A is the area of hatched portion and $\bar{y}$ is the distance of the centroid of that area from the neutral axis. Finally, the shear stress is dependent on the location y from the neutral axis and is expressed as

$$\tau = \frac{VQ}{I_{zz}t} \tag{5.10}$$

where Q is the first moment of the hatched area and I_{zz} is the second moment of the cross-sectional area about the z-axis.

5.3 Shear stress distribution in rectangular cross-section

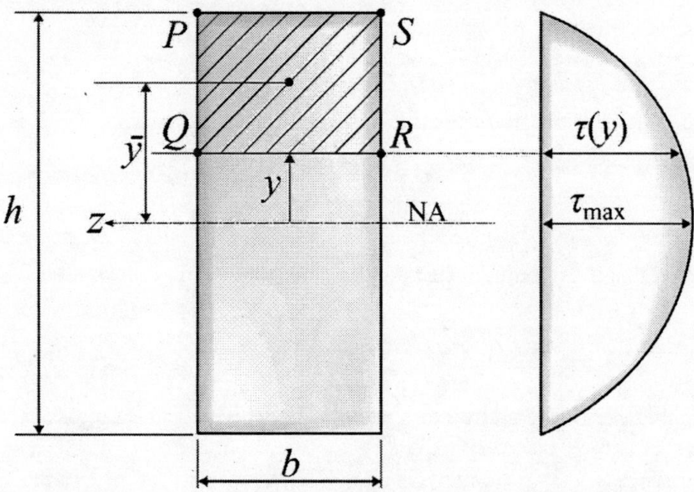

Fig. 5.2 Rectangular cross-section and shear stress profile

Consider the rectangular cross-section of the beam shown in Fig. 5.2. The width and depth of the cross-section are b and h, respectively. To calculate the shear stress at a location y from the neutral axis in a beam with a rectangular cross-section, assume a sub-section $PQRS$ as shown in Fig. **5.2**. Let A be the area of the sub-section *PQRS*. The centroid of area A is at a distance $\overline{y}$ from the neutral axis.

From Eq. (5.10), the expression for shear stress τ is given by

$$\tau = \frac{VQ}{I_{zz}t} \tag{5.11}$$

Area A is given by

$$A = b\left(\frac{h}{2} - y\right) \tag{5.12}$$

The distance from the centroid of the area to the neutral axis is given by

$$\overline{y} = \frac{1}{2}\left(\frac{h}{2} + y\right) \tag{5.13}$$

For the rectangular cross-section, the $I_{zz} = \frac{1}{12}bh^3$. Substituting Eq. (5.12) and (5.13) in Eq. (5.11),

$$\tau = \frac{VQ}{I_{zz}t} = \frac{VA\overline{y}}{I_{zz}t} = \frac{V\frac{b}{2}\left(\frac{h^2}{4} - y^2\right)}{t\frac{bh^3}{12}} = \frac{6V}{bh^3}\left(\frac{h^2}{4} - y^2\right) \tag{5.14}$$

The maximum value of the shear stress is at the neutral axis, i.e., at $y = 0$. It is given by

$$\tau_{\max} = \frac{6V}{bh^3}\left(\frac{h^2}{4} - 0\right) = \frac{3V}{2bh} \tag{5.15}$$

It is to be noted that the maximum stress is 1.5 times the average shear stress.

$$\tau_{\max} = \frac{3}{2}\tau_{\text{mean}} = \frac{3V}{2A_0} \tag{5.16}$$

where A_0 is the area of the entire cross-section. For the rectangular cross-section, it is given by $A_0 = bh$.

Example 5.1: Consider a rectangular cross-sectional beam with dimensions $b = 5$ cm and $h = 15$ cm as shown in Figure. It is subjected to a shear force V of 1 kN. Determine (a) the average and the maximum shear stress, (b) the location from the neutral axis at which the magnitude of the shear stress equals the average shear stress.

Solution: Given $h = 15$ cm, $b = 5$ cm and $V = 1$ kN.

From Eq. (5.15), τ_{max} is given by,

$$\tau_{max} = \frac{3V}{2bh} = \frac{3 \times 1 \times 10^3}{2 \times 50 \times 150}$$

$$\tau_{max} = 0.2 \text{ N/mm}^2$$

For a rectangular section, $\tau_{max} = \frac{3}{2}\tau_{average}$.. Therefore,

$$\tau_{average} = \frac{2}{3}\tau_{max} = \frac{2}{3} \times 0.2 = 0.133 \text{ N/mm}^2$$

The location from the neutral axis at which the magnitude of the shear stress equals the average shear stress can be obtained by equating

$$\frac{6V}{bh^3}\left(\frac{h^2}{4} - y^2\right) = \tau_{average}$$

$$\frac{6 \times 1000}{50 \times 150^3}\left(\frac{150^2}{4} - y^2\right) = 0.133$$

Solving for y, $y = \pm 4.34$ cm

Example 5.2: A beam of rectangular cross-section (depth h, width b) is subjected to a shear force V and bending moment M at a location. Derive the expressions to find out the location of maximum shear stress.

Solution:

Now, considering that the bending moment is M and the shear force is V, at a distance y from the neutral axis, the bending stress and the shear stress is

$$\sigma = -\frac{My}{I}, \quad \tau = \frac{V}{2I}\left(\frac{h^2}{4} - y^2\right)$$

Hence, the maximum shear stress is

$$\tau_{max} = \frac{1}{2}\sqrt{\sigma^2 + 4\tau^2} = \frac{1}{2}\sqrt{\left(\frac{My}{I}\right)^2 + \frac{V^2}{I^2}\left(\frac{h^2}{4} - y^2\right)^2}$$

For the case of $V = 0$, the maximum shear stress will be at $y = h/2$. For $M = 0$, the maximum shear will be at $y = 0$. In other cases, the answer is not so straightforward. The expression for τ_{max} has to be differentiated to find out the minima/maxima. However, instead of differentiating the expression for the maximum shear stress, we can differentiate its square. The following expression is obtained and equated to zero:

$$\frac{2M^2 y}{I^2} - 2y\frac{V^2}{I^2}\left(\frac{h^2}{4} - y^2\right) = 0$$

This gives either $y = 0$ or $y = \sqrt{\frac{h^2}{4} - \frac{M^2}{2V^2}}$. There is no need to take the negative value $y = -\sqrt{\frac{h^2}{4} - \frac{M^2}{2V^2}}$ due to symmetry.

However, it is a constrained problem, y should lie between 0 to $h/2$. Hence, to find out the true location, one needs to compare the values of maximum shear stress at three locations: (i) at $y = 0$, (ii) at $y = h$, and (iii) at $y = \sqrt{\frac{h^2}{4} - \frac{M^2}{2V^2}}$.

5.4 Shear stress distribution in circular cross-section

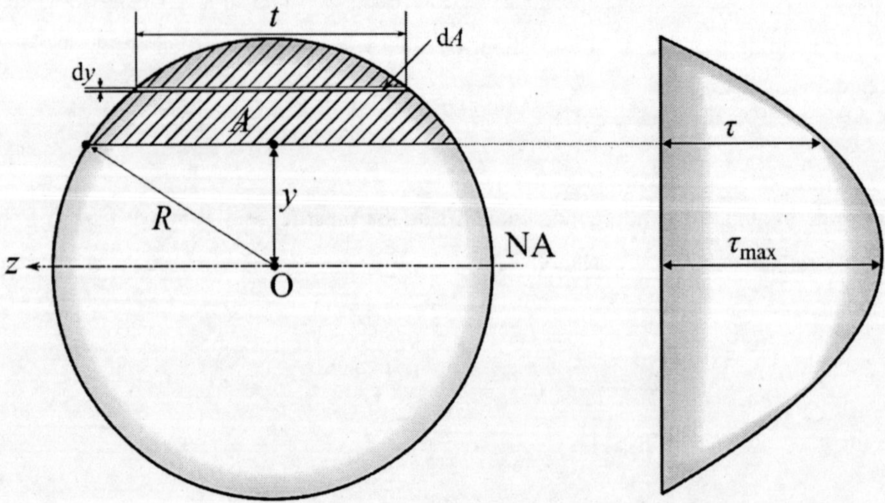

Fig. 5.3 Circular cross-section and shear stress profile

Consider a circular cross-section of the beam with a radius of R as shown in Fig. 5.3. The thickness of the rectangular cross-section and square cross-section t is constant throughout the cross-section but varies in the circular cross-section. To calculate the shear stress at a location y from the neutral axis in a beam with a circular cross-section, let A be the area of the sub-section assumed at the top of the circular cross-section, whose starting point is at y distance from the neutral axis. To determine the shear stress τ at this location, consider that t is the thickness of a thin elemental strip of area dA (Fig. **5.3**). The first moment of area A is given by

$$Q = A\bar{y} = \int_y^R y\mathrm{d}A = \int_y^R yt\mathrm{d}y \tag{5.17}$$

The thickness t at any arbitrary location y can be expressed as

$$t = 2\sqrt{R^2 - y^2} \tag{5.18}$$

Substituting Eq. (5.18) into Eq. (5.17) and integrating Q can be written as

$$Q = A\bar{y} = 2\int_y^R \left(\sqrt{R^2 - y^2}\right) y\mathrm{d}y = \frac{2}{3}(R^2 - y^2)^{3/2} \tag{5.19}$$

For a circular cross-section, $I_{zz} = \dfrac{\pi D^4}{64} = \dfrac{\pi R^4}{4}$. Finally, substituting the expression for t, Q and I_{zz} in Eq. (5.11), the shear stress can be written as

$$\tau = \frac{V\frac{2}{3}(R^2 - y^2)^{3/2}}{\left(\frac{\pi R^4}{4}\right)\left(2\sqrt{R^2 - y^2}\right)} = \frac{4}{3}V\frac{(R^2 - y^2)}{\pi R^4} \tag{5.20}$$

Equation (5.20) provides zero shear stress at $y = R$, which is the top surface of the beam. The shear stress τ is zero. The shear stress τ will be the maximum at $y = 0$, and its magnitude is

$$\tau_{\max} = \frac{4}{3}\frac{V}{\pi R^2}. \tag{5.21}$$

The average shear stress is

$$\tau_{\text{average}} = \frac{V}{\pi R^2}. \tag{5.22}$$

Example 5.3: A beam of circular cross-section diameter D = 150 mm is subjected to shear force V of 2 kN. Determine the (a) average shear stress and maximum shear stress and (b) shear stress at a distance of 30 mm from the neutral axis.

Solution: Given: D = 150 mm, Therefore R = 150/2 = 75 mm. Shear Force V = 5 kN = 5000 N.

(a) From Eq. (5.22), the average shear stress is given by,

$$\tau_{mean} = \frac{V}{\pi R^2} = \frac{5000}{\pi \times (75)^2}$$

$$\tau_{mean} = 0.2829 \text{ N/mm}^2$$

From Eq. (5.21),

$$\tau_{\max} = \frac{4}{3}\tau_{mean} = \frac{4}{3} \times 0.2829$$

$$\tau_{\max} = 0.3772 \text{ N/mm}^2$$

(b) The shear stress at a distance of 30 mm from the neutral axis can be obtained from the Eq. (5.20). It is given by

$$\tau = \frac{4}{3}V\frac{(R^2 - y^2)}{(\pi R^4)} = \frac{4}{3}(5000)\frac{(75^2 - 30^2)}{(\pi 75^4)}$$

$$\tau_{30\text{mm}} = 0.3169 \text{ N/mm}^2$$

5.5 Shear stress in triangular cross-section

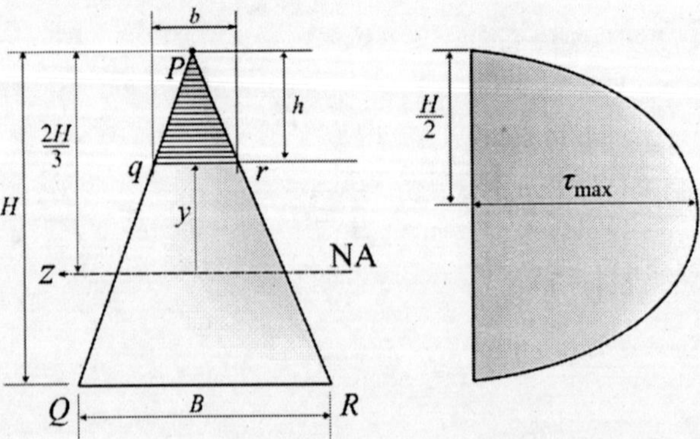

Fig. 5.4 Triangular cross-section and shear stress profile

Fig. **5.4** shows a triangular section denoted by *PQR* that is symmetrical about the $y-$ axis. *H* and *B* are the height and width of the ΔPQR, respectively. The second moment of the area of ΔPQR about the *z*-axis is given by

$$I_{zz} = \frac{BH^3}{36} \tag{5.23}$$

The neutral axis is located at a distance $\frac{2H}{3}$ from the top of the triangular section. From the base, it is at a distance of $\frac{H}{3}$. To calculate the shear stress in a triangular section, assume a sub-section ΔPqr above the neutral axis whose base *pq* is at a distance of *h* from the triangular section's apex point *P*. Let *b* be the base length of the assumed triangular sub-section ΔPqr whose area *A* is given by

$$\frac{1}{2}bh = \frac{1}{2}\frac{Bh}{H}h = \frac{By^2}{2H} \tag{5.24}$$

Since ΔPQR and ΔPqr are similar triangles,

$$\frac{b}{h} = \frac{B}{H}$$
$$b = \frac{Bh}{H} \tag{5.25}$$

This base length *b* is the same as thickness *t*. The centroid of ΔPqr is located at a distance of $\bar{y} = \frac{2H}{3} - \frac{2h}{3}$ from the neutral axis of ΔPQR. Therefore, the first moment of the area ΔPqr is given by

$$Q = A\bar{y} = \left(\frac{Bh^2}{2H}\right)\left(\frac{2H}{3} - \frac{2h}{3}\right) \tag{5.26}$$

Substituting the expression for *t*, *Q* and I_{zz} in Eq. (5.11), the shear stress can be written as

$$\tau = V\frac{\left(\frac{Bh^2}{2H}\right)\left(\frac{2H}{3} - \frac{2h}{3}\right)}{\left(\frac{BH^3}{36}\right)\left(\frac{Bh}{H}\right)} \text{ or,}$$

$$\tau = \frac{12Vh(H-h)}{BH^3} \tag{5.27}$$

From Fig. 5.4, the quantity h can be expressed as

$$h = \frac{2H}{3} - y \tag{5.28}$$

Substituting Eq. (5.28) into Eq. (5.27),

$$\tau = \frac{12V\left(\frac{2H}{3} - y\right)\left(\frac{H}{3} + y\right)}{BH^3} \tag{5.29}$$

At the apex point P, $h = 0$ and therefore, $\tau = 0$. At the neutral axis $y = 0$, the shear stress is

$$\tau = \frac{8}{3}\frac{V}{BH} \tag{5.30}$$

The maximum shear stress, however, occurs at $y = \frac{H}{6}$, given by.

$$\tau_{max} = \frac{3V}{BH} \tag{5.31}$$

Example 5.4: Consider a beam with a triangular cross-section of height H = 350 mm and base length B = 250 mm. It is subjected to a shear force of 5 kN. Determine (a) the shear stress at the neutral axis and (b) the maximum shear stress.

Solution: Given: H = 350 mm and B = 250 mm. The shear force V = 5 kN = 5000 N.

(a) From Eq. (5.30), the shear stress at the neutral axis is

$$\tau = \frac{8}{3}\frac{V}{BH} = \frac{8}{3}\frac{5000}{250 \times 350} = 0.152 \text{ N/mm}^2$$

(b) From Eq. (5.31), the maximum shear stress for a triangular cross-section is given by

$$\tau_{max} = \frac{3V}{BH} = \frac{3 \times 5000}{350 \times 250}$$

$$\tau_{max} = 0.1714 \text{ N/mm}^2$$

5.6 Shear stress distribution in I-section

Fig. 5.5 shows a symmetrical I-section. The I-section comprises two parts: flange and web. While H and B are the depth and width of the entire section, h and b are the depth and width of the web part of the I-section.

Since there is a discontinuity in width between the flange and the web at the junction, the shear stress analysis in the I-section is split into two parts— one for the flange and another for the web.

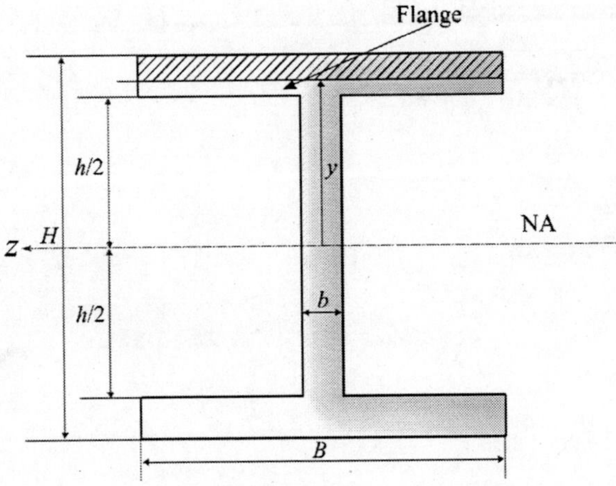

Fig. 5.5 Shear stress in the flange portion of the I-section of a beam

5.6.1 Shear stress in the flange

Assume a sub-section in the flange portion at a distance y from the neutral axis. The width of the sub-section is B, and the depth of the sub-section is $(H-2y)/2$. For the flange portion $t = B$.

The area A_F of the subsection in the flange is

$$A_F = B\left(\frac{H}{2} - y\right) \tag{5.32}$$

The centroid of the subsection $\overline{y}$ is

$$\overline{y} = \left(\frac{H+2y}{4}\right) \tag{5.33}$$

Combining Eqs. (5.32) and (5.33), the first moment of the area of the sub-section is

$$Q = A_F \bar{y} = B\frac{(H^2 - 4y^2)}{8} \tag{5.34}$$

Substituting the expression for t and Q in Eq. (5.11), the shear stress in the flange portion can be written as

$$\tau_F = \frac{V}{I_{zz}B}\frac{B(H^2 - 4y^2)}{8} = \frac{V}{8I_{zz}}(H^2 - 4y^2) \tag{5.35}$$

From Eq. (5.35), the variation of shear stress in the flange is parabolic. It is also clear that the shear stress is zero at the upper edge, i.e., at $y = \frac{H}{2}$. At the lower edge of the flange where $y = \frac{h}{2}$, the shear stress is

$$\tau = \frac{V}{8I_{zz}}(H^2 - h^2) \tag{5.36}$$

5.6.2 Shear stress in the web

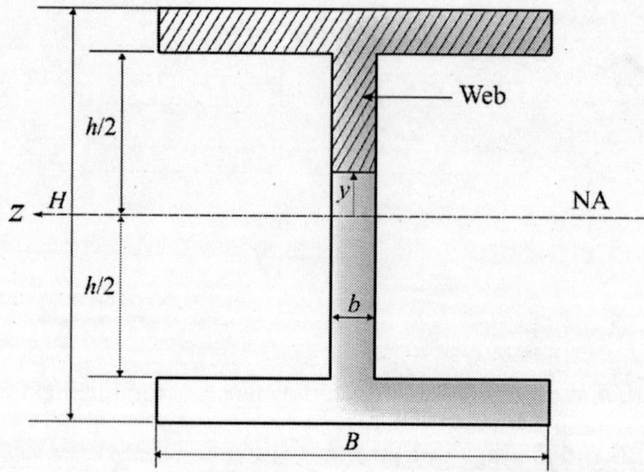

Fig. 5.6 Shear stress in the web portion of the I-section of a beam

For the web portion, the first moment of the area Q has two parts: the first moment of the flange area about the neutral axis plus the first moment of the shaded area of the web about the neutral axis.

$$Q = Q_F + Q_W \tag{5.37}$$

The first term Q_F can be written as

$$Q_F = \left(A\bar{y}\right)_F = B\left(\frac{H}{2} - \frac{h}{2}\right)\left(\frac{H}{2} - \frac{h}{2}\right) = B\frac{\left(H^2 - h^2\right)}{8} \tag{5.38}$$

The second term Q_W will be

$$Q_W = \left(A\bar{y}\right)_W = b\left(\frac{h}{2}-y\right)\frac{\left(\frac{h}{2}+y\right)}{2} = \frac{b}{2}\left(\frac{h^2}{4}-y^2\right) \tag{5.39}$$

Substituting the Eqs. (5.38) and (5.39) in Eq. (5.11),

$$\tau_w = \frac{V}{I_{zz}b}\left[\left(A\bar{y}\right)_F + \left(A\bar{y}\right)_W\right] = \frac{V}{8I_{zz}b}\left[B\left(H^2-h^2\right)+b\left(h^2-4y^2\right)\right] \tag{5.40}$$

The magnitude of the shear stress at the neutral axis ($y = 0$) is

$$\tau = \frac{V}{8I_{zz}b}\left[B\left(H^2-h^2\right)+bh^2\right] \tag{5.41}$$

The shear stress at the neutral axis is also the maximum shear stress. The magnitude of the shear stress in the web near the junction is obtained by setting $y = \frac{h}{2}$ in Eq. (5.40).

$$\tau = \frac{V}{8I_{zz}b}\left[B\left(H^2-h^2\right)\right] \tag{5.42}$$

It is to be noted that at the junction, the ratio of shear stress in the flange to the shear stress in the web is

$$\frac{\tau_F}{\tau_W} = \frac{b}{B} \tag{5.43}$$

The variation of the shear stress in the I-section is shown in Fig. 5.7.

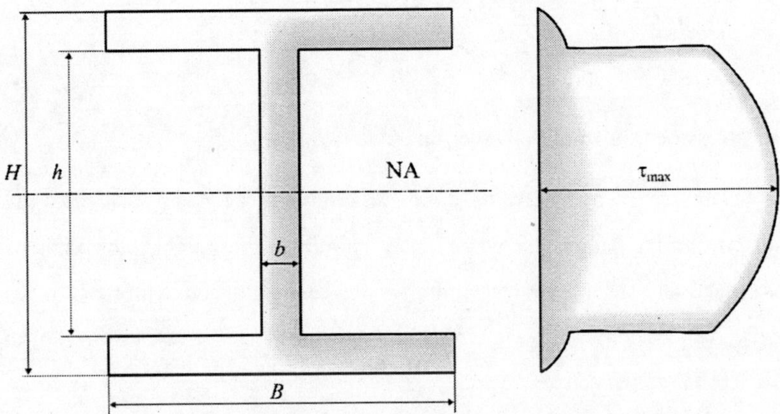

Fig. 5.7 Shear stress variation in the I-section of a beam

Example 5.5: Consider an I-section with rectangular ends with the following dimensions Overall Height $H = 440$ mm, Overall width $B = 200$ mm, Web height $h = 400$ mm, Web thickness $b = 20$ mm.

It is subjected to a shear force of 150 kN. Calculate the maximum shear stress and shear stress at the junction in the web portion.

Solution:

$$I_{zz} = \frac{200 \times 440^3}{12} - \frac{180 \times 400^3}{12} = 459.733 \times 10^6 \text{ mm}^4$$

From Eq. (5.41), the maximum shear stress occurs at the neutral axis and is given by

$$\tau_w = \frac{V}{8I_{zz}t}\left[B\left(H^2 - h^2\right) + bh^2\right]$$

$$\tau_w = \frac{150 \times 10^3}{8 \times 459.733 \times 10^6 \times 20}\left[200\left(440^2 - 400^2\right) + 20 \times 400^2\right]$$

$$\tau_w = 20.23 \text{ N/mm}^2$$

The shear stress in the web portion at the junction is given by,

$$\tau = \frac{V}{8I_{zz}b}\left[B\left(H^2 - h^2\right)\right]$$

$$\tau_w = \frac{150 \times 10^3}{8 \times 459.733 \times 10^6 \times 20}\left[200\left(440^2 - 400^2\right)\right]$$

$$\tau_w = 13.70 \text{ N/mm}^2$$

5.7 Shear stress distribution in T-section

Consider a beam with a T-section, shown in Fig. 5.8. Like the I-section, the T-section comprises two parts: flange and web. Let H and B be the height and width of the entire section, respectively. Moreover, let h and b be the height and width of the web section, respectively. The T-section is symmetrical about the $y-$ axis. Let the centroid of the entire T-section be located at a distance of y_c.

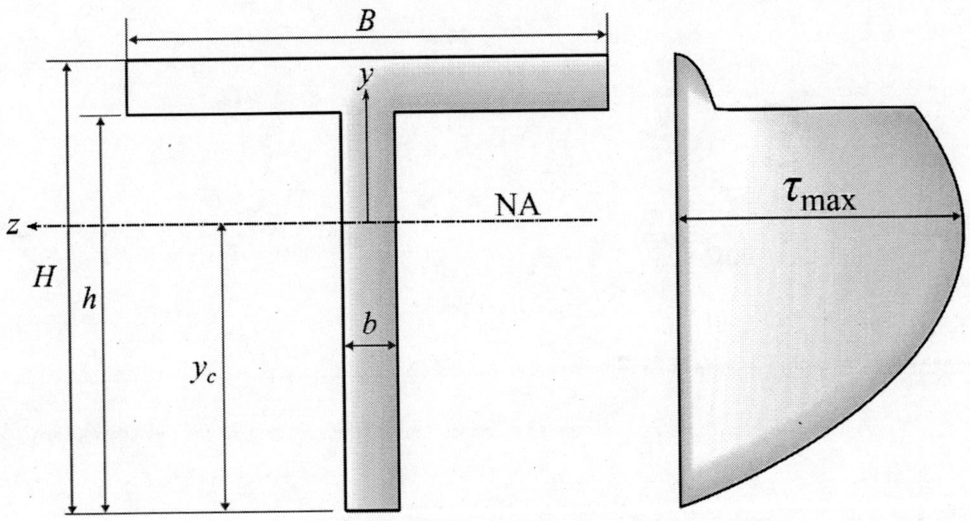

Fig. 5.8 Shear stress variation in the T-section of a beam

The neutral axis is the z–axis passing through the centroid. Following the same procedure as that of finding the shear stress in the flange portion of the I-section in Section 5.6.1, the shear stress τ in the flange portion of the T-section is given by

$$\tau_F = \frac{VQ}{I_{zz}B} \tag{5.44}$$

The first moment of the area of a sub-section in the flange starting from the distance y from the neutral axis can be expressed as

$$Q = B\left[H-(y_c+y)\right]\frac{\left[H-(y_c-y)\right]}{2} = \frac{B}{2}\left[(H-y_c)^2-y^2\right] \tag{5.45}$$

Combining Eqs. (5.44) and (5.45), the shear stress in the flange is

$$\tau_F = \frac{V}{2I_{zz}}\left[(H-y_c)^2-y^2\right] \tag{5.46}$$

The shear stress in the web portion of the T-section can be written as

$$\tau_w = \frac{V}{I_{zz}b}\left[(A\bar{y})_F+(A\bar{y})_W\right] \tag{5.47}$$

where $(A\bar{y})_F = \frac{B}{2}\left\{(H-y_c)^2-(h-y_c)^2\right\}$ and $(A\bar{y})_W = \frac{b}{2}\left\{(h-y_c)^2-(y)^2\right\}$.

Know More

Exercises

Multiple Choice Questions

5.1. The ratio of maximum shear stress to average shear stress in beams of rectangular cross-section is

(a) 1.5

(b) 2

(c) 3

(d) 1

5.2 The maximum shear stress in a beam of a triangular section of base width b and height h subjected to shear force V is given by

(a) $\frac{V}{bh}$

(b) $\frac{3V}{bh}$

(c) $\frac{2V}{bh}$

(d) $\frac{3V}{bh}$

5.3 The ratio of maximum shear stress to average shear stress in beams of circular cross-section is

(a) 1.5

(b) 1

(c) 2

(d) $\frac{4}{3}$

5.4. The side length of a square cross-section is equal to the diameter of the circular cross-section. The ratio of maximum shear stress in square cross-section to circular cross-section beams subjected to the same shear force is

(a) $\frac{9}{16}$

(b) 1

(c) $\frac{9\pi}{32}$

(d) $\frac{\pi}{16}$

5.5. In an I-section beam, the shear stress in the flange close to the junction is x units. The shear stress gets amplified to $10x$ in the web after crossing the junction. The ratio of the web width to that of the flange width is

(a) 0.1

(b) 0.25

(c) 0.05

(d) 0.2

Answers of multiple choice questions

5.1 (a), 5.2 (b), 5.3 (d), 5.4 (c), 5.5 (a).

Practise Problems

5.1. A circular beam of diameter 100 mm has a maximum shear stress of 4 N/mm^2. What is the shear force acting in it? (**Ans.** 23.56 kN)

5.2. A simply supported beam assembly consisting of two rectangular cross-section beams is subjected to a concentrated and uniformly distributed load, as shown in Fig. P1. The beam AB and BC has a depth of b_1 and b_2, respectively. The width of both beams is the same. Find the ratio of b_2 to b_1, if the maximum transverse shear stress in AB and BC are equal. (**Ans.** 4/3)

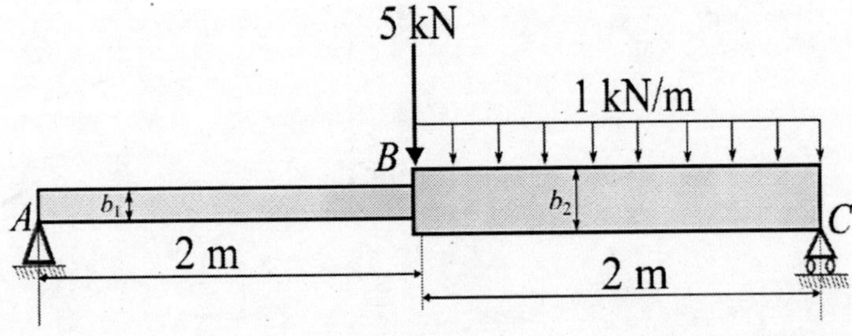

Figure. P1

5.3. A beam of I-section with rectangular ends has an overall height H = 440 mm, overall width B = 200 mm, web height h = 400 mm, and web thickness b = 20 mm. It is subjected to shear force 0f 150 kN. What is the percentage of shear force carried by the web? (**Ans.** 96.3%)

5.4. A triangular cross-section beam is subjected to a uniformly distributed load and a concentrated load, as shown in Figure P2. Find the maximum transverse shear stress acting on the beam's cross-section.

(**Ans.** 0.937 MPa)

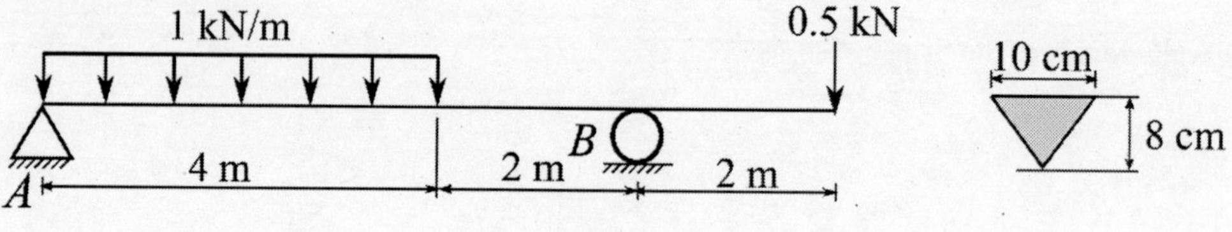

Figure. P2

5.5. A beam of T-shaped cross section (Figure P3) has the dimensions: overall height H = 300 mm, flange width B = 250 mm, web height h = 250 mm, and web width b = 50 mm. The beam is subjected to a load of 150 kN. Calculate the shear stress at (a) the neutral axis, (b) the flange just above the flange-web junction, and (c) the web just below the flange-web junction.

(**Ans.** 14.4 MPa, 2.7 MPa, 13.5 MPa)

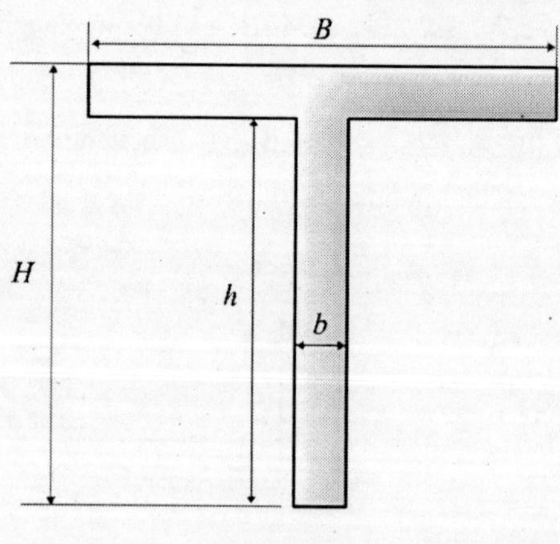

Figure. P3

Unit 6

Deflection and Slope of Beams

UNIT SPECIFICS

Beams will bend when they are subjected to load. Beam deflection occurs when a load causes a beam to change shape from its original, undeformed state to its new, deformed state. Beam deflection is measured with respect to the beam's neutral fiber in the undeformed state since beams are represented two-dimensional objects. The governing differential equation for the beam deflection has been derived in this unit. Three popular approaches, including the double integration method, the moment area method and Macaulay's method, have been used to calculate the deflection and the slope of the beam. In the end, Maxwell's reciprocal theorem was introduced to find the deflection and slope at specific locations of the beam. As with any unit, the current unit end with varieties of multiple-choice questions and practice problems to help the reader attain mastery over the subject.

RATIONALE

In beams, the calculation of deflection serves as a crucial check on serviceability during the design phase. Fracture, finish damage, and improper alignment of fixtures and systems can result from deflection outside of acceptable ranges. Therefore, estimating the deflection under service loading conditions is essential to reduce the service cost, effort and idle time. To this end, this unit's main objective is to find the deflection and slope under various load and support conditions.

PRE-REQUISITES

Mathematics course on differential equations

Bending moment and shear force diagrams (Unit 3) and Theory of simple bending (Unit 4)

UNIT OUTCOMES

After completing this unit, students will be able to

U6-O1: Derive the governing deflection of the beam using the Euler-Bernoulli beam theory

U6-O2: Usage of the double integration method, the moment area method and Macaulay's method to solve for the deflection and slope of the beam under loading

U6-O3: Identifying the location on the neutral fiber where the deflection and slope are maximum

U6-O4: Apply the Maxwell's reciprocal theorem to find the deflection or slope at select locations

Course Outcomes	Expected Mapping with Course Outcomes - CE (1- Weak Correlation; 2- Medium correlation; 3- Strong Correlation)			
	CO-1	CO-2	CO-3	CO-4
U6-O1	2	-	1	-
U6-O2	-	-	-	3
U6-O3	1	-	-	3
U6-O4	-	3	-	2

Course Outcomes	Expected Mapping with Course Outcomes - ME (1- Weak Correlation; 2- Medium correlation; 3- Strong Correlation)	
	CO-1	CO-2
U6-O1	2	-
U6-O2	-	3
U6-O3	1	2
U6-O4	1	2

6.1 Introduction

Deflection is a crucial indicator of a structure's performance. The manner in which structures move and deform has an impact on their uses as well as the kinds of tasks that are best suited to them. A floor system, for instance, needs to be rigid enough to prevent excessive bowing. Even though the floor is entirely secure, people may feel uneasy if it deflects too much.

In this unit, the differential equation governing the deflection of statically determinate beams will be derived; in a statically determinate structure, the reactive forces and moments can be determined from the equilibrium equations alone. Subsequently, three different methods will be described to calculate the deflection and slope of a beam under transverse loading: the double integration method, the moment-area method, and Macaulay's method.

6.2 Euler-Bernoulli beam theory

Euler-Bernoulli beam theory, or classical beam theory, is a simplified model of linear elasticity theory to calculate the deflections and slopes of beams subjected to transverse or lateral loads. This theory was developed circa 1750 CE by Leonhard Euler and Daniel Bernoulli. However, it is popular for analyzing the beam characteristics, i.e., deflection and slope, when the beam deflections are small. The Euler-Bernoulli beam theory uses the following basic assumptions to derive the relationship between the moment, slope, and deflection:

1. Plane sections (cross-sections) remain plane and normal to the axis of the beam after bending. Consider Fig. 6.1, where different planes, such as *a-a'*, *b-b'*, and *c-c'*, are perpendicular to the axis of the beam before deformation. These planes will remain as planes and perpendicular to the axis of the beam after the deformation.
2. The deformations are small. Therefore, the slope of the elastic/deflection curve is small. The elastic curve is the curve adopted by the beam's longitudinal axis when it is bent by any system of forces within its elastic limits.
3. The beam is considered to be linear elastic and isotropic.
4. The effect of rotary inertia shear deformation is neglected.

Further, before deriving the expression for the deflection of the beam, in this unit, it is hypothesized that Young's modulus of the beam is the same in both tension and compression, and the beam is symmetrical about the plane of bending. The beam is initially straight with no imperfections.

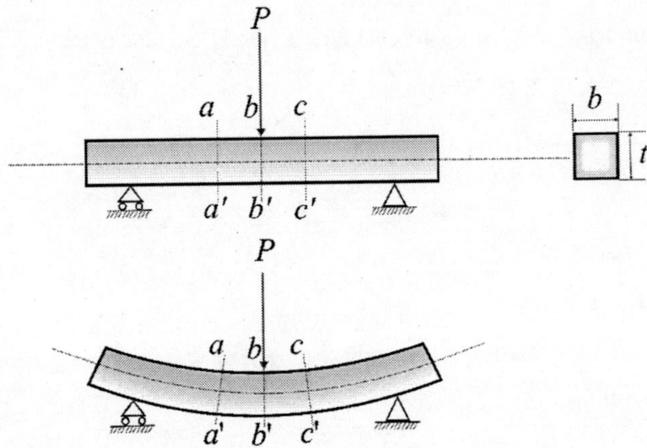

Fig. 6.1 Beam bending under the action of transverse load

Unless the beam receives significant shear or torsional loads in relation to the bending stresses, the first assumption is usually valid for the bending of beams. Shear stress may dominate bending stress if the beam is relatively short and has a higher depth.

Consider a beam whose longitudinal axis is aligned with x – axis. Under the action of the transverse loading, the beam will deform, as shown in Fig. 6.2. The objective is to find out the equation of the elastic curve or the deflection curve $y(x)$.

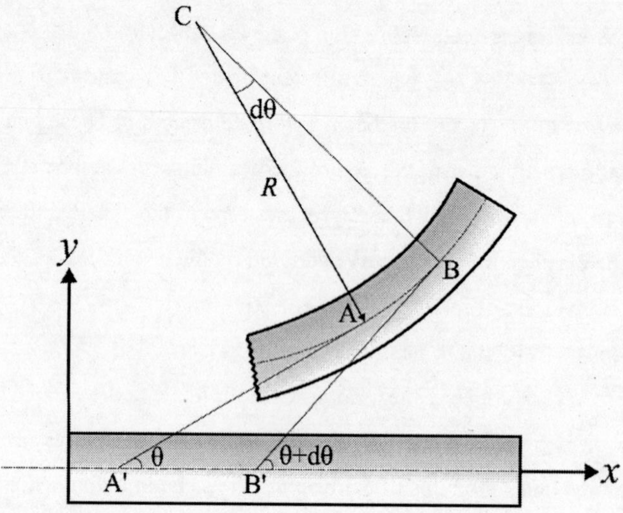

Fig. 6.2 Bending of the beam

In Fig. 6.2, consider the portion AB in the deformed beam. The tangents at locations A and B have a slope θ and $\theta + \mathrm{d}\theta$, respectively. Due to bending, the portion AB will subtend an angle $\mathrm{d}\theta$ at the centre of curvature C. Let the corresponding radius of curvature be R, which is given by

$$\frac{1}{R} = \frac{\dfrac{\mathrm{d}^2 y}{\mathrm{d}x^2}}{\left\{1+\left(\dfrac{\mathrm{d}y}{\mathrm{d}x}\right)^2\right\}^{3/2}} \tag{6.1}$$

Due to the assumption of small deformation, the slope $\theta = \dfrac{\mathrm{d}y}{\mathrm{d}x} \ll 1$. Hence, Eq. (6.1) can be written as

$$\frac{1}{R} = \frac{\mathrm{d}^2 y}{\mathrm{d}x^2} \tag{6.2}$$

From the bending equation

$$-\frac{\sigma}{y} = \frac{M}{I} = \frac{E}{R} \tag{6.3}$$

Substituting the expression of R from Eq. (6.2) into Eq. (6.3)

$$EI\frac{\mathrm{d}^2 y}{\mathrm{d}x^2} = M \tag{6.4}$$

Equation (6.4) relates the expression of the deflection curve with the bending moment. It can be seen from Eq. (6.3) that there is only one non-zero stress component – σ_{xx}. The other stress components are zero. In reality, all the problems in solid mechanics involve three-dimensional (3D) analysis. Solving 3D problems is only possible using computers. However, with reasonable assumptions by engineers, the analysis reduces to 2D or 1D without much loss in accuracy, which can be readily solved using pen and paper. The Euler-Bernoulli theory is a classic example of reducing the 3D nature of the problem to 1D.

σ_{xx} is related to ε_{xx} by the Young's modulus (E). It is given by

$$\sigma_{xx} = E\varepsilon_{xx} = -Ey\frac{\mathrm{d}^2y}{\mathrm{d}x^2} \tag{6.5}$$

Henceforth, σ will be used in place of σ_{xx} and ϵ in place of ϵ_{xx}. Using the Eq. (6.5) and the bending Eq. (6.3)

$$EI\frac{\mathrm{d}^2y}{\mathrm{d}x^2} = M \tag{6.6}$$

The elastic curve is defined by the function $y(x)$, which is measured with respect to the neutral fibre. In the case of a plane beam, it is essential to identify the location of the neutral fibre, which neither contracts nor extends, for the calculations to be based upon that neutral fibre.

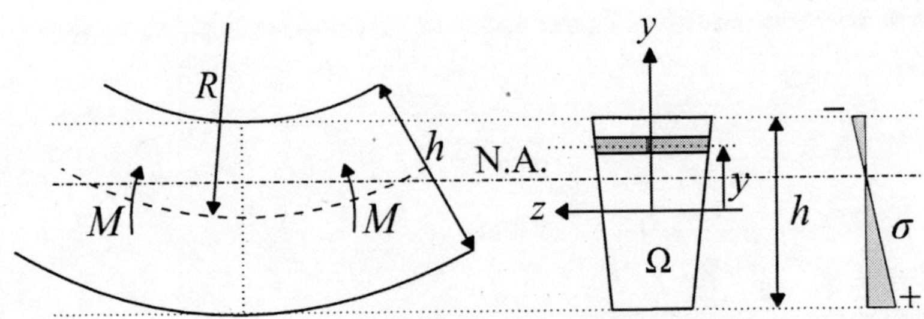

Fig. 6.3 Bending stresses in beam

The longitudinal axis passing through the centroid of the cross-section of the beam is the neutral fibre, as explained in Unit 4. Therefore, it is convenient to choose the x – axis as the neutral fibre (Fig. 6.3). The $x - y$ plane is the plane of loading about which the beam is symmetrical. In reality, the beam is three-dimensional geometry, and therefore, the third axis, i.e. z – axis is orthogonal to $x - y$ plane. The $x - z$ plane is the neutral surface as this surface does not contract nor stretch and, therefore, is a stress-free surface. The intersection of the $x-z$ plane with a cross-section is a line which is called the neutral axis.

Moment of Inertia of the beam

The moment of Inertia (I) of the beam can be calculated using the moment resultant due to σ present on the beam's cross-section. This is written as

$$M = -\iint_{\Omega} \sigma y \mathrm{d}y\mathrm{d}z = \iint_{\Omega} E y^2 \frac{\mathrm{d}^2 y}{\mathrm{d}x^2} \mathrm{d}y\mathrm{d}z \tag{6.7}$$

The top fibre of the beam is compressed due to the positive M convention, which is why the negative sign is inserted in the Eq. (6.7). Eq. (6.7) can be simplified as

$$\begin{gathered} M = EI \frac{\mathrm{d}^2 y}{\mathrm{d}x^2} \\ I = I_{zz} = \iint_{\Omega} y^2 \mathrm{d}y\mathrm{d}z \end{gathered} \tag{6.8}$$

The moment of Inertia — I is the second moment of area about the z – axis i.e. I_{zz}. The term EI is called flexural rigidity of the beam. Flexural rigidity is the resistance given by a structure during bending or the moment necessary to bend a non-rigid structure by one unit of curvature. Flexural rigidity, in this sense, is defined as an inability to bend. The beam's increased flexural stiffness ensures that it would not bend easily.

Recall from Unit 3, from Eq. (3.1), that the shear force, V, is related to the distributed load q as

$$\frac{\mathrm{d}V}{\mathrm{d}x} = -q \tag{6.9}$$

From Eq. (3.3), M is related to V as

$$V = -\frac{\mathrm{d}M}{\mathrm{d}x} \tag{6.10}$$

Substituting Eq. (6.10) into Eq. (6.9)

$$\frac{\mathrm{d}^2 M}{\mathrm{d}x^2} = q \tag{6.11}$$

Finally, after combining Eqs. (6.4) and (6.11), the Euler-Bernoulli beam equation is obtained, describing the deflection of the beam and the applied load.

$$\frac{d^2}{dx^2}\left(EI\frac{d^2y}{dx^2}\right)=q \tag{6.12}$$

Equation (6.12) describes the deflection of a static, uniform beam. However, Eq. (6.4) is preferred for solving the deflection of a beam under transverse loading. For typical beam designs, tabulated equations for the deflection $y(x)$ may be found in engineering handbooks. Deflection may be calculated for more involved scenarios by solving the Euler-Bernoulli equation using the double integration method, moment-area, or Macaulay's method.

6.3 Double integration method

For a beam's elastic deflection curve, the governing second-order differential equation is

$$EI\frac{d^2y}{dx^2}=M(x) \tag{6.13}$$

where the product *EI* is the flexural rigidity, and *M*(*x*) is the moment at section x. The flexural rigidity (*EI*) will be a constant for the prismatic beam. Integrating with respect to x on both sides, we will obtain

$$EI\frac{dy}{dx}=\int M(x)dx+C_1 \tag{6.14}$$

where C_1 is the integration constant. For small deformation, the approximation $\frac{dy}{dx}=\tan\theta\approx\theta(x)$ holds. Using this approximation in the Eq. (6.14)

$$EI\theta(x)=\int M(x)dx+C_1 \tag{6.15}$$

Integrating the Eq. (6.15) with respect to x once again

$$EI\,y(x)=\int\left[\int M(x)dx+C_1\right]dx+C_2 \tag{6.16}$$

where C_2 is the second integration constant. The constants C_1 and C_2 can be determined from the support conditions of the beam

Know More

Example 6.1 A cantilever beam of flexural rigidity EI carries a uniform varying load, as shown in Fig. 6.4. The load intensity (load per unit length) is w at the right end. Find the slope and the deflection at the left end.

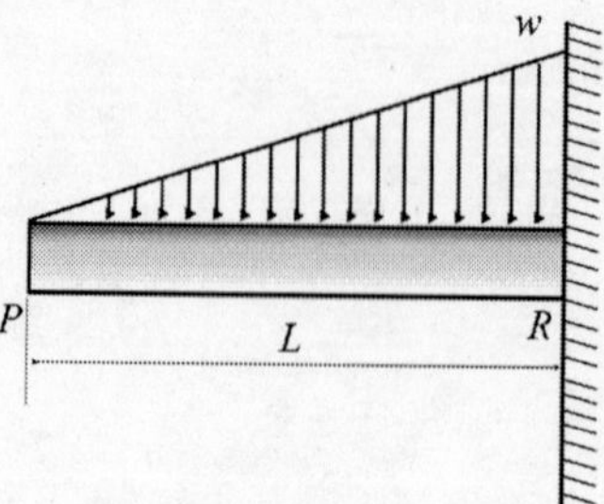

Fig. 6.4 Cantilever beam subjected to uniform varying load

Solution:

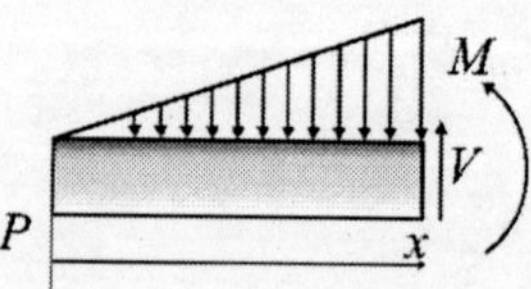

Figure 6.1e1 Free body diagram

Using the free-body diagram (Figure 6.1e1) for a portion PQ of length x of the beam, the moment expression can be written as

$$M(x) = -\frac{wx^3}{6L}$$

The shear force diagram and bending moment diagrams are shown in Figure 6.1e2.

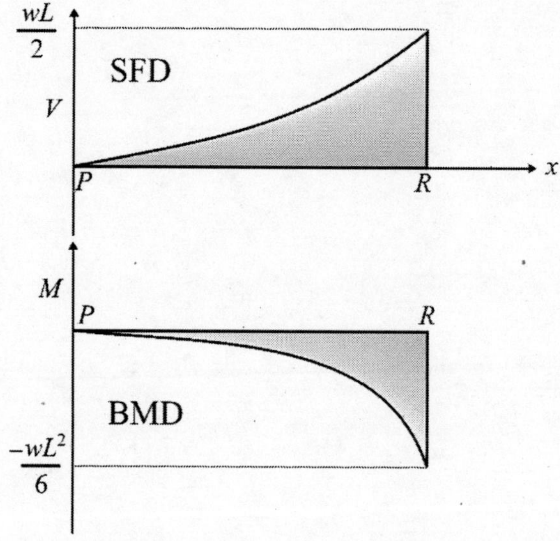

Figure 6.1e2 SFD and BMD for the cantilever beam problem

From Eq. (6.4)

$$EI\frac{d^2y}{dx^2} = -\frac{wx^3}{6L}$$

Integrating with respect to x once, the expression for the slope can be written as

$$EI\frac{dy}{dx} = -\frac{wx^4}{24L} + C_1$$

Now from the fixed-end boundary conditions of the cantilever beam, the slope at $x = L$, i.e. $\frac{dy}{dx} = 0$. Substituting these in the above equation

$$C_1 = \frac{wL^3}{24}$$

This will give the expression for the slope as

$$EI\frac{dy}{dx} = -\frac{wx^4}{24L} + \frac{wL^3}{24}$$

The slope at P can be obtained by putting $x = 0$ in the above equation

$$\theta_P = \left(\frac{\mathrm{dy}}{\mathrm{dx}}\right)_{x=0} = \frac{wL^3}{24EI}$$

Integrating once again with respect to x

$$EI\, y = -\frac{wx^5}{120L} + \frac{wL^3 x}{24} + C_2$$

For the cantilever beam at the right end, i.e., $x = L$, $y=0$. Substituting this in the above equation

$$C_2 = -\frac{wL^4}{30}$$

Therefore, the elastic curve $y(x)$ can be written as

$$y(x) = \frac{1}{EI}\left(-\frac{wx^5}{120L} + \frac{wL^3 x}{24} - \frac{wL^4}{30}\right)$$

Finally, the deflection at P can be obtained by putting $x = 0$ in the above equation.

$$y_P = -\frac{wL^4}{30EI}$$

Example 6.2 A cantilever beam is loaded, as shown in Fig. 6.5. If the spring constant is k, find the deflection in the spring.

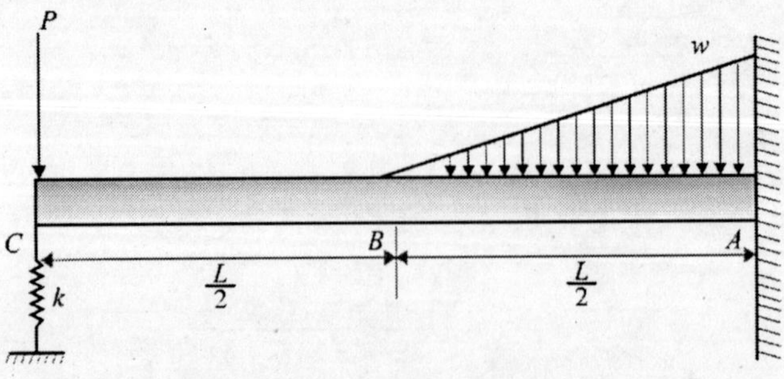

Fig. 6.5 Cantilever beam with a spring support

Solution:

Using the results obtained from Example 6.1, we can write

$$(\theta_B)_w = \frac{wL^3}{192EI} \quad \text{and} \quad (y_B)_w = -\frac{wL^4}{480EI}$$

The free-body diagram of the cantilever structure is shown in Figure 6.2e1.

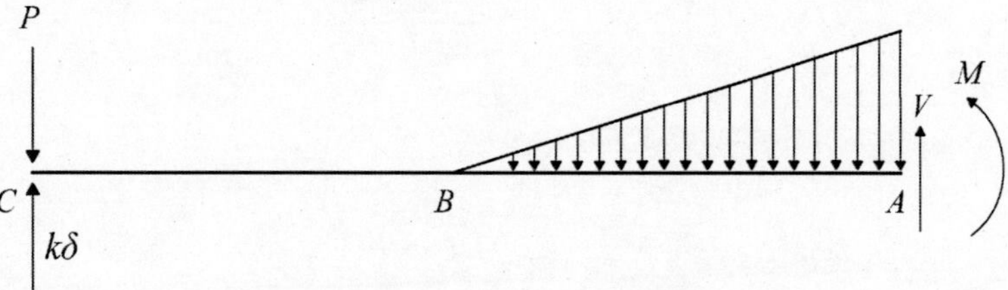

Figure 6.2e1 Free-body diagram

The shear force and bending moment diagrams are shown in Figure 6.2e2. The deflection of the cantilever beam at the left end due to distributed load can be expressed as

$$(y_C)_w = (y_B)_w - \frac{1}{2}(\theta_B)_w L$$

$$(y_C)_w = -\frac{wL^4}{480EI} - \frac{wL^4}{384EI} = -\frac{9wL^4}{1920EI}$$

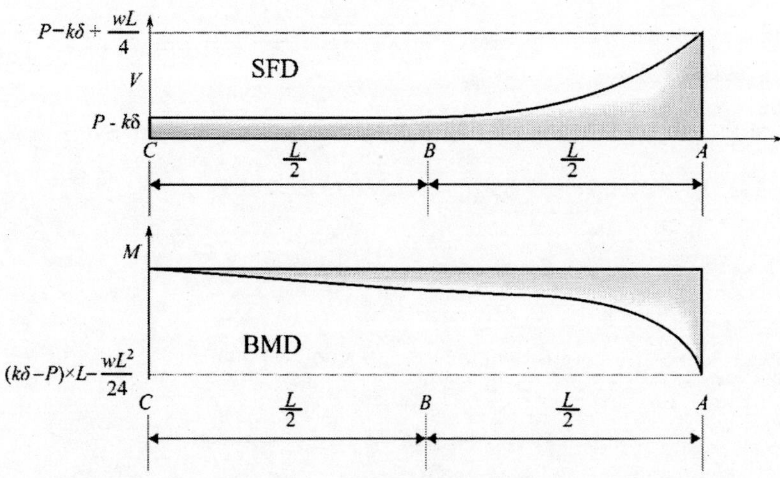

Figure 6.2e2 Shear force and bending moment diagram

Let the magnitude of deflection in the spring be δ. So, the net concentrated load at point C will be given as

$$R = P - k\delta$$

Now from Eq. (6.4)

$$EI\frac{d^2y}{dx^2} = -Rx$$

On integrating, the slope equation is obtained as

$$EI\frac{dy}{dx} = -\frac{Rx^2}{2} + C_1$$

Integrating once more

$$EI\,y = -\frac{Rx^3}{6} + C_1x + C_2$$

Using the boundary conditions: at $x = L,\ y = 0$ and $\frac{dy}{dx} = 0$, we obtain

$$C_1 = \frac{RL^2}{2} \quad \text{and} \quad C_2 = -\frac{RL^3}{3}$$

Substituting the constants in the slope equation and integrating once again with respect to x

$$y(x) = \frac{1}{EI}\left(-\frac{Rx^3}{6} + \frac{RL^2x}{2} - \frac{RL^3}{3}\right)$$

At the left end, $y_C = (y_C)_w + (y_C)_R = -\delta$ where $(y_C)_R$ is the deflection due to R. From the elastic curve, the deflection at C due to net concentrated load is

$$(y_C)_R = -\frac{RL^3}{3EI}$$

Using the principle of superposition, the net deflection at point C is

$$y_C = (y_C)_w + (y_C)_R = -\delta \Rightarrow \delta = \frac{9wL^4}{1920EI} + \frac{(P - k\delta)L^3}{3EI}$$

On simplification,

$$\delta = \frac{9wL^4 + 640PL^3}{1920EI + 640kL^3}$$

6.4 Moment-Area method

The moment-area method uses the area of the beam's curvature to determine the beam's deflection and slope. The curvature κ is given by Eq. (6.25).

$$\kappa = \frac{1}{R} = \frac{\mathrm{d}^2 y}{\mathrm{d}x^2} = \frac{M}{EI} \tag{6.17}$$

The curvature κ is the bending moment divided by the flexural rigidity EI.

6.4.1 First moment-area theorem

For the deflected beam, consider segment AB of the elastic curve as shown in Fig. 6.6 to derive the first moment-area theorem. The flexural stiffness and bending moment determine the beam's curvature. For a beam undergoing small deformation, the curvature at any location is given by

$$\frac{\mathrm{d}^2 y}{\mathrm{d}x^2} = \frac{M}{EI} \tag{6.18}$$

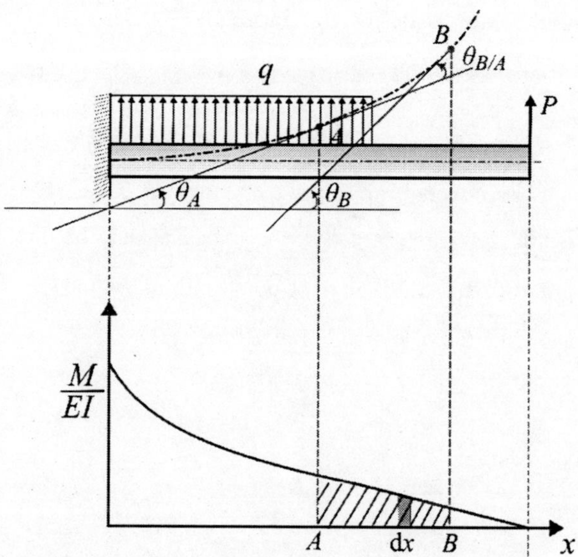

Fig. 6.6 Elastic curve and curvature diagram of beam

Since $\theta = \frac{dy}{dx}$, Eq. (6.18) can be written as

$$\frac{d\theta}{dx} = \frac{M}{EI} \text{ or } d\theta = \frac{M}{EI}dx \tag{6.19}$$

Integrating both sides with respect to x – axis from the location x_A to x_B,

$$\int_{\theta_A}^{\theta_B} d\theta = \theta_B - \theta_A = \theta_{B/A} = \int_{x_A}^{x_B} \frac{M}{EI}dx \tag{6.20}$$

The first moment-area theorem says that the difference in the slopes at any two locations can be obtained by calculating the area of the curvature or the quantity, $\frac{M}{EI}$, between those locations. In an elastic curve, the slope at location *B* with regard to the tangent at point *A* is positive if the tangent at *B* rotates counter-clockwise with respect to the tangent at *A*, and negative otherwise. The procedure for using the first moment-area theorem is as follows

- Draw the beam's curvature or $\frac{M}{EI}$ diagram. This will resemble a normal beam's bending moment diagram if the beam is prismatic.
- Calculate the angle formed by a tangent through the point and another tangent via a different point on the elastic curve and split the $\frac{M}{EI}$ diagram into basic geometric forms (rectangle, triangle, etc.). Then use the first moment-area theorem.

6.4.2 Second moment-area theorem

The second moment-area theorem gives the tangential deviation of point *A* with respect to point *B*. This tangential deviation is denoted by $t_{A/B}$ and may be different from the elastic curve $y(x)$. $t_{A/B}$ is the vertical distance of point *A* from the tangent drawn from *B* on the elastic curve. Consider the figure shown in Fig. 6.7.

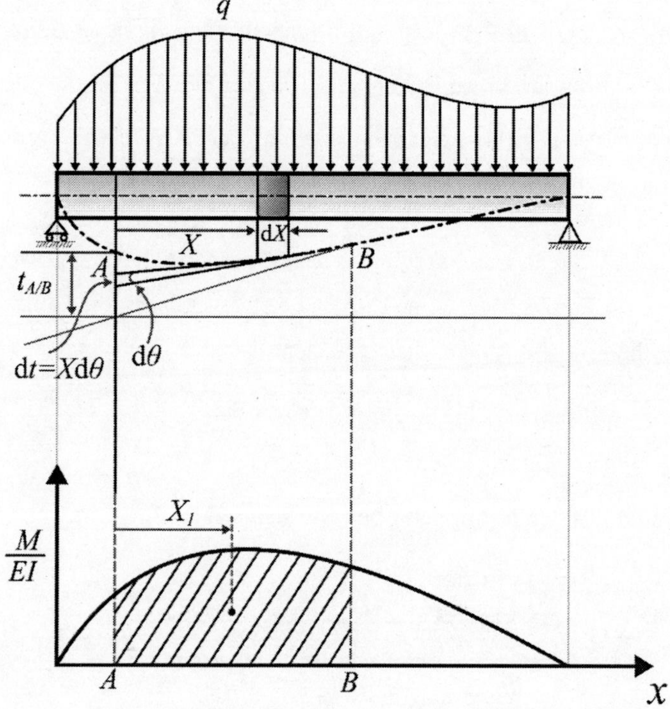

Fig. 6.7 Tangential deviation

The infinitesimal tangential deviation (dt) is given by

$$dt = X d\theta \tag{6.21}$$

Combining Eqs. (6.19) and (6.21),

$$dt = X \frac{M}{EI} dX \tag{6.22}$$

Integrating both sides with respect to x – axis from the location x_A to x_B,

$$t_{A/B} = \int_{x_A}^{x_B} X \frac{M}{EI} dX \tag{6.23}$$

$t_{A/B}$ can be calculated by multiplying the area of the curvature or the quantity, $\frac{M}{EI}$, between those locations and the distance of the centroid (X_1) of that area from location A. To rephrase, the first moment with respect to a vertical axis through A of the area under the curvature diagram between A and B is equal to the tangential deviation of A with respect to B.

The second moment-area theorem is used to find deflections of any point on the beam from the curvature or $\frac{M}{EI}$ diagram. When $\frac{M}{EI}$ diagram's structure prevents it from being broken down into basic geometric forms whose areas and centroids can be calculated in advance, it is more convenient to create the diagram by parts.

The first and second moment-area theorem is handy when the slope is known at some point – the reference point. For instance, in the case of a cantilever beam, the fixed-end point can be considered as the reference point where the slope is zero. Using the second moment-area theorem, the same point can be used to find the deflection of any point on the cantilever beam.

6.4.3 Slope and deflection in the case of unsymmetrical loading

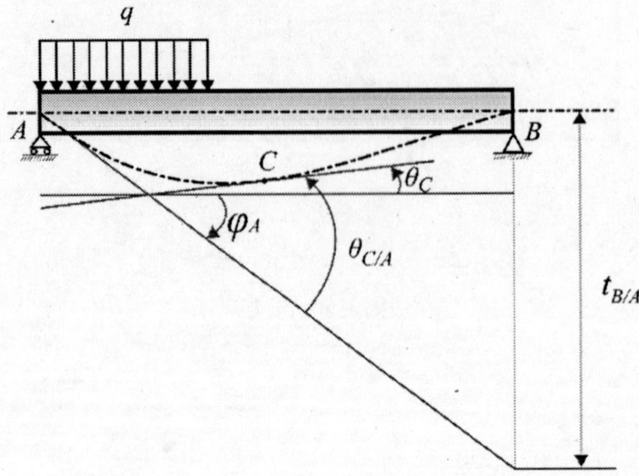

Fig. 6.8 Slope in the unsymmetrical loading on the beam

When the loading or the beam geometry is not symmetrical with respect to the middle section of the beam, as shown in Fig. 6.8, it becomes difficult to use the moment-area theorem, as the slope at any point (reference point) cannot be established. In such a case, the tangential deviation of a beam's endpoint B with respect to the tangent drawn at the beam's start point A can be calculated. Then the slope at point A is

$$\theta_A = \varphi_A = \frac{-t_{B/A}}{L} \tag{6.24}$$

where L is the length of the beam. The negative sign is included to indicate the slope is negative at point A. Alternatively, θ_B can be established by determining $t_{B/A}$.

$$\theta_B = \frac{t_{A/B}}{L} \tag{6.25}$$

The slope at other points can be found with respect to the slope at the reference point – let us say A which is then given by

$$\theta_C = \theta_A + \theta_{C/A} \tag{6.26}$$

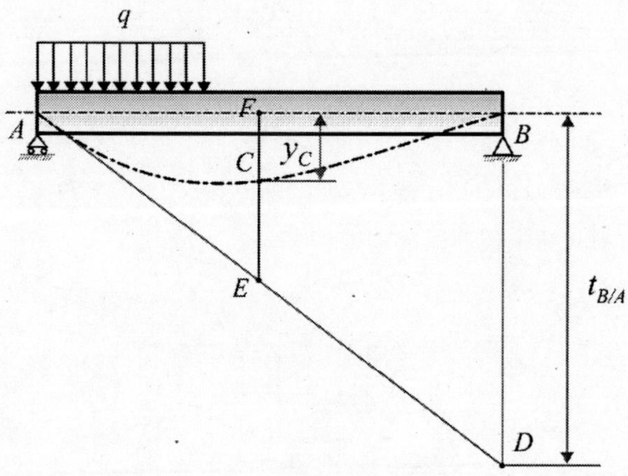

Fig. 6.9 Deflection in the beam subjected to unsymmetrical loading using the moment-area method

Using the concept of similar triangles, the deflection at any given point C, which is at a distance x from the point A, can be obtained as shown in Fig. 6.9.

$$y_C = -(EF - CE) \tag{6.27}$$

where $EF = \frac{x}{L} t_{B/A}$ and $CE = t_{D/A}$.

Example 6.3: Determine the slope and deflection at point B of cantilever beam subjected to a point load and uniformly distributed load (UDL), as shown in Fig. 6.10. Use the moment-area method.

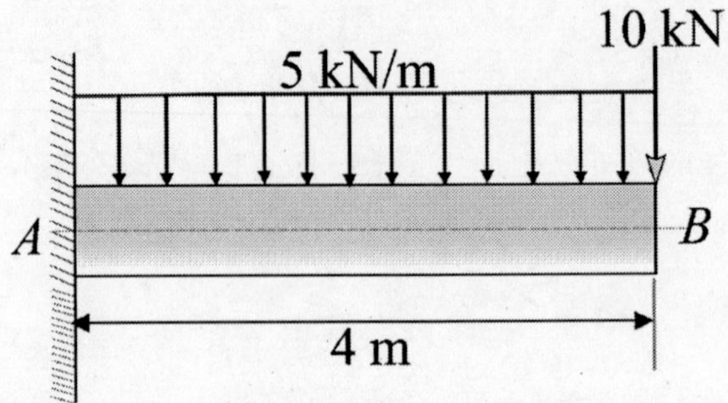

Fig. 6.10 Cantilever beam subjected to a point load and UDL

Solution: After determining the reaction forces from the free-body diagram (Figure 6.3e1(a)), the curvature of the *M*/*EI* diagram is obtained (Figure 6.3e1(b, c)). As the cantilever beam is fixed at point *A*, hence slope will be zero at point *A*, so the tangent of the elastic curve is horizontal (Figure 6.3e1(d)).

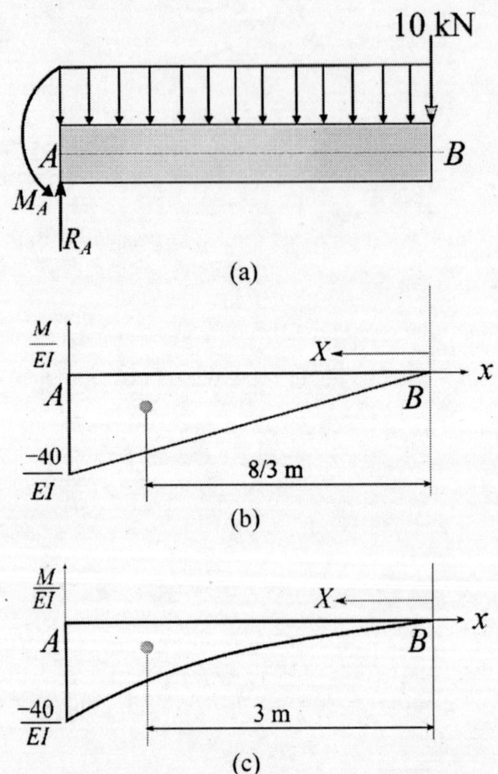

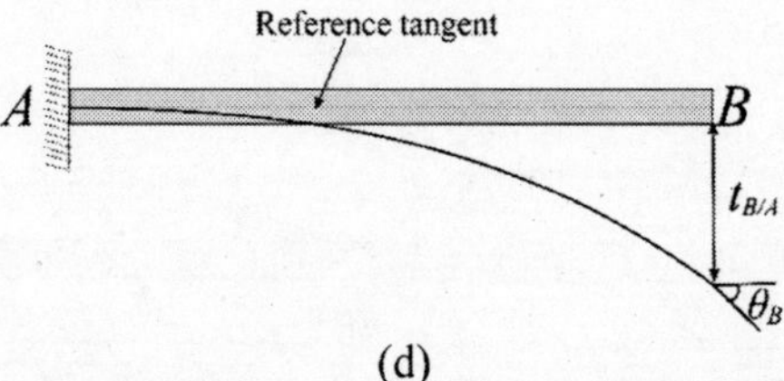

(d)

Figure 6.3e1 Solution procedure: (a) Free-body diagram of the beam (b) *M/EI* diagram due to point load *B* (c) *M/EI* diagram due to UDL on entire span (d) Elastic curve

The first moment-area theorem states that the area between two locations on a *M/EI* diagram is equivalent to the change in slope between those two points on the elastic curve.

Therefore, the change in slope between *A* and *B* i.e., $\theta_B - \theta_A$ = Area of curvature or *M/EI* diagram between *B* and *A*. As $\theta_A = 0$,

$$\theta_{B/A} = \int_{x_A}^{x_B} \frac{M}{EI} \mathrm{d}x$$

$$\theta_B = \frac{1}{2} \times \left[\frac{-40}{EI} \times 4\right] + \frac{1}{3} \times \left[\frac{-40}{EI} \times 4\right] = \frac{-400}{3EI}$$

The negative sign indicates of negative slope of the tangent at location *B*. The second moment-area theorem asserts that the tangential deviation of point *B* from the tangent at *A* is equal to the moment of area of the *M/EI* diagram between *A* and *B*, with respect to *B*. This allows one to calculate the angular deflection at point *B*. Therefore, the deflection at *B* or $t_{B/A}$ is equal to

$$t_{B/A} = \int_{X_B}^{X_A} X \frac{M}{EI} \mathrm{d}X$$

Here, $X_B = 0$ and $X_A = 4$ m since the X is defined from the point B as shown in the Figure 6.3e1(b) and Figure 6.3e1 (d).

$$t_{B/A} = \frac{8}{3} \times \frac{1}{2} \times \left[\frac{-40}{EI} \times 4\right] + 3 \times \frac{1}{3} \times \left[\frac{-40}{EI} \times 4\right]$$

$$= \frac{-1120}{3EI}$$

The deflection at point *B*, in this case is $t_{B/A}$ itself. This could happen because the slope at the fixed support is zero.

Example 6.4: Determine the slope and deflection at the hinge located at *B*, shown in Fig 6.11.

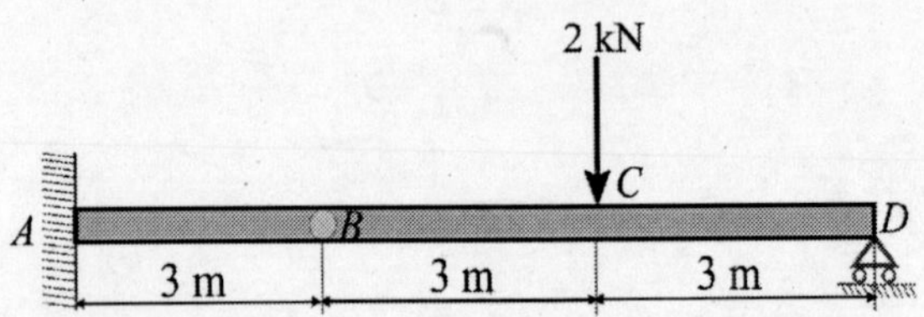

Fig 6.11 Cantilever beam subjected to a point load and UDL

Solution: Based on the free-body diagram (Figure 6.4e1(a)), to produce the beam's curvature diagram, the bending moment M at each point by the flexural rigidity EI (Figure 6.4e1(b). The tangent at end A is selected as the reference tangent since end A is of fixed support (Figure 6.4e1(c)).

From the free body diagram, $R_A = R_B = R_D = 1$ kN.

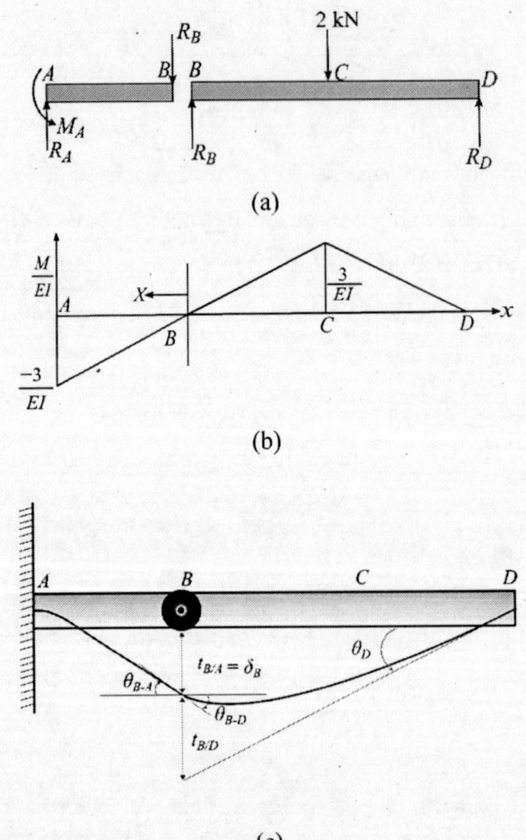

Figure 6.4e1 Solution procedure: (a) Free-body diagram of the beam, (b) M/EI diagram, (c) Elastic curve

As $\theta_A = 0$, applying the first moment area between points *A* and *B* (Figure 6.4E1(b)),

$$\theta_{B/A} = \int_{x_A}^{x_B} \frac{M}{EI} \mathrm{d}x$$

$$\theta_{B/A} = \theta_B = \frac{1}{2} \times \left[\frac{-3}{EI} \times 3 \right] = \frac{-9}{2EI}$$

A negative sign here indicates a negative slope of the tangent at point *B.* One has to note that the slope of the beam at *B* in segments *AB* and *BD* will be different. This is because there is a hinge at location *B*. Therefore, the slope at point *B* is segment *AB*, denoted by θ_{B-A} is

$$\theta_{B-A} = \frac{-9}{2EI}$$

Applying the second moment-area theorem between *A* and *B*

$$t_{B/A} = \int_{X_B}^{X_A} X \frac{M}{EI} \mathrm{d}X$$

$$t_{B/A} = \frac{1}{2} \times \frac{2 \times 3}{3} \times \left[\frac{-3}{EI} \times 3 \right] = \frac{-9}{EI}$$

To find the slope at point *D* (θ_D), taking $L = 3\,\text{m}$ where L is the length of segment *AB*, *BC*, and *CD*, we have

$$\theta_D = \frac{-(t_{B/A} - t_{B/D})}{2L}; t_{B/D} = \frac{1}{2} \times \frac{3}{EI} \times 2L \times L$$

Therefore, θ_D is given by

$$\theta_D = \frac{(t_{B/A} + t_{B/D})}{2 \times 3}$$

$$\theta_D = \frac{1}{6} \left[\frac{9}{EI} + \frac{1}{2} \times \frac{3}{EI} \times 6 \times 3 \right]$$

$$= \frac{6}{EI}$$

Now to find the slope at the hinge point B as we approach from point D can be found by applying again the first moment-area theorem but between the points B and D

$$\theta_D - \theta_B = \frac{1}{2} \times \left[\frac{3}{EI} \times 2 \times 3 \right]$$

$$\theta_B = \frac{6}{EI} - \frac{9}{EI}$$

$$= \frac{-3}{EI}$$

The slope at point B as one approaches from D, denoted by θ_{B-D}, is

$$\theta_{B-D} = \frac{-3}{EI}$$

The negative sign indicates the clockwise direction.

Example 6.5: Fig. 6.12 shows a non-prismatic simply supported beam. The beam supports a concentrated load that acts in the middle of the span of the beam. Find out the deflection at the centre and slopes at endpoints.

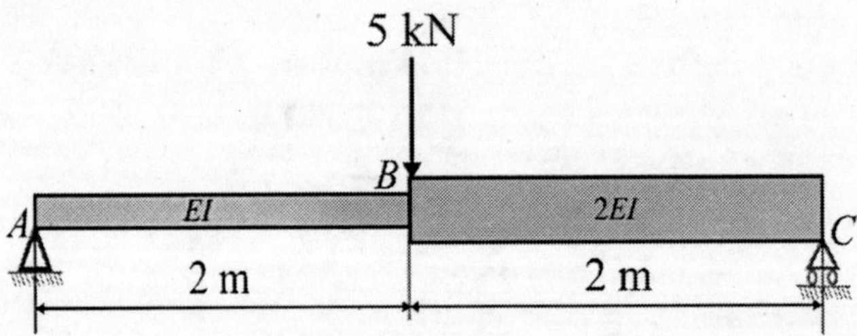

Fig. 6.12 Cantilever beam subjected to a point load and UDL

Solution: Based on the free-body diagram in Figure 6.5e1(a), the M/EI diagram can be drawn (Figure 6.5e1(b)).

From the free-body diagram, it can be established $R_A = R_C = 2.5$ kN.

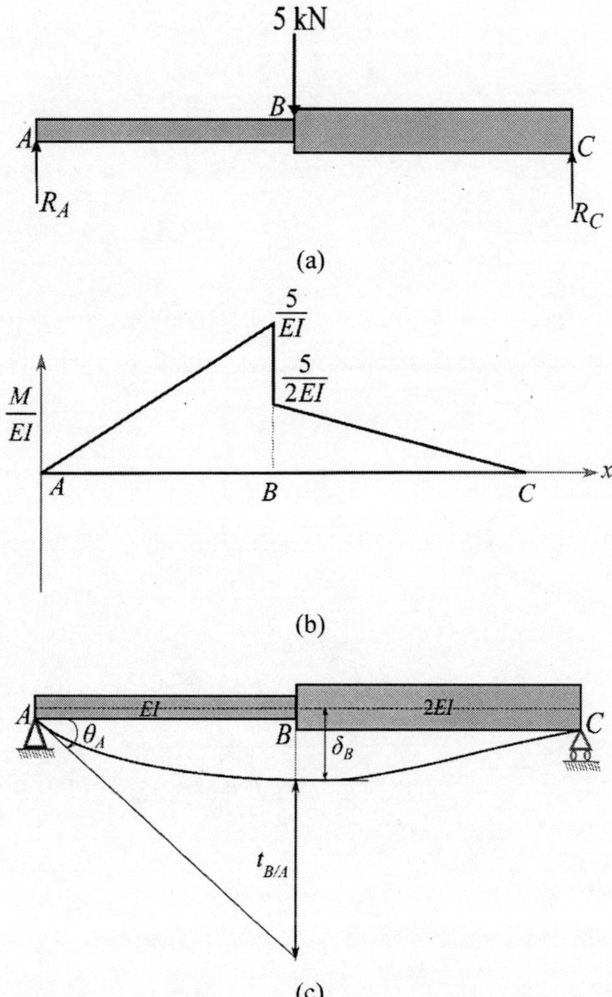

Fig. 6.5e1 Solution procedure: (a) Free-body diagram of the beam (b) *M/EI* diagram (c) Elastic curve

Though the loading is symmetrical, the beam geometry is not symmetrical with respect to the middle plane. Therefore, the slope at A i.e., θ_A is determined before proceeding ahead. It is obtained by using the equation

$$\theta_A = \frac{-t_{C/A}}{2L},$$

where $L = 2\,\text{m}$. The $t_{C/A}$ is given by

$$t_{C/A} = \frac{1}{2}\times 2\times\frac{5}{EI}\times\left(2+\frac{2}{3}\right)+\frac{1}{2}\times 2\times\frac{5}{2EI}\times\left(2\times\frac{2}{3}\right)$$

$$\theta_A = \frac{-t_{C/A}}{2L} = \frac{\left(\frac{50}{3EI}\right)}{2L}$$

$$\theta_A = \frac{-25}{6EI}$$

Negative sign here indicates of a negative slope of the tangent at point *A*. To find the slope at the point *B*, the first moment-area theorem between *A* and *B* is used, which is given by

$$\theta_B - \theta_A = \frac{1}{2}\times 2\times\frac{5}{EI}$$

Hence, $\theta_B = \frac{5}{6EI}$. In order to find the deflection at point *B*, Eq. (6.27) is used. It is given by

$$\delta_B = -\left(\frac{L}{2L}\times t_{C/A} - t_{B/A}\right)$$

Considering the Figure 6.5e1(c), the tangential deviation of *B* with respect to *A* can be obtained by

$$t_{B/A} = \frac{1}{2}\times 2\times\frac{5}{EI}\times\frac{2}{3} = \frac{10}{3EI}$$

$$\delta_B = -(\frac{L}{2L}\times t_{C/A} - t_{B/A})$$

$$= -\left(\frac{1}{2}\times\frac{50}{3EI} - \frac{10}{3EI}\right)$$

$$= \frac{-5}{EI}$$

Negative sign indicates the downward deflection at point *B*.

6.5 Macaulay's method

It is understood that the integration provides an efficient way to compute the slope and deflections of the beam throughout its length. However, this is effective only when the bending moment can be represented by an analytical equation throughout the length of the beam. If a beam is subjected to two or more discontinuous load functions, then it requires more than one equation for the bending moment, which upon integration twice, leads to constants that are twice the number of analytical forms. Therefore, the boundary conditions at the supports themselves will not be sufficient and will result in mathematical complexity to solve. These challenges will be overcome by employing the discontinuity functions, which are referred to as Macaulay's functions or singularity functions. To explain the distributed loadings on the beam, W. H. Macaulay, a mathematician proposed the functions which can be expressed as:

$$\langle x-a\rangle^n = \begin{cases} (x-a)^n & \text{when } x \geq a \\ 0 & \text{when } x < a \end{cases} \tag{6.28}$$

where x defines the location along the beam, and a is the position where the distributed loading initiates. These functions are valid only for the values $n \geq 0$. Upon indefinite integration, the Macaulay functions can be written as follows:

$$\int \langle x-a\rangle^n \,\mathrm{d}x = \frac{\langle x-a\rangle^{n+1}}{n+1} + C \tag{6.29}$$

Recall the Euler-Bernoulli's beam equation (6.12) given by

$$\frac{\mathrm{d}^2}{\mathrm{d}x^2}\left(EI\frac{\mathrm{d}^2 y}{\mathrm{d}x^2}\right) = q \tag{6.30}$$

Consider a simply supported beam subjected to UDL, as shown in Fig 6.13a.

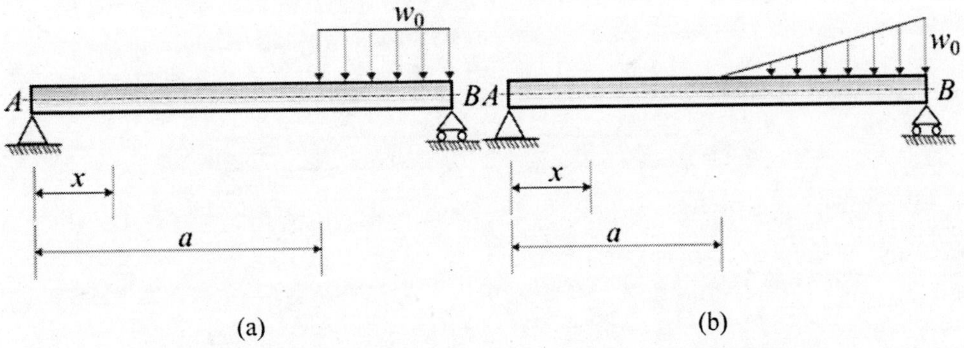

Fig 6.13 Simply supported beam subjected to (a) UDL, (b) UVL

The loading function q can be expressed as

$$q = -w_0\langle x-a\rangle^0 = \begin{cases} -w_0 & \text{when } x \geq a \\ 0 & \text{when } x < a \end{cases} \tag{6.31}$$

The loading function q involves only the external forces and moments as if the boundaries are extended hypothetically. The reactions forces and moments at the supports are not considered in q

Equation (6.31) can be substituted into Eq. (6.30) and integrated four times to obtain the elastic curve $y(x)$. Integrating four times involves four constants of integration. Appropriate conditions have to be employed to solve the four unknowns. Establishing the bending moment function $M(x)$ in terms of Macaulay's functions and using the Eq. (6.6) involves only two constants of integration, which is more convenient.

For a simply supported beam which is subjected to a linearly varying load, as shown in Fig 6.13b, the loading function q can be expressed as

$$q = -w_0 \langle x-a \rangle^1 = \begin{cases} -w_0(x-a) & \text{when } x \geq a \\ 0 & \text{when } x < a \end{cases} \tag{6.32}$$

Therefore, uniform loading is defined for $n = 0$ and linearly varying load for $n = 1$.

When a concentrated force P is acting at a location a from point A (Fig. 6.14), then q can be expressed as

$$q = -P\langle x-a \rangle^{-1} \tag{6.33}$$

For $n = -1$, the loading function q is defined as the concentrated force.

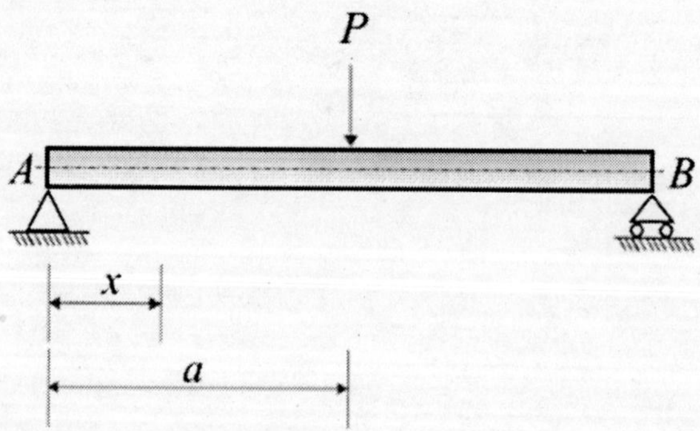

Fig. 6.14 Simply supported beam subjected to concentrated force P

For $n = -2$, it represents the concentrated moment. When a concentrated moment M_0 is acting at a location a from point A (Fig. 6.15), then q can be expressed as

$$q = -M_0 \langle x-a \rangle^{-2} \tag{6.34}$$

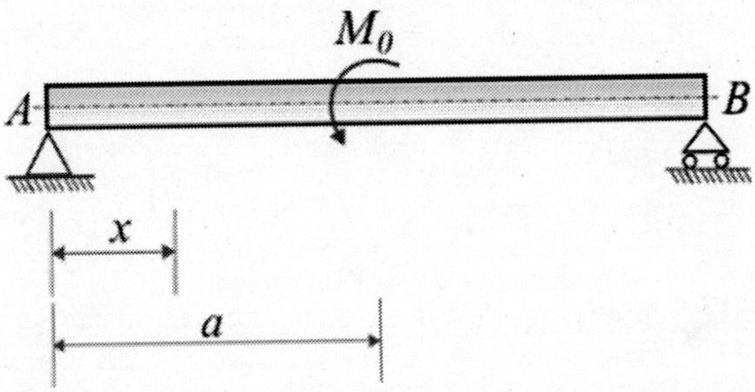

Fig. 6.15 Simply supported beam subjected to concentrated force M_0

It should be noted here that an anticlockwise moment generates a negative sign in the loading function.

Following the rules of operational calculus, the singularity functions upon integration can be written as,

$$\int \langle x-a \rangle^{n} \mathrm{d}x = \langle x-a \rangle^{n+1} + C \quad \text{for } n < 0 \tag{6.35}$$

The rules of integration depend on the power exponent n. Use the normal rules of integration, when the power exponent is greater than or equal to zero.

$$\begin{aligned}
&\int \langle x-a \rangle^{-2} \mathrm{d}x = \langle x-a \rangle^{-1} + C \\
&\int \langle x-a \rangle^{-1} \mathrm{d}x = \langle x-a \rangle^{0} + C \\
&\int \langle x-a \rangle^{0} \mathrm{d}x = \langle x-a \rangle^{1} + C \\
&\int \langle x-a \rangle^{1} \mathrm{d}x = \frac{1}{2}\langle x-a \rangle^{2} + C \\
&\int \langle x-a \rangle^{2} \mathrm{d}x = \frac{1}{3}\langle x-a \rangle^{3} + C \\
&\int \langle x-a \rangle^{3} \mathrm{d}x = \frac{1}{4}\langle x-a \rangle^{4} + C
\end{aligned} \tag{6.36}$$

Example 6.6: A simply supported beam with a uniform cross-section is 10 m long and carries concentrated loads at points B and C, as shown in Fig. 6.16. Taking the flexural rigidity of the beam as $EI = 2.5 \times 10^8$ N. m^2, find i) maximum deflection and ii) the deflection at the points B and C of the beam.

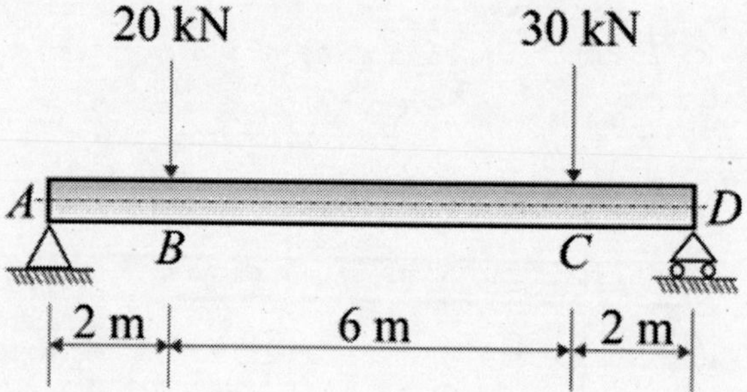

Fig. 6.16 Simply supported beam subjected to concentrated forces

Solution: Let R_A and R_D are the vertical reactions at supports A and D (Fig. 6.6e1)

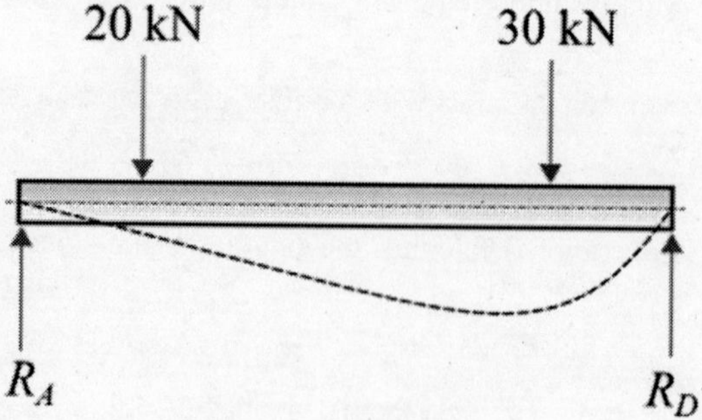

Fig. 6.6e1 Free-body diagram

$\sum F_y = 0 \Rightarrow R_A + R_D = 50$ kN

Taking a moment about A,

$$R_D \times 10 = 30 \times 8 + 20 \times 2$$
$$R_D = 28 \text{ kN}$$
$$\therefore R_A = 22 \text{ kN}$$

The loading function q, which takes account of the external forces and moments can be written as

$$q = -20\langle x-2\rangle^{-1} - 30\langle x-8\rangle^{-1}$$

We know that from Eq. (6.9) that $\frac{dV}{dx} = -q$ or $V = -\int q dx$ and obtain

$$V(x) = 20\langle x-2\rangle^{0} + 30\langle x-8\rangle^{0} + c_1$$

At $x = 0, V = -R_A \Rightarrow c_1 = -22$. Therefore,

$$V(x) = 20\langle x-2\rangle^0 + 30\langle x-8\rangle^0 - 22$$

From Eq. (6.10), it is known $\frac{dM}{dx} = -V$ or $M = -\int V dx$. Therefore,

$$M(x) = -20\langle x-2\rangle^1 - 30\langle x-8\rangle^1 - 22x + c_2$$

At $x = 0, M = 0 \Rightarrow c_2 = 0$. Therefore,

$$M(x) = 22x - 20\langle x-2\rangle^1 - 30\langle x-8\rangle^1$$

Following the usual procedure of finding the bending moment expression, it is convenient to directly construct the bending moment expression $M(x)$, in terms of the Macaulay's functions, without involving determination of c_1 and c_2. Then,

$$EI\frac{d^2y}{dx^2} = 22x - 20 < x-2 > -30 < x-8 >$$

$$EI\frac{dy}{dx} = 11x^2 - 10 < x-2 >^2 - 15 < x-8 >^2 + C_1$$

$$EIy = \frac{11}{3}x^3 - \frac{10}{3} < x-2 >^3 - 5 < x-8 >^3 + C_1x + C_2$$

At $x = 0, y = 0 \Rightarrow C_2 = 0$

At $x = 10, y = 0 \Rightarrow 0 = \frac{11}{3}(10)^3 - \frac{10}{3} < 10-2 >^3 - 5 < 10-8 >^3 + C_1(10)$

$$\therefore C_1 = -192$$

Hence, deflection at 'x' is rewritten as

$$EIy = \frac{11}{3}x^3 - \frac{10}{3} < x-2 >^3 - 5 < x-8 >^3 - 192x$$

(i) The maximum deflection of the beam: Let us assume that the location of the maximum deflection of the beam exists between the points B and C and equate the slope at that section to zero,

$$EI\frac{dy}{dx} = 11x^2 - 10 < x-2 >^2 - 192 = 0$$

Solving, gives $x = 7.038$ m

$\therefore$At $x = 7.038$ m the maximum deflection is calculated as,

$$EIy_{max} = \frac{11}{3}(7.038)^3 - \frac{10}{3} < 7.038 - 2 >^3 - 192(7.038)$$

$$y_{max} = -\frac{499.274 \times 10^3}{EI} = \frac{-499.274 \times 10^3}{2.5 \times 10^8}$$

$$y_{max} = -1.997 \text{ mm}$$

(ii) At $x = 2$ m, the deflection y_B is calculated as

$$EIy_B = \frac{11}{3}(2)^3 - 192(2)$$

$$y_B = -\frac{354.67 \times 10^3}{EI} = -\frac{354.67 \times 10^3}{2.5 \times 10^8}$$

$$y_B = -1.418 \text{ mm}$$

At $x = 8$ m, the deflection y_C is calculated as

$$EIy_C = \frac{11}{3}(8)^3 - \frac{10}{3} < 8 - 2 >^3 - 5 < 8 - 8 >^3 - 192(8)$$

$$y_C = \frac{-378.67 \times 10^3}{EI} = \frac{-378.67 \times 10^3}{2.5 \times 10^8}$$

$$y_C = -1.514 \text{ mm}$$

Example 6.7: A cantilever beam shown in Fig. 6.17 is subjected to a uniformly distributed load of intensity *w* throughout its length *L*, and its free end, point *B*, rests on a simply supported beam of the same material and cross-section. Find the force experienced by the cantilever beam at its free end.

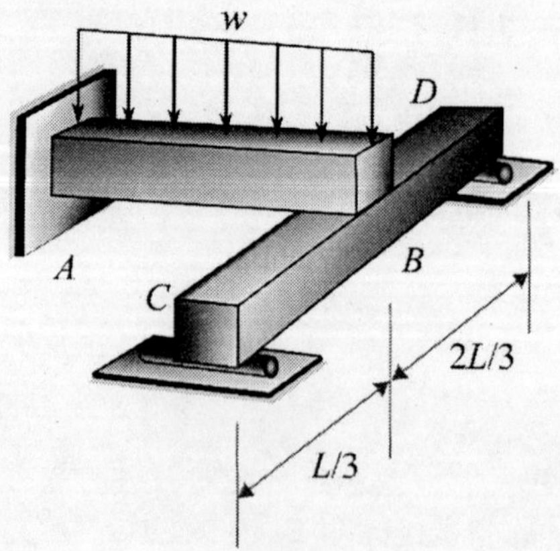

Fig. 6.17 Cantilever beam resting on a simply supported beam

Solution:

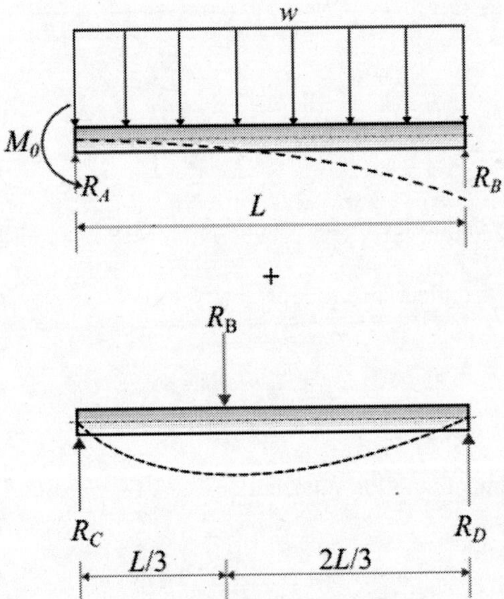

Fig. 6.7e1 Elastic curve of cantilever beam and simply supported beam

Let R_B be the common reaction force between the cantilever and simply supported beam (Fig. 6.7e1); the bending moment at any section of the cantilever beam is given as

$$M(x) = R_A x - M_0 - \frac{wx^2}{2}$$

$$\therefore EI\frac{d^2y}{dx^2} = R_A x - M_0 - \frac{wx^2}{2}$$

$$EI\frac{dy}{dx} = \frac{R_A x^2}{2} - M_0 x - \frac{wx^3}{6} + C_1$$

$$EIy = \frac{R_A x^3}{6} - \frac{M_0 x^2}{2} - \frac{wx^4}{24} + C_1 x + C_2$$

For the cantilever beam, at the fixed support i.e., at $x = 0$, $\frac{dy}{dx} = 0 \Rightarrow C_1 = 0$ and at $x = 0$, $y = 0 \Rightarrow C_2 = 0$

Substituting the constants in the deflection equation

$$EIy = \frac{R_A x^3}{6} - \frac{M_0 x^2}{2} - \frac{wx^4}{24}$$

i.e., $$EIy = \frac{(wL - R_B)x^3}{6} - \frac{\left(\frac{wL^2}{2} - R_B L\right)x^2}{2} - \frac{wx^4}{24}$$

Therefore, at the free end, $y_B = \frac{R_B L^3}{3EI} - \frac{wL^4}{8EI}$

Considering the simply supported beam which is subjected to R_B at $x = \frac{L}{3}$ from point C. The bending moment and the deflection equation at any section are given by,

$$M(x) = R_C x - R_B < x - \frac{L}{3} >$$

From the force and moment equilibrium equations, $R_C = \frac{2R_B}{3}$ and $R_D = \frac{R_B}{3}$. Hence,

$$EI\frac{d^2y}{dx^2} = \frac{2R_B}{3}x - R_B < x - \frac{L}{3} >$$

$$EI\frac{dy}{dx} = \frac{R_B x^2}{3} - \frac{R_B}{2} < x - \frac{L}{3} >^2 + C_3$$

$$EIy = \frac{R_B x^3}{9} - \frac{R_B}{6} < x - \frac{L}{3} >^3 + C_3 x + C_4$$

However,

$$\text{at } x = 0, y = 0 \Rightarrow C_4 = 0$$

$$\text{at } x = L, y = 0 \Rightarrow 0 = \frac{R_B L^3}{9} - \frac{R_B}{6}\left(\frac{2L}{3}\right)^3 + C_3 L$$

$$C_3 = -\frac{5R_B L^2}{81}$$

Substituting C_3 and C_4 in the deflection equation, we get,

$$EIy = \frac{R_B x^3}{9} - \frac{R_B}{6} < x - \frac{L}{3} >^3 - \frac{5R_B L^2}{81}x$$

The deflection at $x = \frac{L}{3}$ from point 'C' is $y_B = \frac{-4R_B L^3}{243EI}$

Since the cantilever beam's free end rests at the point 'B' of the simply supported beam, they undergo the same deflection at that location

$$\therefore (y_B)_{\text{Cantilever}} = (y_B)_{\text{Simply supported}}$$

$$\frac{R_B L^3}{3EI} - \frac{wL^4}{8EI} = -\frac{4R_B L^3}{243EI}$$

$$\therefore R_B = \frac{243}{680} wL$$

Example 6.8: For a simply supported beam shown in Fig. 6.18, determine (i) reactions at the supports *A* and *C*, (ii) the equation of the elastic curve, and (iii) the maximum deflection of the beam using Macaulay's method. (Assume flexural rigidity of the beam as $EI = 2.5 \times 10^8\ \text{N.m}^2$).

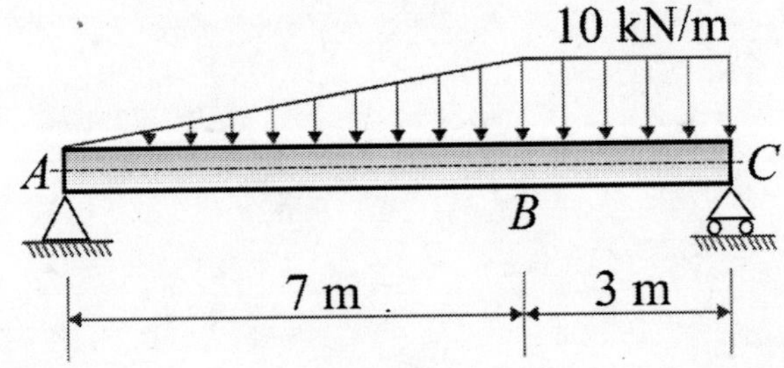

Fig. 6.18 Simply supported beam subjected to distributed loading

Solution:

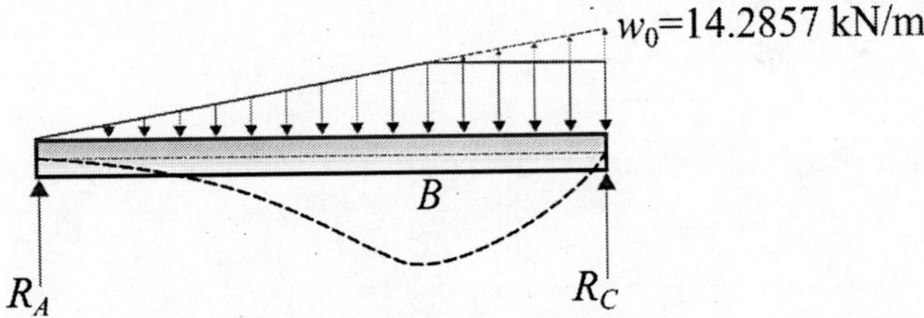

Fig. 6.8e1 Simply supported beam

(i) Let us find the reaction forces R_A and R_C at points A and C (Fig. 6.8e1). Taking the sum of the equilibrium of vertical forces equal to zero,

$$\sum F_V = 0 \Rightarrow R_A + R_C = \frac{1}{2} \times 10 \times 7 + 10 \times 3$$

$$R_A + R_C = 65\ \text{kN}$$

Taking moments about A,

$$R_C \times 10 = 10 \times 3 \times \left(\frac{3}{2} + 7\right) + \frac{1}{2} \times 10 \times 7 \times \frac{2 \times 7}{3}$$

$$\therefore R_C = 41.833 \text{ kN}$$

$$\therefore R_A = 23.167 \text{ kN}$$

(ii) The linearly varying load in the section AB is amended to point C, shown in Fig. 6.8e1. Therefore, the intensity at point C is

$$\frac{7}{10} = \frac{10}{w_0}$$

$$w_0 = 14.2857 \text{ kN/m}$$

The bending moment at any section 'x' along the length of the beam is

$$EI\frac{d^2y}{dx^2} = 23.167x - \frac{14.2857x^3}{60} + \frac{4.2857(x-7)^3}{18}$$

$$EI\frac{dy}{dx} = \frac{23.167x^2}{2} - \frac{14.2857x^4}{240} + \frac{4.2857}{72}(x-7)^4 + C_1$$

$$EIy = \frac{23.167x^3}{6} - \frac{14.2857x^5}{1200} + \frac{4.2857x^4}{360}(x-7)^5 + C_1x + C_2$$

At point A, i.e., $x = 0, y = 0 \Rightarrow C_2 = 0$

At point B, i.e., $x = 10 \text{ m}, y = 0 \Rightarrow 0 = \frac{23.167}{6}(10)^3 - \frac{14.2857}{1200}(10)^5 + \frac{4.2857}{360}(10-7)^5 + C_1(10)$

$$C_1 = -267.165$$

Substitute the constants C_1 and C_2 in the deflection and slope equations. We obtain

$$y = \frac{1}{EI}\left[\frac{23.167x^3}{6} - \frac{14.2857x^5}{1200} + \frac{4.2857}{360}(x-7)^5 - 267.165x\right]$$

$$\frac{dy}{dx} = \frac{1}{EI}\left[\frac{23.167x^2}{2} - \frac{14.2857x^4}{240} + \frac{4.2857}{72}(x-7)^4 - 267.165\right]$$

(iii) At maximum deflection, slope is zero and from the problem, the maximum deflection occurs in section AB.

$$\therefore \frac{23.167x^2}{2} - \frac{14.2857x^4}{240} - 267.165 = 0$$

Solving the above 4th degree polynomial equation, gives $x = 5.17$ m

Substitute $x = 5.17$ m in the deflection equation, results in

$$y_{max} = \frac{10^3}{2.5 \times 10^8}\left[\frac{23.167}{6}(5.17)^3 - \frac{14.2857(5.17)^5}{1200} - 267.165(5.17)\right]$$

$$y_{max} = -3.397 \text{ mm}$$

The maximum deflection, slope, and the elastic curve's equation for familiar beam problems are provided in Table 6.1.

6.6 Maxwell-Betti's law of reciprocal deflection

The Maxwell-Betti's law of reciprocal deflections shows that when a unit load is applied to an elastic structure at two places in succession, the displacements at those sites are identical in magnitude. For a perfectly stable elastic body, the Maxwell-law Betti's of reciprocal deflection states that the linear displacement at point *A* caused by a unit force applied at point *B* is identical in magnitude to the linear displacement at point *B* caused by a unit load delivered at point *A*. Let us consider a beam that has been sequentially subjected to the loads P_1 and P_2 at points 1 and 2 (Fig. 6.19) to demonstrate the Maxwell-Betti's law of reciprocal deflections, as shown in Fig. 6.20

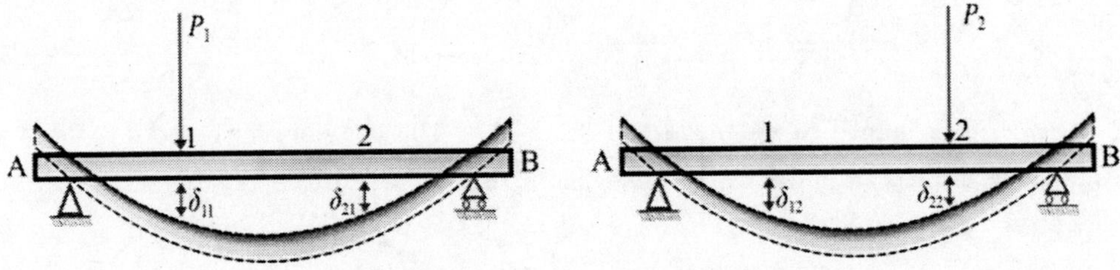

Fig. 6.19 Simply supported beam subjected to concentrated loads

In the first case, P_1 is applied at point 1 followed by P_2 at point 2. The forces are applied gradually and not suddenly. Then, the work done at point 1 caused by a load P_1 is

$$W_1 = \frac{1}{2} P_1 \delta_{11} \tag{6.37}$$

where δ_{11} is the deflection at point 1 due to the load P_1. Now when P_2 is applied, the work is done both by P_1 as well as P_2 since P_1 is still acting at point 1. The work done will be therefore,

$$W_2 = P_1 \delta_{12} + \frac{1}{2} P_2 \delta_{22} \tag{6.38}$$

where δ_{12} and δ_{22} are the deflections at point 1 and 2, respectively, caused due to the gradual application of load P_2. The total work done would be

$$W_1 + W_2 = \frac{1}{2} P_1 \delta_{11} + P_1 \delta_{12} + \frac{1}{2} P_2 \delta_{22} \tag{6.39}$$

In the second case, we reverse the application of the loads. Initially, the load P_2 at point 2 is applied, followed by P_1 at point 1. The work done at point 2 due to the gradual application of load P_2 is

$$W_1' = \frac{1}{2} P_2 \delta_{22} \tag{6.40}$$

With P_2 still in its place, when P_1 is applied gradually at point 1, then the work done will be

$$W_2' = P_2 \delta_{21} + \frac{1}{2} P_1 \delta_{11} \tag{6.41}$$

The total work done will be

$$W_1' + W_2' = \frac{1}{2} P_2 \delta_{22} + P_2 \delta_{21} + \frac{1}{2} P_1 \delta_{11} \tag{6.42}$$

The work done in the first and the second case will be the same since the order of application of forces for linear elastic structures. Equating (6.39) and (6.42), we obtain

$$\frac{1}{2} P_1 \delta_{11} + P_1 \delta_{12} + \frac{1}{2} P_2 \delta_{22} = \frac{1}{2} P_2 \delta_{22} + P_2 \delta_{21} + \frac{1}{2} P_1 \delta_{11} \tag{6.43}$$

Eq. (6.43) implies $P_1 \delta_{12} = P_2 \delta_{21}$. If the loads $P_1 = P_2 = 1$, then $\delta_{12} = \delta_{21}$.

Table 6.1 Deflections and slopes of beam under different loading conditions (similar tables are available in different books)

Beam configuration	Deflection curve	Maximum deflection	Slope at the end	Elastic curve equation
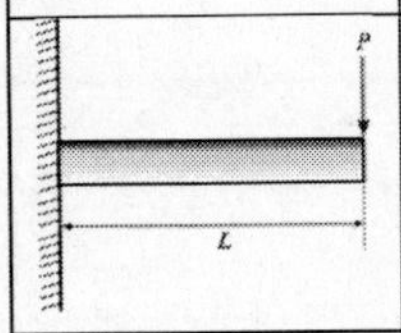	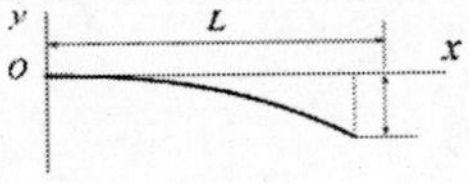	$-\frac{PL^3}{3EI}$	$-\frac{PL^2}{2EI}$	$y=\frac{P}{6EI}(x^3-3Lx^2)$
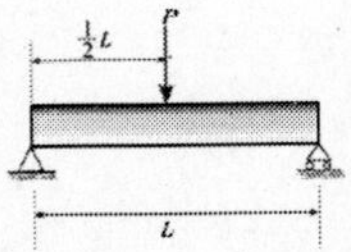	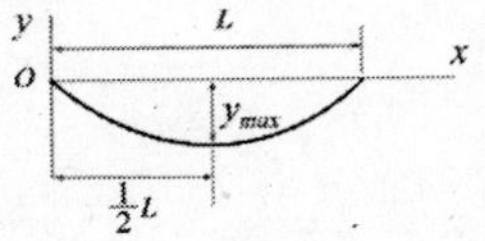	$-\frac{PL^3}{48EI}$	$\pm\frac{PL^2}{16EI}$	For $x \le \frac{1}{2}L$: $y=\frac{P}{48EI}(4x^3-3Lx^2)$
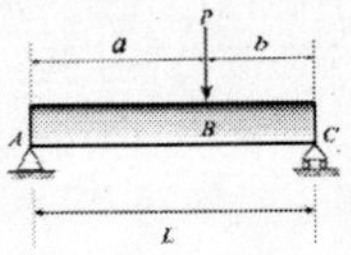	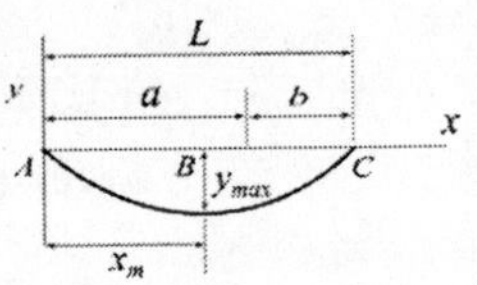	For $a>b$: $-\frac{Pb(L^2-b^2)^{3/2}}{9\sqrt{3}EIL}$ at $x_m=\sqrt{\frac{L^2-b^2}{3}}$	$\theta_A=-\frac{Pb(L^2-b^2)}{6EIL}$ $\theta_C=\frac{Pa(L^2-a^2)}{6EIL}$ $\theta_B=\frac{Pab(a-b)}{3EIL}$	For $x<a$: $y=\frac{Pb}{6EIL}[x^3-(L^2-b^2)x]$ At $x=a$: $y=-\frac{Pa^2b^2}{3EIL}$ For $x \ge a$: $y=\frac{1}{EI}\left[\frac{Pbx^3}{6L}-\frac{P(x-a)^3}{6}+\ldots\left(\frac{Pab(a-b)}{3L}-\frac{Pa^2b}{2L}\right)x\right]$
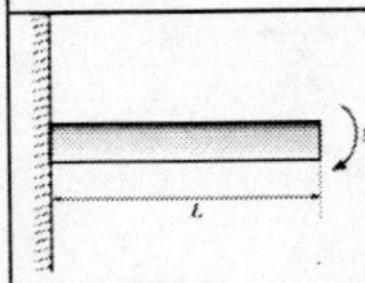	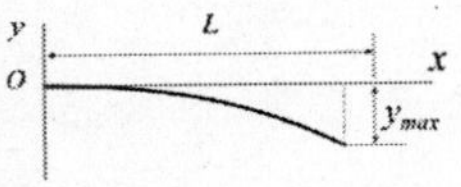	$-\frac{ML^2}{2EI}$	$-\frac{ML}{EI}$	$y=-\frac{M}{2EI}x^2$
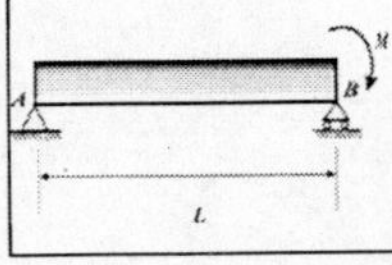	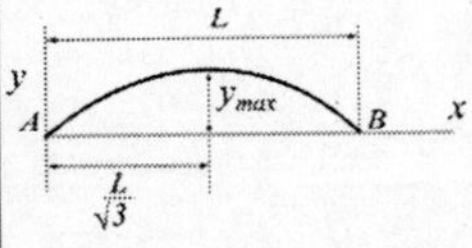	$\frac{ML^2}{9\sqrt{3}EI}$	$\theta_A=+\frac{ML}{6EI}$ $\theta_B=-\frac{ML}{3EI}$	$y=-\frac{M}{6EIL}(x^3-L^2x)$

Beam configuration	Deflection curve	Maximum deflection	Slope at the end	Elastic curve equation
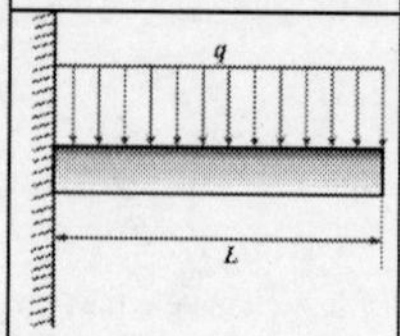	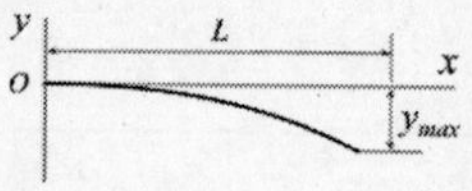	$-\frac{qL^4}{8EI}$	$-\frac{qL^3}{6EI}$	$y=-\frac{q}{24EI}(x^4-4Lx^3+6L^2x^2)$
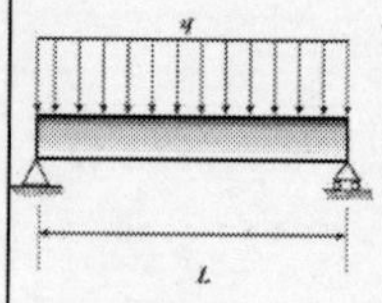	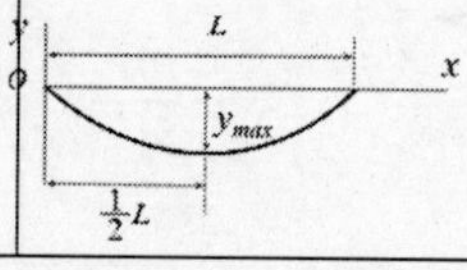	$-\frac{5qL^4}{384EI}$	$\pm\frac{qL^3}{24EI}$	$y=-\frac{q}{24EI}(x^4-2Lx^3+L^3x)$

Example 6.9: For the cantilever beam subjected to concentrated forces, as shown in Fig. **6.20** (a) and (b), determine (i) the deflection at B (δ_{BC}) due to P using the known methods used to find the deflection and (ii) the deflection at C (δ_{CB}) due to Q using the Maxwell-Betti's reciprocal law of deflection. Take the flexural rigidity as EI.

Solution: (i) The deflection at the point B due to load P can be obtained from the Table 6.1 as

$$\delta_{BC} = \frac{Pa^2}{6EI}(a - 3L)$$

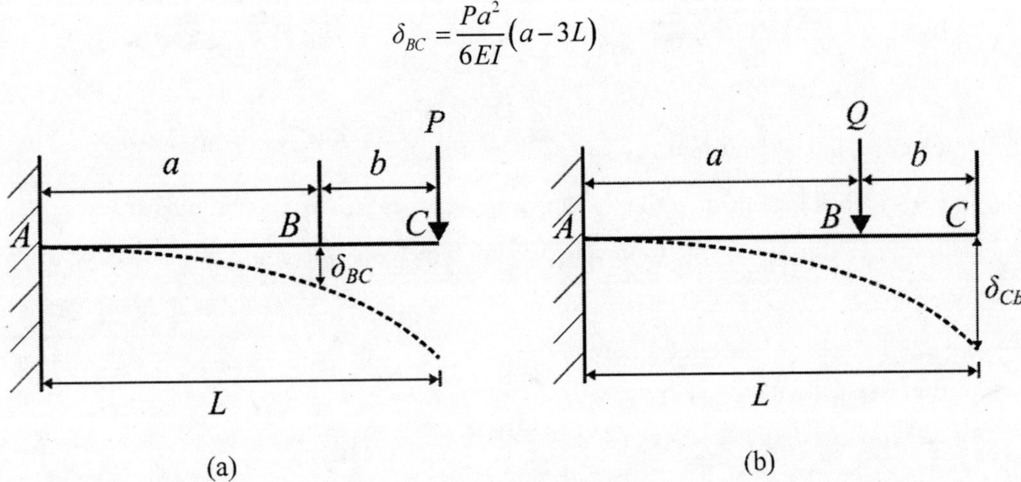

Fig. 6.20 Cantilever beam subjected to concentrated force (a) P at the free end (b) Q at the intermediate location

(ii) Using the Maxwell-Betti's reciprocal law of deflection, we can write

$$P\delta_{CB} = Q\delta_{BC}$$

Therefore, δ_{CB} is

$$\delta_{CB} = \frac{Qa^2}{6EI}(a - 3L)$$

While it is simple to establish δ_{BC} using the known procedures, δ_{CB} is not obtained with ease. However, with the usage of Maxwell-Betti's reciprocal law of deflection, δ_{CB} is easily obtained.

Know More

Exercises

Multiple Choice Questions

6.1. Lateral loading on a simply supported beam caused it to deflect above the allowable limit. Among the following options, which one will cause less deflection to occur?

a) Increase the flexural rigidity
b) Decrease the flexural rigidity
c) Increase the span of the beam
d) Use another material with a lower modulus of elasticity

6.2. A cantilever beam supports a concentrated load at the middle. Then which of the following is true?

a) The maximum bending stress occurs at the free end
b) The slope of the elastic curve is constant between the free end and the point of application of the concentrated load
c) The slope of the deflection curve is maximum at the fixed end
d) Shear stress remains constant across the span of the beam

6.3. If the area of M/EI diagram between points A, located at $x = 0$, and B, located at $x = 1$, is negative, then which one of the following is true?

a) Slope at tangent A is higher than slope at tangent B

b) Slope at tangent A is lower than slope at tangent B

c) Slopes at A and B are zero

d) Slopes at A and B are equal

6.4. For the analysis of beams, Macaulay's method is suitable for the beams with

a) multiple concentrated loads only

b) multiple distributed load intensities only

c) multiple concentrated and multiple distributed loadings

d) None as it does not offer any advantage

6.5. In the figure, the moment function in terms of Macaulay's function is given by

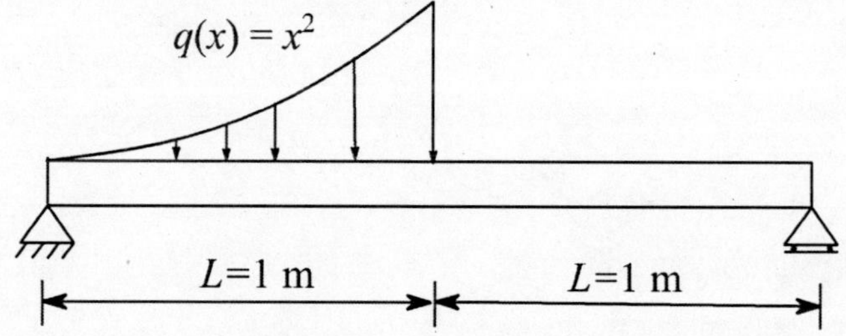

a) $M(x) = \frac{5}{24}x - \frac{<x-0>^3}{6} + \frac{<x-L>^3}{6}$

b) $M(x) = \frac{5}{24}x - \frac{<x-0>^4}{12} + \frac{<x-L>^4}{12}$

c) $M(x) = \frac{5}{24}x - \frac{<x-0>^4}{12} + \frac{<x-L>^4}{12} + \frac{<x-L>^3}{6}$

d) $M(x) = \frac{5}{24}x - \frac{<x-0>^4}{12} + \frac{<x-L>^4}{12} + \frac{<x-L>^3}{3} + \frac{<x-L>^2}{2}$

6.6. A simply supported beam carries a uniformly distributed load of 20 kN/m over the length of 1 m. What is the maximum deflection in the beam, if flexural rigidity is 200 kN.m^2?

a) 4 mm

b) 0.26 mm

c) 1.3 mm

d) 2.6 mm

6.7. Which of the following is a valid differential equation for finding the deflection of a beam?

a) $\frac{dy}{dx} = \frac{M}{EI}$

b) $\frac{d^2y}{dx^2} = \frac{MI}{E}$

c) $\frac{dy}{dx} = \frac{ME}{I}$

d) $\frac{d^2y}{dx^2} = \frac{M}{EI}$

6.8. The curvature at any point in the beam is

a) directly proportional to the bending moment

b) directly proportional to the shear force

c) inversely proportional to the bending moment

d) inversely proportional to the shear force

6.9. The maximum deflection of the cantilever beam (flexural rigidity – EI) of length l subjected to a concentrated moment (M) at its free end will be equal to

a) $\frac{ML^2}{3EI}$

b) $\frac{ML^3}{3EI}$

c) $\frac{ML^3}{2EI}$

d) $\frac{ML^2}{2EI}$

6.10. The reciprocal theorem of Maxwell is valid for structures

a) that are linear or non-linear elastic

b) that are plastic

c) having a linear force-displacement relation

d) whose support should be unyielding

Keys: 6.1-(a), 6.2-(b), 6.3-(a), 6.4-(c), 6.5-(d), 6.6-(c), 6.7-(d), 6.8-(a), 6.9-(d), 6.10-(c)

Practice Problems

6.1. Determine the minimum value of the coefficient of friction between the beam and the block (Fig. P1) such that the block does not slip.

[**Ans:** $\frac{MgL^2}{2EI}$]

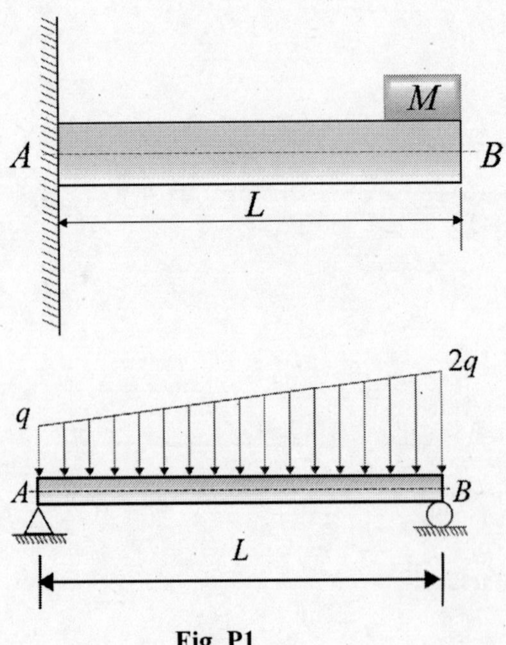

Fig. P1 **Fig. P2**

6.2. Find the deflection at the centre of the simply supported beam as shown in Fig. P2. Consider a constant flexural rigidity of the beam as *EI*.

[**Ans:** $-\dfrac{5}{256EI}qL^4$]

6.3. A simply supported beam with a uniform load on the mid-span is shown in Fig. P3. Using the moment-area method, calculate the slope and deflection at (a) the end-points and (b) 2 m distance from the end *A*. Take *E*=210 GPa. [**Ans: a)** $\theta_A = -0.0419$ rad, $y_A = 0$, $\theta_B = 0.0419$ rad, $y_B = 0$, **b)** $\theta_{2A} = -0.0305$ rad, $y_{2A} = -76.143$ mm]

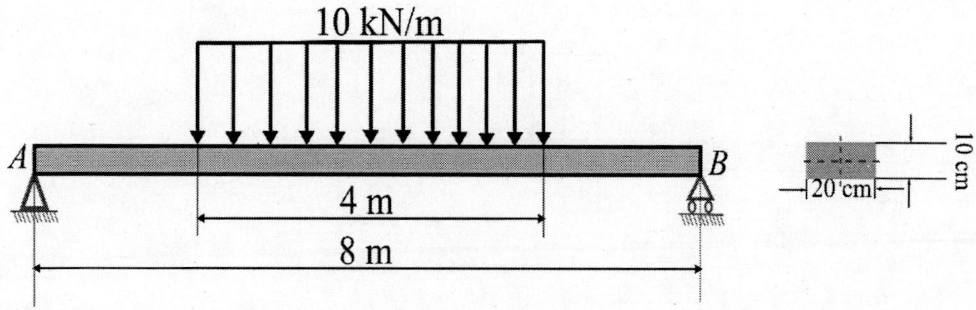

Fig. P3

6.4. A cantilever beam with a uniformly varying load on the entire span is shown in Fig. P4. Using the moment-area method, calculate the slope and deflection at (a) the free end (b) point *B*. Take *E*=200 GPa. [**Ans: a)** $\theta_C = -0.0159$ rad, $y_C = -58.3568$ mm **b)** $\theta_B = -0.0099$ rad, $y_B = -8.1298$ mm]

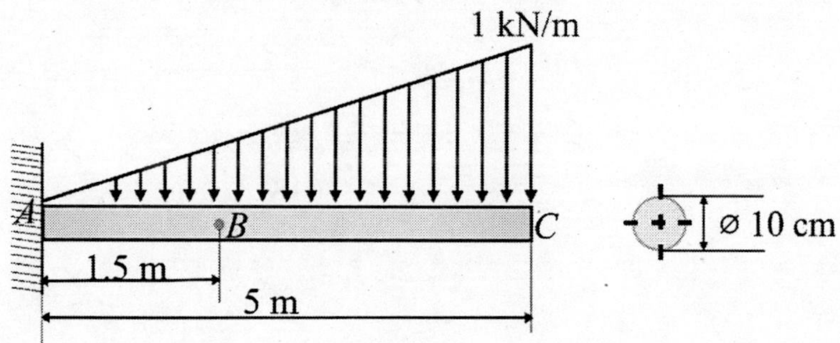

Fig. P4

6.5. A simply supported beam with a uniform distributed load (UDL) is shown in Fig. P5. Using the moment-area method, calculate the slope and deflection at the mid-span of the UDL. Take *E*=200 GPa. [**Ans:** $\theta = -0.0044$ rad, $y = -21.2749$ mm]

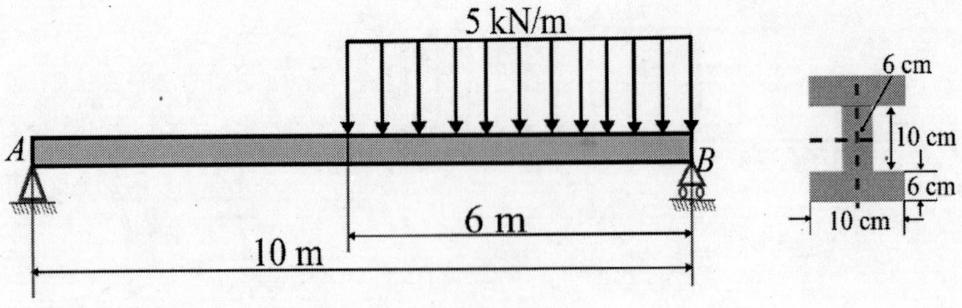

Fig. P5

6.6. A simply supported beam of length 10 m is subjected to a parabolic load of intensities $q/4$ and q at the locations shown in the Fig. P6. Using Macaulay's method, find the magnitude of the intensity q such that the midsection of the beam touches support B, positioned 5 mm below it. Take $E = 200$ GPa, $I = 25 \times 10^7$ mm^4.

[**Ans:** $q = 1.613$ kN/m]

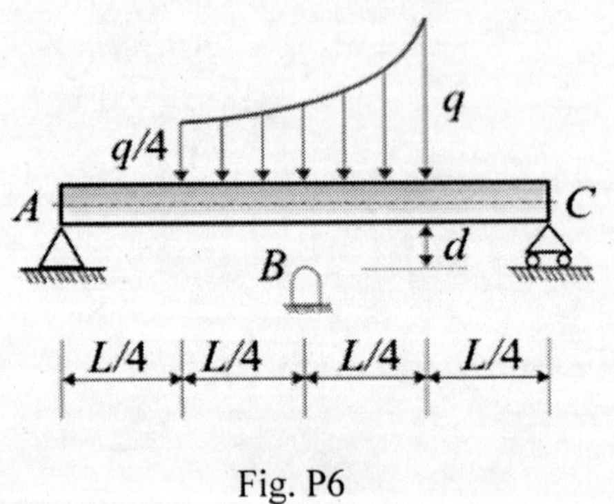

Fig. P6

6.7. A slightly curved overhanging beam of length 10 m is simply supported at B and C, as shown in the Fig. P7. Using the Macaulay's method, determine the magnitude of the moments M_A and M_B required to move the beam from its initial curvature to the position of the level of supports. Take: $y_A = -10$ mm, $y_B = -5$ mm, $EI = 2.5 \times$

10^6 N.m^2. [**Ans:** M_A = 9.6 kN/m, M_D = 7.2 kN/m]

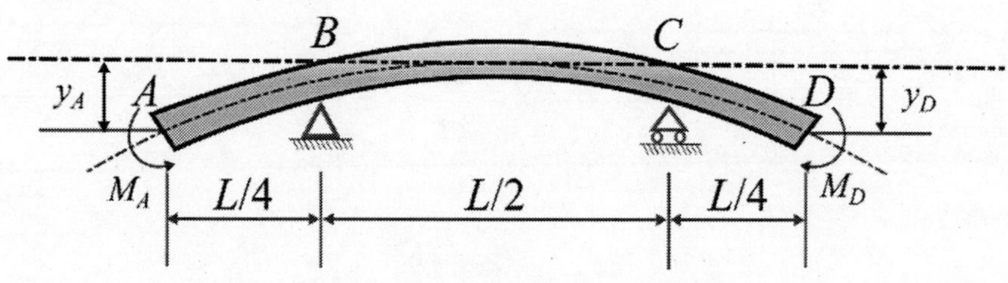

Fig. P7

6.8. Using the Macaulay's method, find the maximum deflection (in terms of $w, L,$ and EI) of a simply supported beam of length L, which carries the linearly varying loads as shown in the Fig. P8.

[**Ans:** $-0.00791wL^4 / EI$]

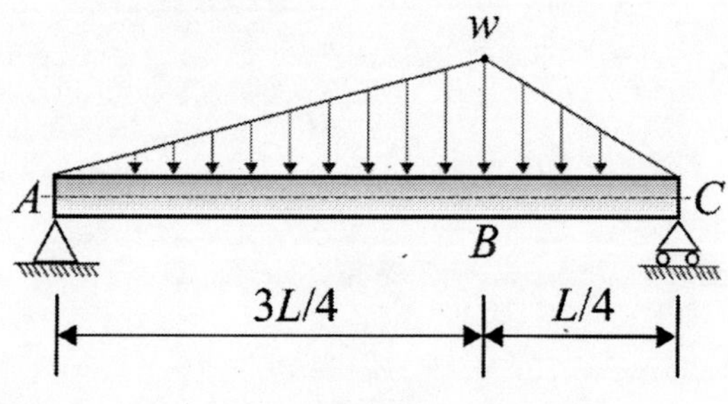

Fig. P8

6.9. For the simply supported beam subjected to concentrated forces, as shown in Fig.P9 (a) and (b), verify the Maxwell-Betti's reciprocal law of deflection using the deflection data given in the Table 6.1. Take the flexural rigidity as EI.

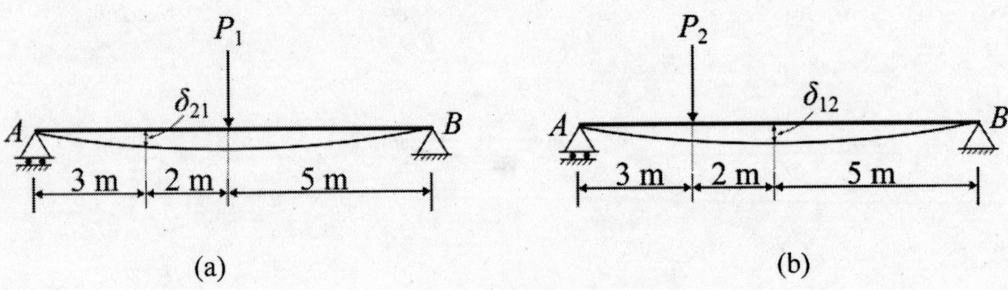

Fig. P9

Unit 7

Torsion of Circular Shafts

UNIT SPECIFICS

A structure can be twisted by the application of torque, which is a twisting moment. Torsion is the name given to the twist that occurs to a structure when it is subjected to the application of torques on either side of the body but in opposing rotational directions. Torque induces a stress pattern distributed over the object's cross-section, as opposed to the axial loads that generate a stress pattern averaged across the cross-section. Analysis of the circular cross-sectioned structures, often known as rods or shafts, is the major focus of this unit. The torsion equation is derived for the solid circular shaft, and the concept is extended to the hollow circular shaft and stepped shaft. Emphasis is given to the analysis of circular shaft subjected to combined twisting and bending moments. An example problem is solved to determine the principle stresses and the maximum stress under combined loading of torsion and bending. The unit finally ends with the analysis of close-coiled-helical springs based on the torsion equation.

RATIONALE

Torsion occurs when torque is applied to any shaft, regardless of whether the shaft is in motion or stationary. The former can occur in the case of driving shafts of engines and motors, and the latter can occur for bolts. When the shaft is subjected to a torque, it twists, and thus, there is a relative rotation of one end with respect to the other, resulting in shear stress across the cross-section. In such a scenario, excess shear stress can cause failure in the specimen. In most situations, there are combined loads on the shafts, including twisting, bending and axial loads. The effect of combined loading on the principal stresses and the maximum shear has to be considered during the design stages.

PRE-REQUISITES

Simple stresses and strains (Unit 1)

UNIT OUTCOMES

After completing this unit, students will be able to

U7-O1: Derive the torsion equation for the circular shaft

U7-O2: Derive the expression for variation of shear stress in solid, hollow and stepped circular shafts

U7-O3: Determine the principal stresses and the maximum shear stress under conbined torsion and bending of circular shafts

U7-O4: Analysis of the close-coiled-helical springs for deflection and stresses.

Course Outcomes	Expected Mapping with Course Outcomes - CE (1- Weak Correlation; 2- Medium correlation; 3- Strong Correlation)			
	CO-1	CO-2	CO-3	CO-4
U7-O1	1	2	-	3
U7-O2	-	3	-	2
U7-O3	-	3	2	1
U7-O4	-	2	2	3

Course Outcomes	Expected Mapping with Course Outcomes - ME (1- Weak Correlation; 2- Medium correlation; 3- Strong Correlation)	
	CO-1	CO-2
U7-O1	1	3
U7-O2	2	-
U7-O3	3	3
U7-O4	2	3

7.1 Introduction

There are several examples of when a component is subjected to a load that has the tendency to twist it. Such a type of load is called torsion. Shafts are often used in machines to transfer motion from the motor to the gearbox or other places; they typically experience cyclic torsional loading over long periods of time. Torque on these shafts is the component of the moment vector along the longitudinal axis of the shaft, which has a tendency to rotate one cross-section relative to the cross-section. It is essential to ensure that a component does not fail in torsion, particularly when a risk to human life is involved. For example, the propeller shaft of a boat should be properly designed to bear torsional stresses. The wings of an aircraft are also subjected to torsional loads besides other types of loads. It is essential that a wing does not fracture due to torsion.

The cross-section of the shaft or a member under torsional load can be of any shape. Usually, the shafts are of circular cross-sections, which is the focus of the present unit. In the case of the shafts of non-circular cross-sections, torsion also causes the cross-section warping. This means that all the points in a cross-sectional plane do not undergo the same longitudinal displacement; some portion of the cross-section bulges out, and some portion gets depressed. Warpage is not observed in the circular shafts. This is intuitively obvious. A circular cross-section has perfect symmetry about the longitudinal axis. Hence, there is no reason why a particular portion of the cross-section will bulge with respect to another portion. Fig. 7.1 shows the torsion of the circular and non-circular shafts. Analysis of such non-circular shafts is dealt with in the course on advanced solid mechanics topics. Here, we shall confine to the torsion of the circular shaft.

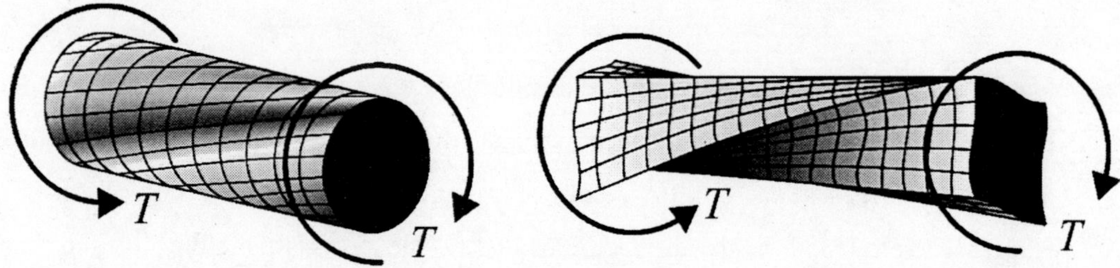

Fig. 7.1 Torsion of shafts

7.2 Strains and Stresses Due to Torsion

Torsion is also referred to as a twisting moment. The twisting moment vector is along the longitudinal axis of the shaft, and it causes in-plane rotation of the cross-sections. The stress analysis of a circular shaft under pure torsional loads involves some reasonable assumptions. During deformation, there is no distortion of the cross-sections; they stay flat, and the radius R does not change. Moreover, the length L of the shaft stays unchanged. Accordingly, we can assume that after the deformation, (a) the cross-sections remain as plane due to torsion, (b) the axis of the shaft continues to remain normal to the cross-section, (c) the distances between the cross-sectional planes remain constant and, (d) the cross-sections undergo pure shear in plane-strain conditions. In the forthcoming analysis, the shaft material is assumed to be isotropic and homogenous.

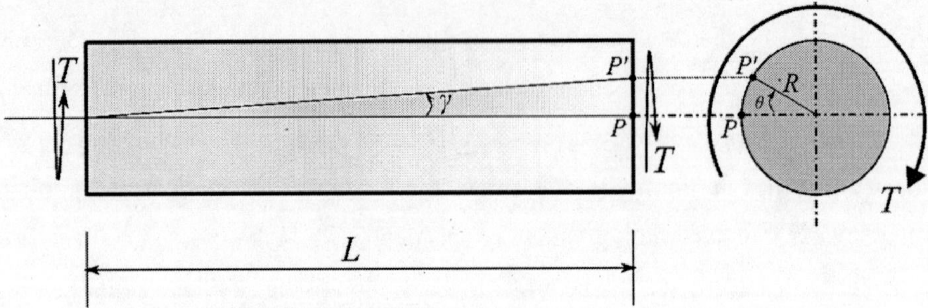

Fig. 7.2 Twisting of a circular shaft under torsion T

Figure. 7.2 shows the twisting of a solid shaft of length L and outer radius R, subjected to torque T. The point P on the surface of the shaft in the undeformed configuration has moved to a new location P' in the deformed configuration under the action of torsional load T. The arc length or the distance travelled by the point is therefore $L\gamma$. The same distance can be measured by observing the rotation (angle of twist - θ) of the radial line about the axis of the cylindrical shaft. It is given by $R\theta$. Hence,

$$L\gamma = R\theta$$

$$\gamma = \frac{R\theta}{L} \tag{7.1}$$

Here, γ is the shear strain experienced by any element on the skin of the outer surface. If τ is the shear stress and G is the shear modulus, then the shear strain is given by

$$\gamma = \frac{\tau}{G} \tag{7.2}$$

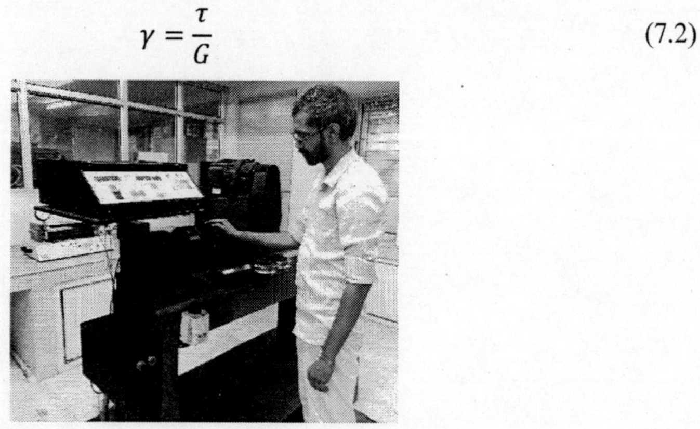

Fig. 7.3 Torsion tester

Shear stresses are generated during torsion. The modulus of rigidity, commonly known as shear modulus, is the term used to describe stiffness under shear stress. The modulus of rigidity is determined in a laboratory using the torsion tester (Fig. 7.3). In a torsion test, the cylindrical specimen is held between two jaws in a lathe type of machine. One end is held fixed, and the other end is subjected to torque, and its effect on the angular rotation of the end is recorded. Then we can plot torque versus twist angle.

Combining Eqs. (7.1) and (7.2), we get

$$\frac{\tau}{R} = \frac{G\theta}{L} \tag{7.3}$$

In fact, the same derivation can be applied to any point located at a radius r since G, θ, and L do not vary on a cross-section. Therefore, we can express Eqs. (7.3) as

$$\frac{\tau(r)}{r} = \frac{G\theta}{L} \tag{7.4}$$

Equations. (7.4) implies that the shear stress $\tau(r)$ is directly propotional to the radius r. The variation of shear stress on a cross-section is shown in Fig. 7.4. The maximum value of shear stress occurs at the periphery of the cross-section. The minimum value of zero occurs at the center.

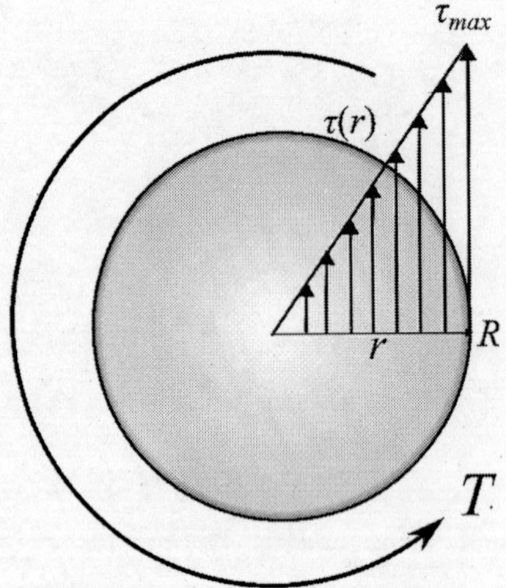

Fig. 7.4 Shear stress variation with r

To summarize, due to the torsional load T, the circular or cylindrical shaft undergoes twisting, as shown in Fig. 7.5. Consequently, the shear stresses are generated, and their nature is demonstrated on a shaft element.

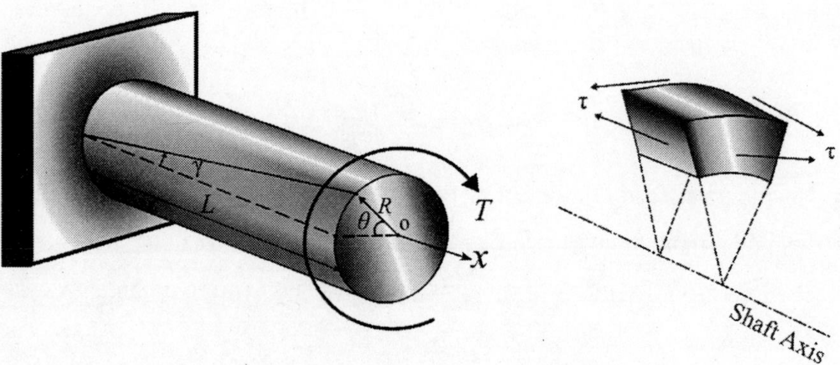

Fig. 7.5 Twisting of the circular shaft

The relation between the shear stresses and the external loading T can be determined from the moment equilibrium condition along the x – axis. Consider the scenario shown in Fig. 7.6. The net twisting moment about the x – axis can be obtained by calculating the resultant moment, which is none other than the external torsional load T. This can be expressed as

$$T = \int_A r\mathrm{d}F = \int_A r\tau(r)\mathrm{d}A \tag{7.5}$$

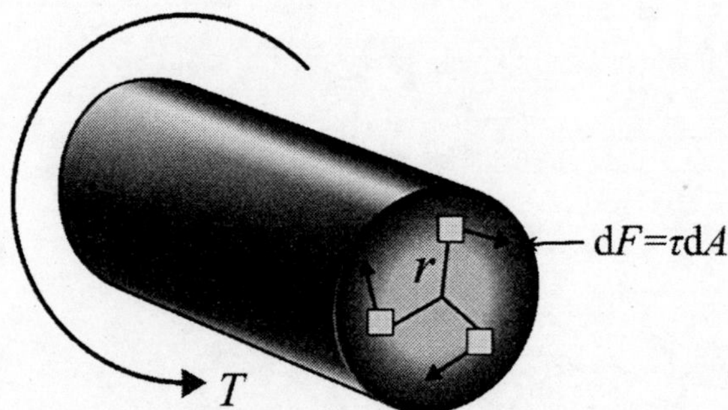

Fig. 7.6 Forces due to shear stress on an infinitesimal element on the cross-section

Combining Eqs. (7.4) and (7.5), we get

$$T = \int_A r^2 \frac{G\theta}{L} \mathrm{d}A = \frac{G\theta}{L} \int_A r^2 \mathrm{d}A = \frac{GJ\theta}{L} \tag{7.6}$$

where J is the polar second moment of the area of the cross-section. This is also referred to as the polar moment of inertia of the cross-sectional area. In the SI system, the consistent units are T [N. m], G [Pa], $J[\mathrm{m}^4]$, θ [rad], and $L[\mathrm{m}]$. Combining Eqs. (7.4) and (7.6), one can write

$$\frac{T}{J} = \frac{\tau}{r} = \frac{G\theta}{L} \tag{7.7}$$

The angle of twist θ is related to the torque T by

$$\frac{T}{\theta} = \frac{GJ}{L} \tag{7.8}$$

The quantity $\frac{GJ}{L}$ is called the 'torsional stiffness of the shaft. It is defined as the torque required to twist a circular shaft by a unit radian.

For the solid circular cross-section, $J = \frac{\pi R^4}{2}$ and for a hollow shaft, it is $J = \frac{\pi}{2}(R_{out}^4 - R_{in}^4)$. R_{out} and R_{in} is the outer and inner radius of the hollow shaft, respectively. Eqs. (7.4) is also applicable to the hollow shaft, for which the shear stress distribution is shown in Fig. 7.7. The maximum shear stress for the solid and hollow circular shafts are

$$\text{Solid circular shaft: } \tau_{max} = \frac{2T}{\pi R^3} \tag{7.9a}$$

$$\text{Hollow circular shaft: } \tau_{max} = \frac{2TR_{out}}{\pi(R_{out}^4 - R_{out}^4)} \tag{7.9b}$$

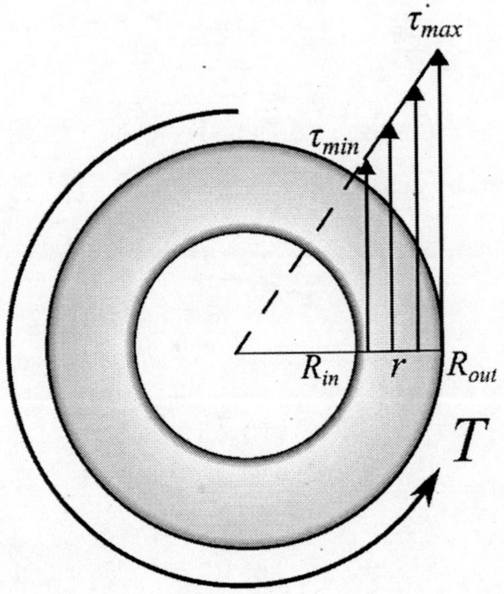

Fig. 7.7 Shear stress variation in a hollow shaft due to torsion

The power delivered by the shaft rotating with a fixed angular velocity ω being actuated by a twisting moment T is given by

$$P = T\omega = T(2\pi f) \tag{7.9}$$

where P is the power, T is the torque, and f is the frequency of the rotation.

Example 7.1 A solid shaft of a length of 3 m is subjected to a torque of 10 kN.m. The shear modulus of the shaft is $G = 80$ GPa. Find out the minimum diameter of the shaft to ensure that the angle of twist is less than 1°. What is the value of the maximum shear stress to the torsional load?

Solution: The angle of twist in terms of torque and given parameters, using Eq. (7.7), is given by

$$\theta = \frac{TL}{GJ}$$

Now, $T =$ 10 kN.m, $L =$ 3m, $G =$ 80 GPa. The polar moment of inertia for the solid shaft of radius r is given by

$$J = \frac{\pi R^4}{2}$$

For the angle of twist to be less than

$$\frac{\pi}{180} \leq \frac{10 \times 10^3 \times 3}{\frac{\pi R^4}{2}(80 \times 10^9)}$$

The minimum radius is, therefore $R =$ 60.81 mm. Hence, the minimum diameter is 121.62 mm.

For the solid shaft, as per Eq. (7.9a), the maximum shear stress occurs at the periphery of the circular cross-section. It is given by

$$\tau_{max} = \frac{2T}{\pi R^3} = \frac{2 \times 10 \times 10^3}{\pi (0.0608)^3}$$

The magnitude of the maximum shear stress is 28.32 MPa.

Example 7.2 A solid propeller shaft of length 10 m is required to transmit a power of 6 MW at 5 Hz. The maximum allowable shear stress is 80 MPa, and the maximum allowable angle of twist is 2°. What is the minimum diameter of the shaft for safe operation?

Solution: The twisting moment T that is acting on the propeller shaft can be found using Eq. (7.9). It is given by

$$T = \frac{P}{2\pi f} = \frac{6 \times 10^6}{2\pi \times 5} = 190.985 \text{ kN. m}$$

From Eq. (7.9a)a, the minimum radius required to sustain a load of 80 MPa is given by

$$R^3 = \frac{2T}{\pi \tau_{max}} = \frac{2 \times 190.985 \times 10^3}{\pi \times 80 \times 10^6} = 1.521 \text{ mm}$$

$$R = 0.115 \text{ m}$$

As per the maximum shear stress condition, the minimum radius of the shaft is 0.115 m. However, there is another condition on the angle of twist. The minimum radius as per the angle of twist condition for a solid circular shaft can be obtained using Eq. (7.7). It is given by

$$R^4 = \frac{2TL}{\pi G \theta} = \frac{2 \times 190.985 \times 10^3 \times 10}{\pi \times 80 \times 10^6 \times 2 \times \left(\frac{\pi}{180}\right)} = \frac{3819700}{8772981.69} = 0.435 \text{ m}$$

$$R = 0.812 \text{ m}$$

Based on the two conditions, the radius of the shaft has to be the maximum of obtained values of R, which in this case is 0.812 m. Therefore, the minimum diameter is 1.624 m.

7.3 Analysis of stepped shaft

When the shaft has non-uniform cross-sections, then Eq. (7.7) cannot be used to determine the angle of twist. For example, a shaft shown in Fig. 7.8 has three regions of different diameters. It also has torsional loads at multiple locations.

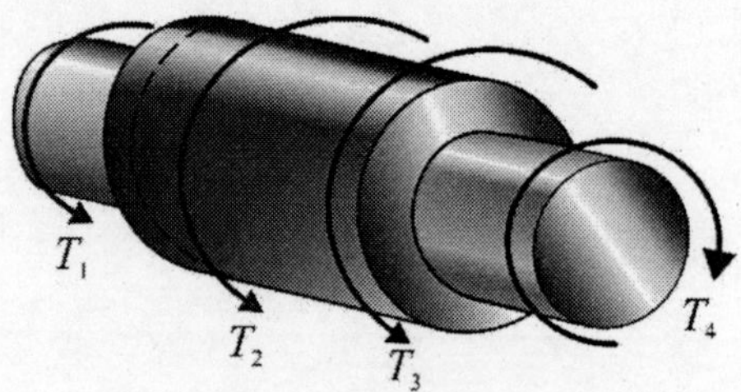

Fig. 7.8 Shaft with different cross-sections and multiple loads

Shafts containing different cross-sections and multiple loads need to be analyzed section-wise. A new section needs to be considered whenever there is a discontinuity geometry/material or the torsional load experienced by the shaft. A discontinuity in geometry is encountered when there is a sudden change in the diameter of the cross-section. A material discontinuity corresponds to a sudden change in the shear modulus. In Fig. 7.8 there are four sections that are displayed in Fig. 7.9.

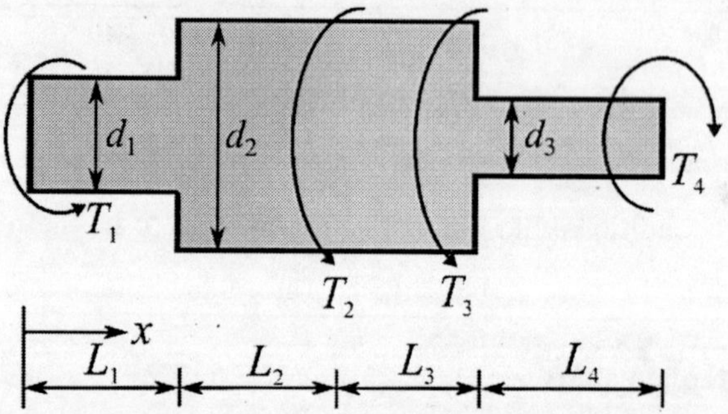

Fig. 7.9 Sections for stepped shaft analysis

The first section is of length L_1 that comprise the left portion of the shaft of diameter d_1. This section experiences a torque of magnitude T_1. After $x = L_1$, there is a discontinuity in the cross-section diameter; therefore, the next portion after $x = L_1$ belongs to the second section until there is a discontinuity in the diameter or the torsional loading. The second section of diameter d_2 and length L_2 experiences a torque of magnitude T_1 as well. At a location $x = L_1 + L_2$, an external torque T_2 is present, and therefore the third section begins at this location until the location at $x = L_1 + L_2$ until $x = L_1 + L_2 + L_3$. The third section is of length L_3 of diameter d_2 and is subjected to torsional loading of magnitude $T_1 + T_2$. Finally, the fourth section will be of length L_4 starting from $x = L_1 + L_2 + L_3$ until the end.

The direction of the torque is positive if it is aligned along the +ve x – axis (the right-hand thumb rule is implied). The direction is along the negative x – axis if a clockwise torque is acting on the shaft. If the shaft (Fig. 7.9) is in equilibrium, then the moment balance along the x – axis gives

$$T_4 = T_1 + T_2 + T_3 \tag{7.10}$$

If we identify the sections in the circular shaft with different cross-sections and multiple torsional loads, then the net angle of twist can be found using

$$\theta = \sum_{i=1}^{n} \frac{T_i L_i}{G_i J_i} \tag{7.11}$$

where i is the section number, n is the total number of sections and T_i is the torque acting on the section i. L_i, G_i and J_i are the length, shear modulus, and polar moment of inertia of the ith section of the shaft, respectively.

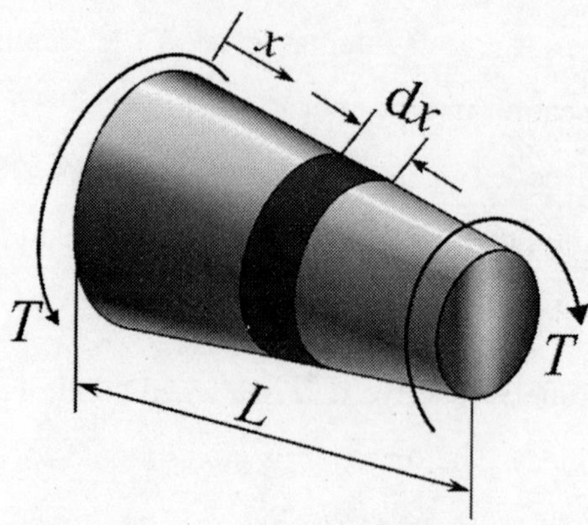

Fig. 7.10 Shaft with varying diameter

The same concept can be extended to a shaft of varying diameter, as shown in Fig. 7.10. If diameter can be expressed in terms of a continuous function of x, then the polar moment of inertia can also be expressed in terms of a continuous function of x. In such a scenario, the differential change in the angle of twist and, therefore, the net angle of twist can be written as

$$\frac{d\theta}{dx} = \frac{T}{GJ(x)} \tag{7.13a}$$

$$\theta = \int_0^L \frac{T dx}{GJ(x)} \tag{7.13b}$$

Example 7.3 Consider the pulley-shaft system shown in Fig. 7.11. The shaft has a diameter of 10 cm and a shear modulus of 80 GPa. Two pulleys A and B support a load of 1 kN and 2 kN, respectively, along the directions indicated in the figure. The diameter of the pulleys A and B are 30 cm and 20 cm respectievely. The entire shaft is supported on journal bearings at the ends that offer negligible resistance to rotation. Assuming the thickness of pulleys to be small, determine (a) the value of torque T to maintain this load, (b) the angle of twist between B and A, (c) the angle of twist between C and B, and (d) the angle of twist between C and A. Take the distance between A and B as $L_{AB} = 0.5$ m and the distance between B and C as $L_{BC} = 0.25$ m.

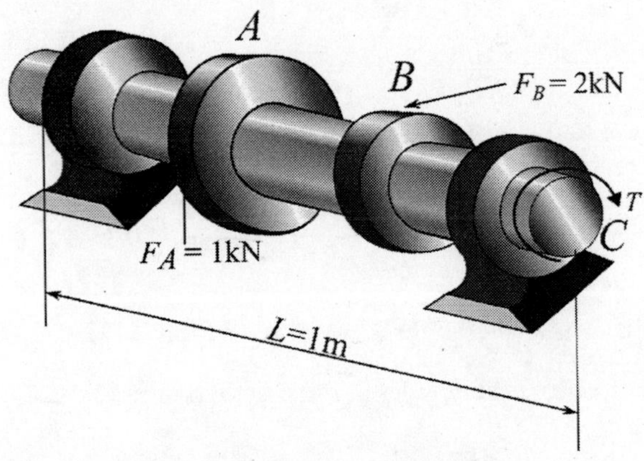

Fig. 7.11 Pulley shaft system

Solution: (a) Given $F_A = 1\ kN, F_B = 2\ kN, R_A = \frac{D_A}{2} = 0.3\ m$ and $R_B = \frac{D_B}{2} = 0.2\ m$, consider the equilibrium of the couple along the axis of the shaft to obtain T

$$F_B \times R_B = F_A \times R_A + T$$

$$T = 0.1\ \text{kN.m}$$

(b) The angle of twist in the section AB can be obtained using Eq. (7.7). It is given by

$$\theta_{B/A} = \frac{T_{AB}L_{AB}}{GJ}$$

$\theta_{B/A}$ stands for the angle of twist at location B with respect to the location A. The polar moment of inertia J for the shaft, which is of solid circular cross-section, is $J = \frac{\pi R^4}{2} = \frac{\pi \times 0.1^4}{2} = 1.571 \times 10^{-4}$ m^4. The torque on the section AB i.e. T_{AB} is equal to $F_B \times R_B$ or

$T_{AB} = 0.3$ kN. m. The length of section AB is provided in the question – $L_{AB} = 0.5$ m. Therefore,

$$\theta_{B/A} = \frac{0.3 \times 10^3 \times 0.5}{80 \times 10^9 \times 1.571 \times 10^{-4}} = 1.19 \times 10^{-4} \text{ rad } \circlearrowleft$$

(c) The angle of twist in the section BC is given by

$$\theta_{C/B} = \frac{T_{BC} L_{BC}}{GJ} = \frac{0.1 \times 10^3 \times 0.25}{80 \times 10^9 \times 1.571 \times 10^{-4}} = 0.198 \times 10^{-4} \text{ rad } \circlearrowright$$

It is to be noted that while the angle of twist in section AB i.e. $\theta_{B/A}$ is oriented in the counter-clockwise direction, the $\theta_{C/B}$ is in the clockwise direction.

(d) The angle of twist between C and A is given by

$$\theta_{C/A} = \theta_{C/B}\,(\circlearrowright) + \theta_{B/A}\,(\circlearrowleft) = 0.992 \times 10^{-4} \text{ rad } \circlearrowleft$$

7.4 Deflection of shafts fixed at two ends

When a shaft is rigidly fixed at the two ends, as shown in Fig. 7.12, the torques that are exerted by the supports at locations A and B cannot be found using the moment equilibrium equation along the axis of the shaft since there are two unknowns and only one equilibrium condition. Such a problem comes under the category of statically indeterminate problems. If the torques at the supports cannot be obtained, the angle of twist and the shear stress cannot be determined.

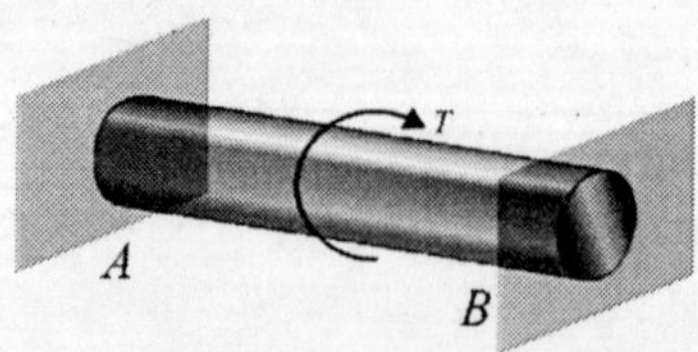

Fig. 7.12 Shaft fixed at two ends

In addition to the equilibrium equation, a compatibility equation is invoked to solve for two unknowns. In this case, the compatibility equation is that the magnitude of the angle of twist at the point of application of the external torque T as one approaches the location of the T from A and B should be equal.

Example 7.4 For the problem shown in Fig. 7.13, the length of the shaft is L, the shear modulus is G and its polar moment of inertia is J. Determine the torques at the supports A and B. Also, find the angle of twist at location C with respect to the A.

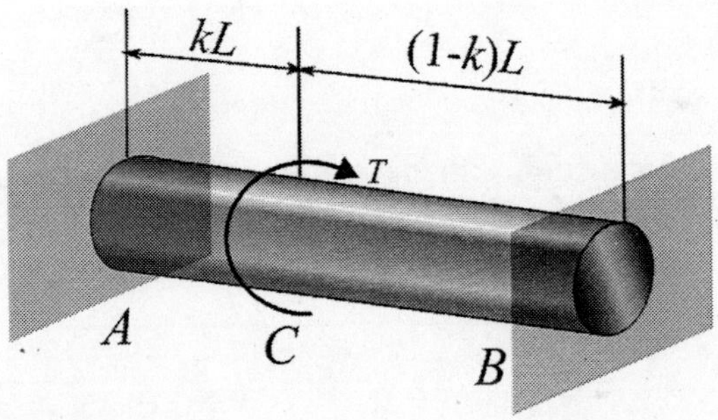

Fig. 7.13 Shaft fixed at two ends subjected to external torque T

Solution: The free-body diagram of the shaft is

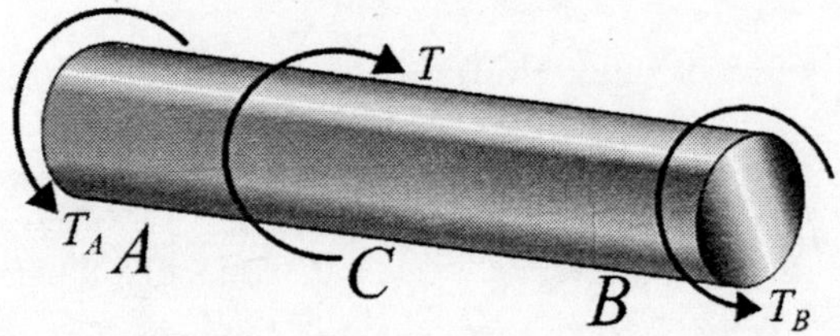

The moment equilibrium equation along the axis of the shaft is given by

$$T_A + T_B = T$$

There are two unknowns viz., T_A and T_B. To solve both unknowns, in addition to the equilibrium condition, the compatibility condition is invoked; for now, the signs (sense) of T_A and T_B are ignored. The compatibility condition can be expressed as

$$\frac{T_A L_{AC}}{GJ} = \frac{T_B L_{CB}}{GJ}$$

Thus,

$$T_A = \frac{T_B L_{CB}}{L_{AC}} = T_B\left(\frac{1}{k} - 1\right),$$

where k denotes the ratio of the length of segment AC to the total length. When this expression is used in conjunction with the equilibrium condition, $T_A + T_B = T$, we get

$$T_A = T(1 - k)$$

$$T_B = Tk$$

The angle of the twist $\theta_{C/A}$ can be written as

$$\theta_{C/A} = \frac{T_{AC} L_{AC}}{GJ} = \frac{TLk(1-k)}{GJ} \circlearrowright$$

7.5 Combined loading on circular shafts – Torsion and Bending

Many machine parts and civil structures are subjected to combined loading, both torsional and bending moments. Fig. 7.1a shows a circular shaft subjected to pure torsional loads. Fig. 7.1b depicts a typical element subjected to pure shear.

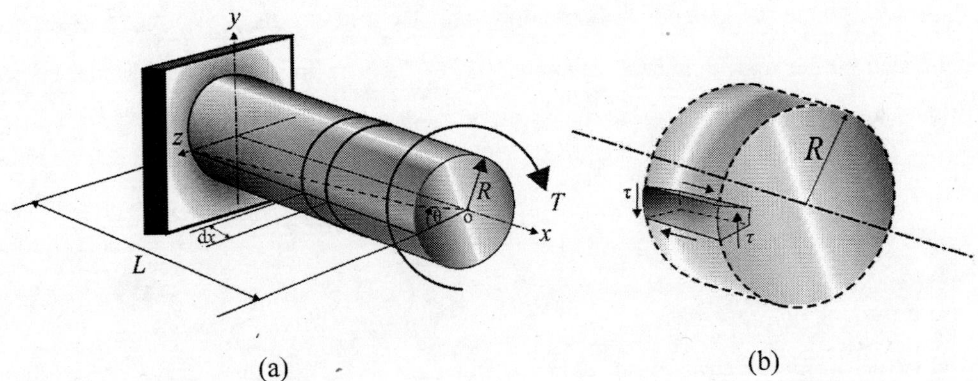

Fig. 7.14 (a) Shaft subjected to torsional load, (b) shear stress on the shaft element

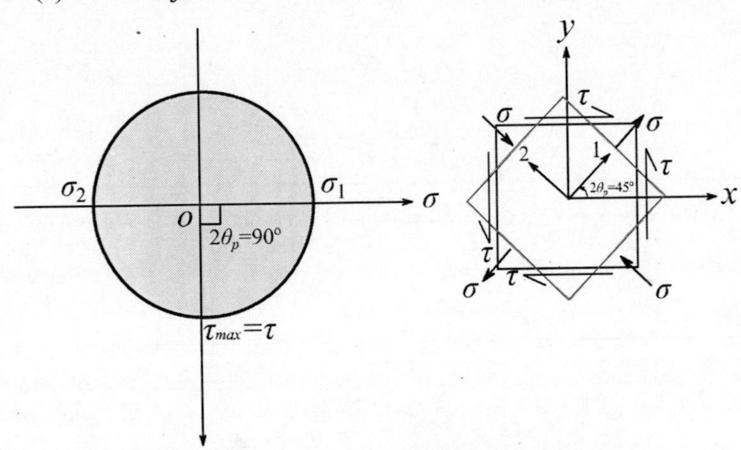

Fig. 7.15 Mohr's circle for the shaft element

If we draw the Mohr's circle for the above configuration, it will have a radius of τ with the center of the Mohr's circle at the origin of $\sigma - \tau$ axes, as shown in Fig. 7.15. Therefore, $\sigma_1 = -\sigma_2 = \tau$. A pure shear case can be considered as a biaxial tension-compression case. The principal axes are oriented at an angle of 45° with the reference axes.

In addition to the twisting moments, if bending moments are also present, then the normal stresses in the shaft's element will be non-zero. This scenario is shown in

Fig. 7.16(a). Due to the bending moment M_y and M_z on the shaft, the normal stresses are generated on the shaft's element, as shown in Fig. 7.16(b). In such a scenario, the center of the Mohr's circle will not lie at the origin of $\sigma - \tau$ axes.

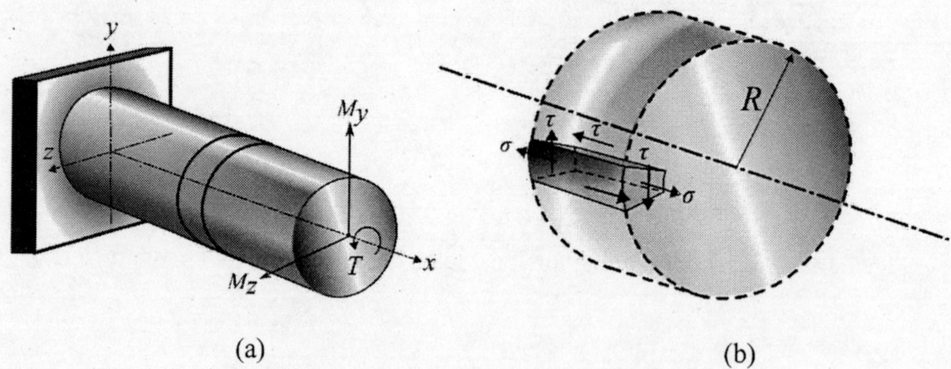

Fig. 7.16 (a) Combined torsion and bending moment, (b) normal and shear stress on the shaft element due to combined loading

Consider a case when a circular shaft is subjected to twisting moment (torque) – T, bending moment (about the z – axis) – M, and axial thrust – P. Due to the twisting moment, the shear stress is given by

$$\tau(r) = \frac{Tr}{J} \tag{7.12}$$

where r and J are the radial location and polar moment of inertia of the cross-section, respectively. Due to the bending moment, the bending stress is given by

$$\sigma_b = -\frac{My}{I_{zz}} \tag{7.13}$$

where y is the distance from the neutral surface and I_{zz} is the second moment of inertia of the cross-section about the z-axis. The direct stress due to the axial thrust is given by

$$\sigma_d = \frac{P}{A} \tag{7.14}$$

where A is the area of the cross-section. Under combined loading, the principal stresses and the maximum shear stress will occur on the periphery of the cross-section where the radial location is R. It is given by

$$\sigma_{1,2} = \frac{\sigma_d + \sigma_b}{2} \pm \sqrt{\left(\frac{\sigma_d - \sigma_b}{2}\right)^2 - \tau^2} \tag{7.15}$$

$$\tau_{max} = \frac{1}{2}\sqrt{(\sigma_d - \sigma_b)^2 + 4\tau^2}$$

For a circular shaft of radius R, the maximum shear stress, bending stress, and axial stress (axial stress will be constant) would be

$$\tau^{max} = \frac{2T}{\pi R^3}$$
$$\sigma_b^{max} = \frac{4M}{\pi R^3} \tag{7.16}$$
$$\sigma_d = \frac{P}{\pi R^2}$$

Then, using the first expression of the Eq. (7.15), the major principal stress (σ_1) will be

$$\sigma_1 = \frac{1}{2}\left[\frac{P}{\pi R^2} + \frac{4M}{\pi R^3}\right] + \frac{1}{2}\left[\sqrt{\left(\frac{P}{\pi R^2} - \frac{4M}{\pi R^3}\right)^2 - \left(\frac{4T}{\pi R^3}\right)^2}\right] \quad or \tag{7.17}$$

$$\sigma_1 = \frac{2}{\pi R^3}\left[\left(\frac{Pr}{4} + M\right) + \sqrt{\left(\frac{Pr}{4} - M\right)^2 + T^2}\right]$$

Using the second expression of the Eq. (7.15), the maximum shear stress will be

$$\tau_{max} = \frac{2}{\pi R^3}\left[\sqrt{\left(\frac{Pr}{4} - M\right)^2 + T^2}\right] \quad (7.18)$$

If the axial thrust P is zero, then the major principal stress will become

$$\sigma_1 = \frac{2}{\pi R^3}\left[M + \sqrt{M^2 + T^2}\right] \quad (7.19)$$

The equivalent bending moment for a shaft that is subjected to the combined twisting moment (T) and bending moment (M) is given by

$$M_{eq} = \frac{1}{2}\left[M + \sqrt{M^2 + T^2}\right] \quad (7.20)$$

Likewise, the equivalent torsional load or twisting moment is given by

$$T_{eq} = \sqrt{M^2 + T^2} \quad (7.21)$$

Example 7.5 A shaft shown is subjected to $F_y = 50$ kN. Detemine the principal stresses and its orientation wih respect to $y - z$ axes at locations 1 and 2: location 1 coordinates is $(-200\text{ mm}, 0\text{ mm}, 25\text{ mm})$ and location 2 coordinates – $(-200\text{ mm}, 25\text{ mm}, 0\text{ mm})$. Consider the effect of shear stress developed due to shear force as well.

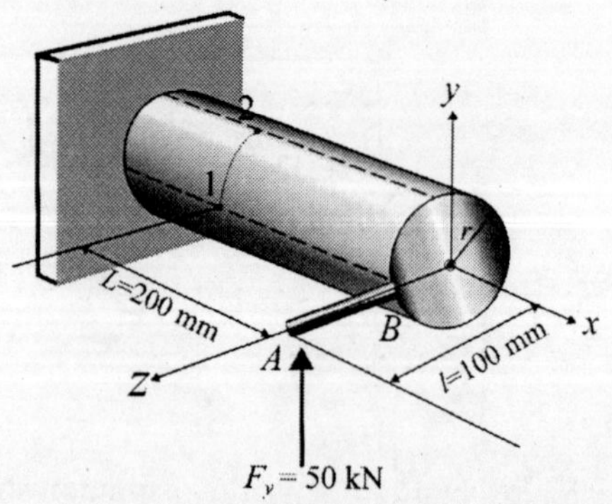

Fig. 7.17 Combined loading on the shaft

Solution: Given $F_y = 50$ kN, and therefore, the shear force on the shaft $V = F_y = 50$ kN. The torsional load acting on the shaft is given by

$$T = F_y l = (50 \text{ kN})(100 \text{ mm}) = 5000 \text{ kN} \cdot \text{mm} \circlearrowright$$

The bending moment about the $z-$ axis is given by

$$M_z = F_y L = (50 \text{ kN})(200 \text{ mm}) = 10000 \text{ kN} \cdot \text{mm}$$

For both locations 1 and 2,

$$A = \pi r^2 = \pi(25)^2 = 1963.4954 \text{ mm}^2$$

$$I_y = I_z = \frac{1}{4}\pi r^4 = \frac{1}{4}\pi(25)^4 = 306796.1575 \text{ mm}^4$$

$$J = \frac{1}{2}\pi r^4 = \frac{1}{2}\pi(25)^4 = 613592.3151 \text{ mm}^4$$

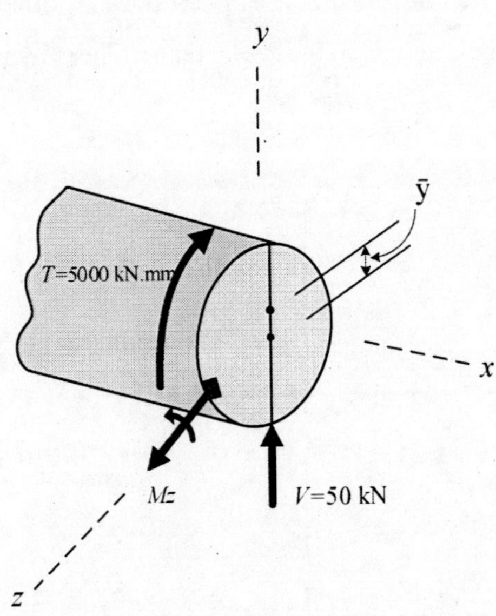

At location 1:

$$Q = A'\bar{y} = \left(\frac{1}{2}\pi r^2\right)\left(\frac{4r}{3\pi}\right) = \frac{2}{3}r^3 = \frac{2}{3}(25)^3 = 416.667\ \text{mm}^3$$

$$t = 2c = 2(25) = 50\ \text{mm}$$

The bending stress at location 1 $(-200\ \text{mm}, 0\ \text{mm}, 25\ \text{mm})$ due to bending moment is zero as this location lies on the neutral axis i.e. $\sigma_x = 0$ MPa. But, there will be shear stress due to shear force and torsion. They are given by

$$\tau_{xy}^V = \frac{VQ}{I_z t} = \frac{(50 \times 10^3)(416.667)}{(306796.1575)(50)} = 1.358\ \text{MPa}\ \uparrow$$

$$\tau_{xy}^T = \frac{Tr}{J} = \frac{(5000)(25)}{(613592.315)} = 203.718\ \text{MPa}\ \uparrow$$

$$\tau_{xy} = \tau_{xy}^V + \tau_{xy}^T = 1.358 + 203.718 = 205.076\ \text{MPa}$$

If we draw the Mohr's circle, the principal planes will be oriented at an angle of 45° and 135° with respect to the $x-$ axis in the $x-y$ plane. The principal stresses would be $\sigma_1 =$ 205.076 MPa and $\sigma_2 = -205.076$ MPa.

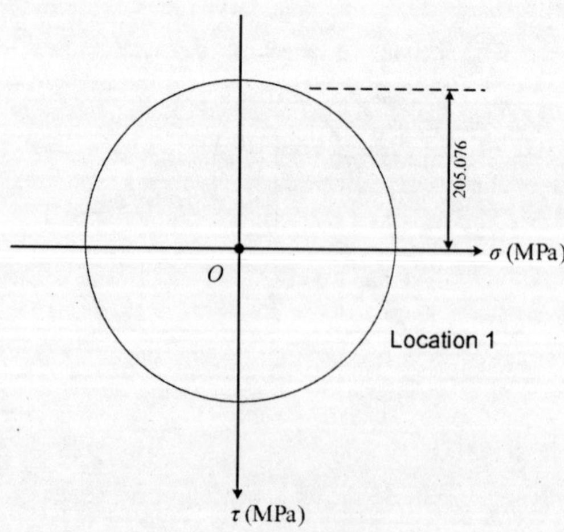

At location 2:

The normal stress at location 2 – $(-200\text{ mm}, 25\text{ mm}, 0\text{ mm})$ will be

$$\sigma_x = -\frac{M_z y}{I_z} = -\frac{(10000 \times 10^3)(25)}{(306796.1575)} = -814.87\text{ MPa}$$

The shear stress will be

$$\tau_{xz}^T = \frac{Tr}{J} = \frac{(5000)(25)}{(613592.3151)} = 203.72\text{ MPa}$$

There will be no shear stress due to the shear force V at location 2. The Mohr's circle at location 2 will be

The center of the Mohr's circle C would be at $(-407.435,0)$ MPa because

$$OC = CD = \left|\frac{OD}{2}\right| = \frac{814.87}{2} = 407.435\text{ MPa}$$

The radius of the Mohr's circle R is

$$R = \sqrt{203.72^2 + 407.435^2} = 455.53\text{ MPa}$$

Therefore, $\tau_{max} = R = 455.527$ MPa. The principal direction is given by

$$\tan 2\theta_p = \frac{2\tau_{xy}}{(\sigma_x - \sigma_y)} = \frac{2 \times 203.72}{(-814.87)} = -0.5$$

$$2\theta_p = 153.43° \; or \; \theta_p = 76.72°$$

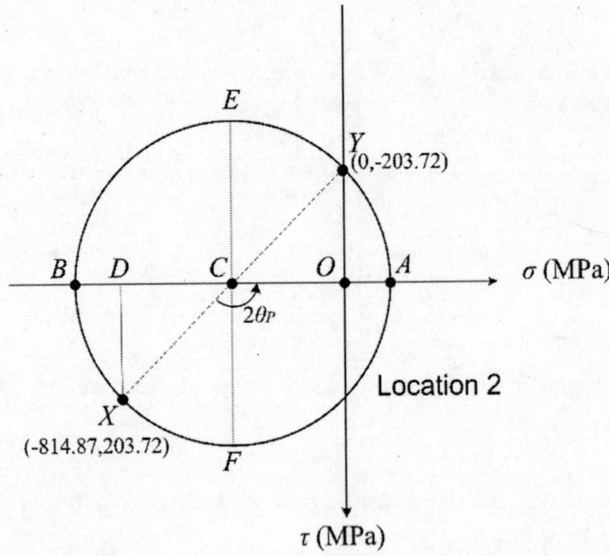

The principal plane corresponding to the major principal stress is oriented at an angle of 76.72° counter-clockwise with respect to the $x-$ axis. The principal stresses are given by

$$\sigma_1 = R - OC = 455.527 - 407.4365 = 48.09 \text{ MPa}$$

$$\sigma_2 = OC - R = -407.4365 - 455.527 = -862.96 \text{ MPa}$$

7.6 Analysis of close-coiled-helical springs

Mechanical springs are widely used in many machines. They behave as flexible joints between the connected parts. The springs are used in applications involving cushioning in impact loads, force measurement in spring balances, energy storage, and maintaining contact between moving parts, such as in the cam-follower mechanism.

In this section, we focus on the analysis of a close-coiled-helical spring subjected to the load F as shown in Fig. 7.18a. The spring can be subjected to tensile or compressive load. The wires are of circular cross-sections with a constant wire diameter (d). The spring is characterized by number of active turns (N_a), wire-diameter (d), coil diameter (D) and the shear modulus (G). The wire-diameter of a coil or a turn is shown in Fig. 7.18b.

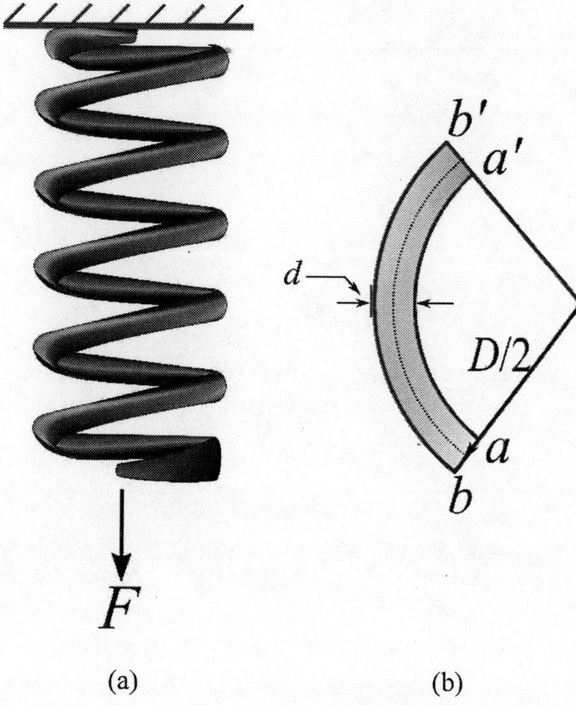

Fig. 7.18 (a) Close-coiled-helical spring, (b) wire-diameter – d of a coil

The pitch (p) of a spring is the distance between the centers of neighboring coils, which is analogous to the threads (lead) on a bolt or screw. When constructing springs, it is advised that the engineer indicate the number of active coils, as the pitch is frequently mistaken with the gap or the distance between the coils. An inactive turn or coil is located at each end of the spring; consequently, active turns consist of all coils that are not located at the spring's ends.

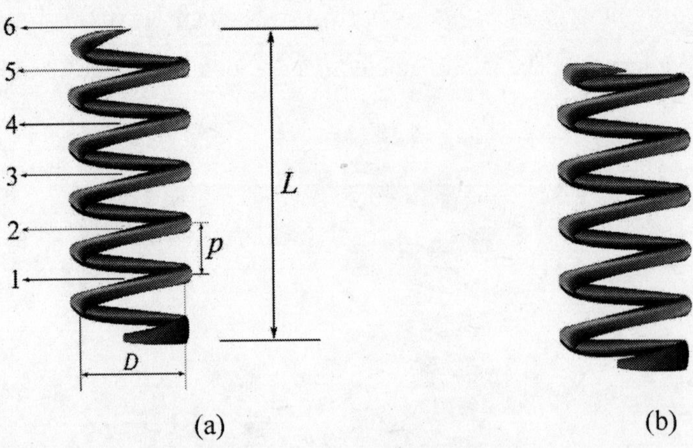

Fig. 7.19 (a) Active turns and the pitch (expanded view along the length), and (b) Representation of close-coiled-helical spring

Fig. 7.19(a) shows the length (L), pitch (p) and the numbering of the turns of a close-coiled-helical spring. The coil at either end of the spring can be considered dead (Ref: Fig. 7.19(b)). The pitch of the spring is given by

$$p = \frac{(L - N_d d)}{N_a} \tag{7.22}$$

where N_d is the number of dead coils and N_a is the number of active turns. In Fig. 7.19(a), the number of active turns would be four; the total coils are six, and the dead coils are 2.

Imagine a cut section of a coil when the spring is subjected to a tensile force shown in Fig. 7.20. Since the spring is under static equilibrium, the force and moment balance relations indicate that there is no horizontal force on a wire's cross-section. Only shear force (V) exists and is equal to the applied force F. There will be no bending moment, instead there will be a twisting moment (T) of magnitude $\frac{FD}{2}$. It is assumed that the external force is acting at the center of the circular spring, and the coils are parallel to each other so that no bending moment would arise at any cut part of the spring.

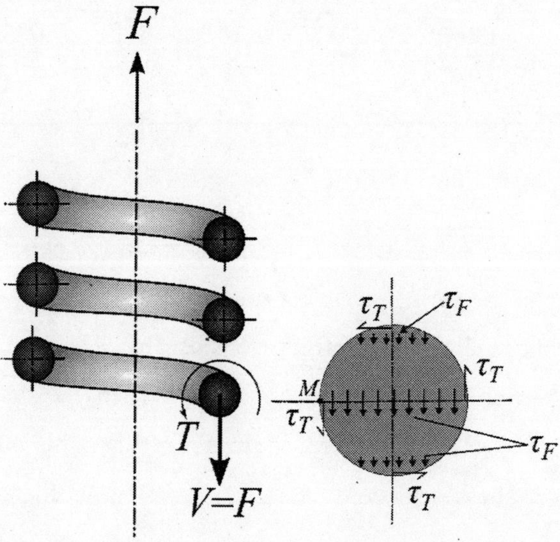

Fig. 7.20 Cut section of a coil when spring is subjected to a tensile force

The polar moment of inertia of the wire of the spring is $J = \frac{\pi d^4}{32}$. The shear stress due to torsional load T at the periphery of the wire's cross-section is

$$\tau_T = \frac{Tr}{J} = \frac{\frac{FD}{2} \times \frac{d}{2}}{\left(\frac{\pi d^4}{32}\right)} = \frac{8FD}{\pi d^3} \tag{7.23}$$

The average shear stress on the cross-section due to the shear force $V = F$

$$\tau_F = \frac{F}{\left(\frac{\pi d^2}{4}\right)} = \frac{4F}{\pi d^2} \tag{7.24}$$

Therefore, the shear stress at the periphery, which is maximum at the point M is given by

$$\tau_{max} = \tau_T + \tau_F = \frac{8FD}{\pi d^3} + \frac{4F}{\pi d^2} \tag{7.25}$$

Rearranging the Eq. (7.25), we can express τ_{max} as

$$\tau_{max} = \frac{8FD}{\pi d^3}\left(1 + \frac{1}{\frac{2D}{d}}\right) = \frac{8FD}{\pi d^3}\left(1 + \frac{1}{2C}\right); C = \frac{D}{d} \tag{7.26}$$

C is called as spring index. The term $\left(1 + \frac{1}{2C}\right)$ is called a shear correction factor and is denoted by 'K_s'

In springs with a small spring index C, the shear strain (γ) experienced by a segment close to the center of the spring is more than the shear strain experienced by the outer segment. This is called the curvature effect. Consider Fig. 7.18b. Imagine due to torsional load T, the cross-section gets rotated by an angle θ. Then, the shear strain in the inner segment $a - a'$ will experience more shear strain than the outer segment $b - b'$. Therefore, the shear stresses torsional loading T will be depedent on radius and polar angle of the cross-section.

Equation (7.26) is modified to take into account the curvature effect. The modified equation is written as

$$\tau_{max} = K_w \frac{8FD}{\pi d^3} \tag{7.27}$$

where K_w is the Wahl's correction factor that includes both the shear stress effect due to shear force and the curvature effect. K_w is given by

$$K_w = \frac{0.615}{C} + \frac{4C - 1}{4C - 4} \tag{7.28}$$

Deflection of close-coiled-helical springs

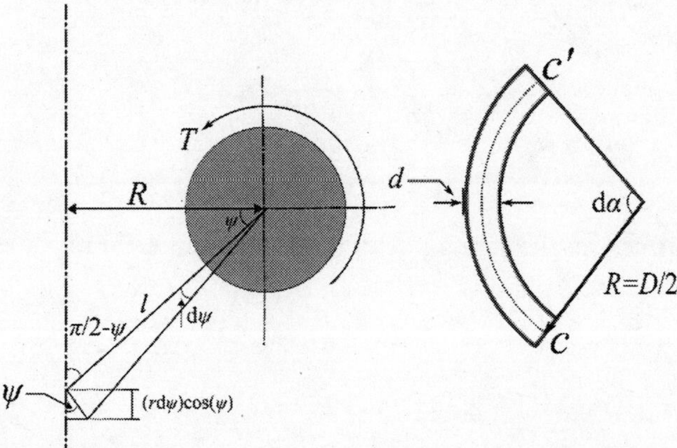

Fig. 7.21 Deflection due to torsional load on a cross-section

A wire's cross-section (Fig. 7.21) is considered to determine the deflection due to load F on a close-coiled-helical spring. Due to torsional load T, let the cross-section rotate by an amount $\mathrm{d}\psi$. Then, the vertical deflection due to the rotation would be

$$\mathrm{d}\delta = l\mathrm{d}\psi \cos\psi = l\mathrm{d}\psi \times \frac{R}{l} = \frac{D\mathrm{d}\psi}{2} \tag{7.29}$$

The horizontal component of the deflection will cancel out due to the symmetry of the helical spring. Using Eq.(7.13a)**Error! Reference source not found.**, the change in angular displacement $\mathrm{d}\psi$ considering a small portion of helical spring of arc length $\mathrm{d}s = R\mathrm{d}\alpha$ (Fig. 7.21), can be written as

$$\mathrm{d}\psi = \frac{T\mathrm{d}s}{GJ} = \frac{TR\mathrm{d}\alpha}{GJ} = \frac{F \times \frac{D}{2} \times \frac{D}{2} \times \mathrm{d}\alpha}{G \times \frac{\pi d^4}{32}} = \frac{8FD^2}{G\pi d^4}\mathrm{d}\alpha \tag{7.30}$$

Combining Eqs. (7.29) and (7.30), we get

$$\mathrm{d}\delta = \frac{4FD^3}{G\pi d^4}\mathrm{d}\alpha \tag{7.31}$$

The net deflection along the line of action of external force F would be

$$\delta = \int_0^{2\pi N_a} \frac{4FD^3}{G\pi d^4} d\alpha$$
$$\delta = \frac{8FD^3 N_a}{Gd^4} \tag{7.32}$$

The effective stiffness or the spring rate of the helical spring will be, therefore,

$$K = \frac{F}{\delta} = \frac{Gd^4}{8D^3 N_a} \tag{7.33}$$

Example 7.6 A rail car weighing 2000 kg and traveling at 1.5 m/s collides with a bumper made of two helical springs of spring index 6. The springs are compressed by 150 mm during the process. The springs are made of steel alloy with a shear modulus of 90 GPa. If the allowable shear stress of the steel alloy is 90 MPa, determine the design parameters of the spring.

Solution: The kinetic energy of the rail car gets converted to the potential energy of the helical springs during the collision process. Given $m = 2000\ \text{kg}, v = 1.5\ \text{m/s}$ and $\delta = 150\ \text{mm}$.

If K is the spring rate of the helical springs, then using the principle of conservation of energy, we can write

$$\frac{1}{2}mv^2 = 2 \times \frac{1}{2}K\delta^2 \rightarrow K = \frac{mv^2}{2\delta^2} = \frac{2000 \times 1.5^2}{2 \times 0.15^2} = 100\ \text{kN/m}$$

Using Eq. (7.33), we can write

$$F = K\delta_y = 100000 \times 0.15 = 15\ \text{kN}$$

The Wahl's correction factor – K_w can be obtained from Eq. (7.28). The K_w is a function of the spring index which is given as $C = 6$.

$$K_w = \frac{0.615}{C} + \frac{4C - 1}{4C - 4} = 1.2525$$

The maximum shear stresses that the cross-section of a wire experiences is given by Eq. (7.27). It is

$$\tau_{max} = K_w \frac{8FD}{\pi d^3} = K_w \frac{8FCd}{\pi d^3} = 1.2525 \frac{8 \times 15000 \times 6d}{\pi d^3} = \frac{0.287}{d^2} \text{ MPa}$$

The allowable shear stress is 90 MPa, and therefore, $\tau_{max} \leq 90$ MPa. From the above equation,

$$\frac{0.287}{d^2} \leq 90 \rightarrow d \geq 56.5 \text{ mm}$$

The wire diameter (d) has to be a minimum of 56.5 mm. Since the spring index is 6, the coil diameter has to be a minimum of 338.82 mm. To get the active coils, Eq. (7.33) is used.

$$100 \times 1000 = \frac{Gd^4}{8D^3 N_a} = \frac{90 \times 10^9 \times 0.0565^4}{8 \times 0.33882^3 \times N_a} \rightarrow N_a = 29.5 \approx 30$$

So, thirty active coils are needed in the helical spring to avoid damage to the rail car.

Know

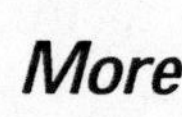

Exercises

Multiple Choice Questions

7.1. A helical spring gets deflected by 10 mm under the action of 500 kN force. If two such helical springs are connected in parallel, what will be the deflection under the action of 250 kN?

(a) 2.5 mm

(b)10 mm

(c) 5 mm

(d) 4 mm

7.2. A helical spring has a spring index of 6 with a wire diameter of 5 mm. The maximum shear stress developed in the spring is 250 MPa. What is the force (F) acting on the spring?

(a) 235 N

(b) 327 N

(c) 470 N

(d) 800 N

7.3. A shaft is subjected to a twisting moment of 4 kN.m and a bending moment of 3 kN.m. What is the magnitude of the equivalent bending moment?

(a) 8 kN.m

(b) 10 kN.m

(c) 2 kN.m

(d) 4 kN.m

7.4. In a hollow shaft subjected to a torque, the shear stress developed is

(a) Minimum near the inner radius.

(b) Minimum near the outer radius.

(c) Midline between the inner and the outer radius

(d) Remains constant everywhere.

7.5 If a modification to a shaft subjected to torsion results in torsional strength improvement, the modification could be

(a) Decrease the diameter of the shaft

(b) Drill a hole in the shaft

(c) Reduce the length of the shaft

(d) Increase the diameter of the shaft

7.6 Consider a small square plate element on the outer surface of the shaft subjected to torsion. At what angle relative to the axes of the plate element does the element experience only the normal stresses?

(a) 45°

(b) 90°

© 25°

(d) 22.5°

7.7 For a circular shaft subjected to constant torque, keeping the angle of twist constant, if the volume is doubled, then

(a) Shear stress will be halved

(b) Shear stress will reduce by $\sqrt{2}$ times

(c) Shear stress will increase by 2 times

(d) There will be no change in the magnitude of the shear stress

7.8 If the shaft of radius 2 mm develops maximum shear stress of 210 MPa, what would be the torque applied?

(a) 4.6 N m

(b) 2.6 N m

(c) 6.2 N m

(d) 5.3 N m

7.9 If two shafts shown below of the same length and material are subjected to the same torque T, then the angle of twist will be

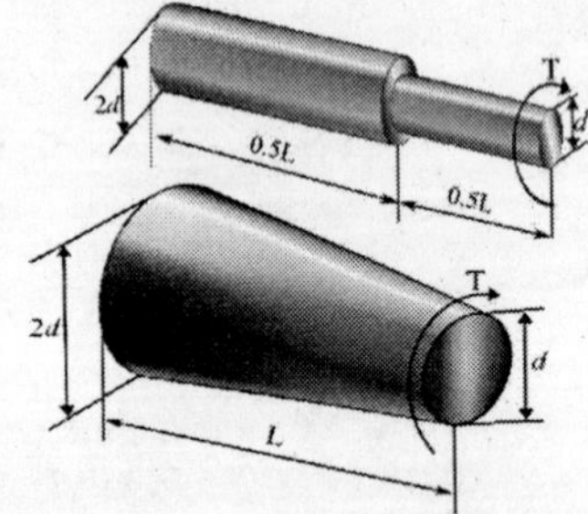

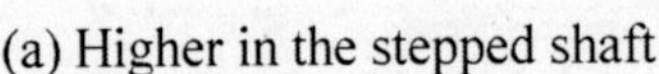

(a) Higher in the stepped shaft

(b) Higher in the tapered shaft

(c) Same in both shaft

(d) Zero in both shafts

7.10 A hollow tube of outer diameter 10 cm and inner diameter 8 cm undergoes an angular test of 0.01 radians under the action of 1kN.m torsional load. If the length of the shaft is 1m, then the shear modulus (GPa) of the shaft's material is

(a) 210 GPa

(b) 90 GPa

(c) 17.25 GPa

(d) 35 GPa

Answers of multiple choice questions

7.1 (a), 7.2 (b), 7.3 (d), 7.4 (a), 7.5 (d), 7.6 (a), 7.7 (b), 7.8 (d), 7.9 (a), 7.10 (c)

Numerical Problems

7.1. Steel alloy with a 200 MPa permissible shear stress is used to make a solid shaft. Find the greatest torque T that can be transferred, assuming that the shaft's diameter is 30 mm. If a 20 mm diameter hole was to be drilled through the shaft, what would be the maximum torque that can be transferred?

(**Ans.** 1.06 kN.m, 0.85 kN.m)

7.2. Consider the pulley-shaft system shown in Figure P2. The shaft has a diameter of 10 cm and a shear modulus of 80 GPa. A pulley B supports a load of 1 kN along the direction indicated in the figure. The diameter of the pulley B is 30 cm. The entire shaft is supported on journal bearings at the ends that offer negligible resistance to rotation. Assuming the thickness of pulleys to be small, determine (a) the value of torque T to maintain this load, (b) the angle of twist between B and A, (c) the angle of twist between C and B, and (d) the angle of twist between C and A. Take the distance between A and B as L_{AB} = 0.5 m.

(**Ans.** 50 N.m, 0°, 0.0018°, 0.0018°)

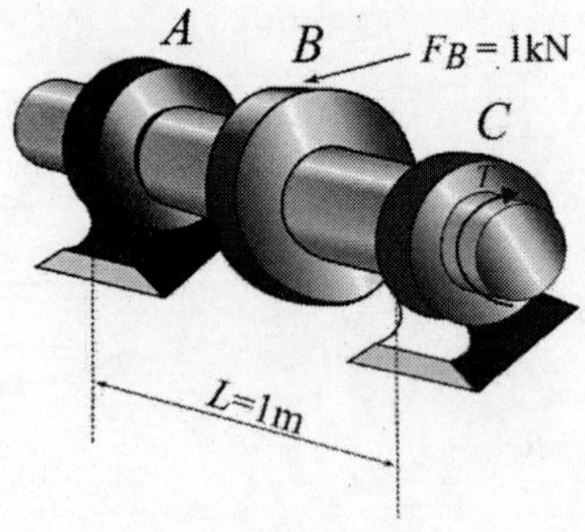

Figure P7.2

7.3. A generator receives power from a turbine, as shown in Figure P3, through a solid steel shaft 3 m long. The shaft has a diameter of 40 mm and transmits power at 100 rev/min. The allowable shear stress is 75 MPa, and the shear modulus of the shaft is 100 GPa. Then what is the maximum power that can be transmitted and the corresponding angle of twist? (**Ans.** 9.87 MW, 0.645°)

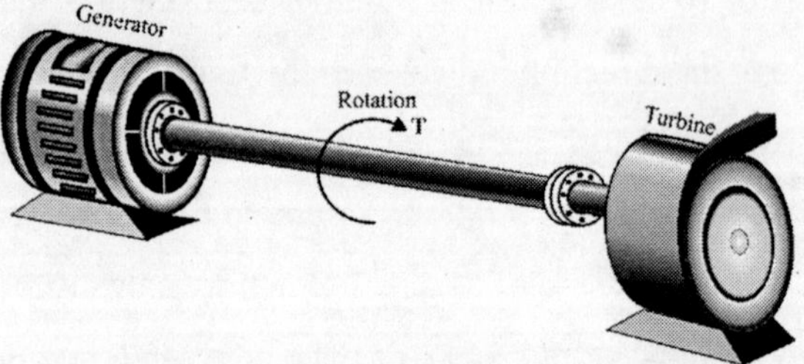

Figure P7.3

7.4. A circular shaft of uniform radius r and length L is subjected to a counter-clockwise torque intensity $t(x) = cx$ as shown in Figure P4. Determine the angle of twist at location B with respect to A. Take the shear modulus as G.

(**Ans.** $\frac{2CL^3}{3\pi G r^4}$)

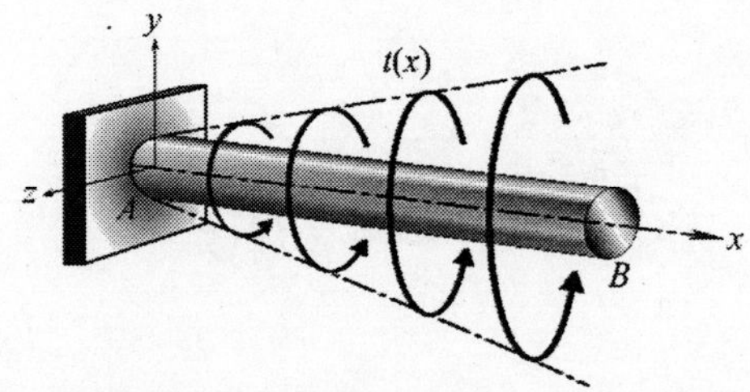

Figure P7.4

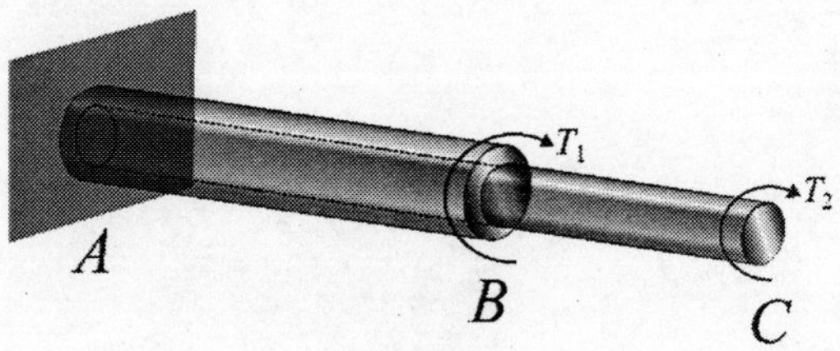

Figure P7.5

7.5. A stepped shaft made of the same material with $G = 100$ GPa is fixed at one end, as shown in Figure P5. Shaft AB is a hollow shaft with $r_{in} = 25$ mm and $r_{out} = 40$ mm. Shaft BC is a solid shaft of $r = 25$ mm. The length of shaft AB and BC is 0.8 m and 0.5 m, respectively. If $T_1 = 2$ kN. m and $T_2 = 1$ kN. m, determine the net angle of twist at location B and C with respect to A.

(**Ans.** 0.4°, 0.86°)

7.6. Stiff supports support the composite shaft seen in Figure P6. The diameter of the bronze section AB is 75 mm, and the allowable shear stress is less than 60 MPa. The diameter of the steel section BC is 50 mm, and the allowable shear stress is less than 120 MPa. The shear modulus of bronze and stress section is 40 GPa and 83 GPa, respectively. If the length of the AB is 0.8 m and BC is 0.5 m, calculate the maximum allowable torque. (**Ans.**7.44 kN.m)

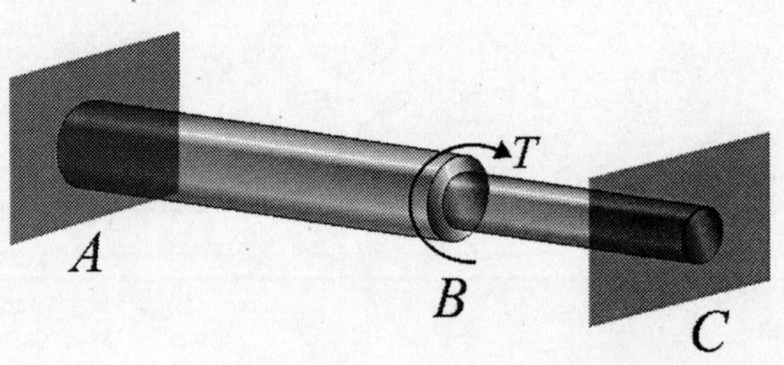

Figure P7.6

Follower
Cam
100 mm
50 mm

7.7. A cam-follower mechanism is shown in Figure P7. A helical spring enables the roller follower to be held

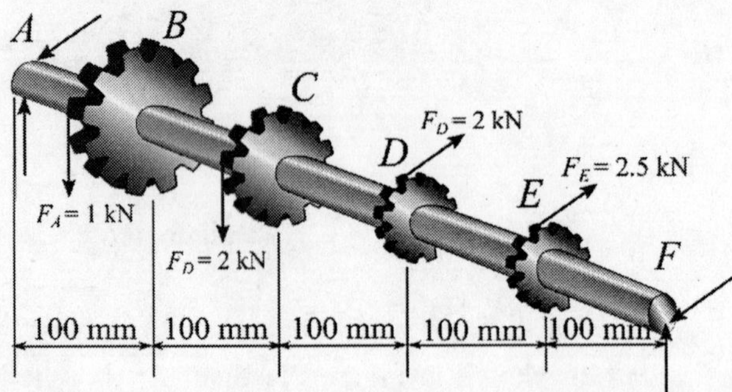

against the cam. Due to the cam's rotation, the force experienced by the spring varies from 200 N to 600 N. Determine the number of active coils, wire diameter, and a coil diameter of the spring if the allowable shear stress is 160 MPa. The shear modulus of the spring is 80 GPa, and the spring index is 6. (**Ans.** $N_a = 50$, 8.47 mm, 50.82 mm)

7.8. The shaft *AF* transmits 50 kW at 500 rpm. The free-body diagram of the shafts and gears is shown in Figure P8. The radius of the gear B, C, D, and E is 100 mm, 60 mm, 30 mm, and 30 mm, respectively. Find the smallest shaft diameter if the allowable shear stress is 120 MPa. (**Ans.** 13.2 mm)

Figure P7.7

Figure P7.8

Unit 8

Thin and thick cylinders and spheres

UNIT SPECIFICS

Pressure vessels are used in a variety of applications, such as the aircraft industry, chemical industry, and thermal and nuclear power plants. A pressure vessel is a steel container to hold fluids at a pressure very different from the atmospheric conditions. This unit analyses the cylindrical and spherical pressure vessels for the stresses developed due to internal pressure. The analysis differs depending on the ratio of the wall-thickness of the pressure vessel to its radius. It is rigorous if the ratio is comparatively higher. The unit ends with the derivation of deformations in shells due to internal pressure.

RATIONALE

Stress analysis is essential to keep the pressure vessel from exploding or bursting. Leakage or rupture failures can occur if a vessel develops cracks or is otherwise damaged. Rupture failures are significantly more likely to be catastrophic, resulting in loss of life and extensive property damage. For this reason, a significant amount of focus should be placed on applying analytical methodologies to estimate their operating stresses.

PRE-REQUISITES

Mathematics course on differential equations

Simple stresses and strains (Unit 1)

UNIT OUTCOMES

After completing this unit, students will be able to

U8-O1: Derive the formulae for hoop stress and longitudinal stress in thin-walled cylindrical and spherical pressure vessel

U8-O2: Calculate the strains in thin-walled cylindrical and spherical pressure vessels due to internal pressure

U8-O3: Analysis of thick-walled cylindrical pressure vessel for stresses, strains and displacement

U8-O4: Analysis of thick-walled spherical pressure vessel for stresses, strains and displacement

Course Outcomes	Expected Mapping with Course Outcomes - CE (1- Weak Correlation; 2- Medium correlation; 3- Strong Correlation)			
	CO-1	CO-2	CO-3	CO-4
U8-O1	3	2	1	1
U8-O2	-	2	-	2

U8-O3	-	2	1	2
U8-O4	-	2	1	2

Course Outcomes	Expected Mapping with Course Outcomes - ME (1- Weak Correlation; 2- Medium correlation; 3- Strong Correlation)	
	CO-1	CO-2
U8-O1	3	1
U8-O2	1	3
U8-O3	3	3
U8-O4	3	3

8.1 Introduction

Pressure vessels serve the function of storage tanks and are used to store compressed liquids or gases at pressures significantly different from ambient pressure. They can be of any shape, although cylinders and spheres are the most commonly employed forms in the oil industry, the petrochemical industry, and gas reservoirs. Due to the high pressure inside the pressure vessel, the companies in these industries demand a fail-safe design. Likewise, pressure vessels such as the fuselage of the aircraft and soda cans must be designed and manufactured to fulfil specific structural integrity requirements.

Leakage or rupture failures may happen from pressure vessels that are fractured or damaged. Poisonings, asphyxia, and explosions are potential health and safety risks associated with leaky vessels. On the other hand, rupture failures may be far more severe and inflict substantial harm to people and property. Therefore, analytical and experimental approaches should be used to avoid pressure vessel failure under service loading conditions.

The cylindrical and spherical vessels can be classified into two types based on the wall thickness — thin-walled and thick-walled. Pressure vessels are generally regarded as thin-walled if the ratio of the radius r to the thickness of the wall t exceeds 10. In thin-walled pressure vessels — both cylinder and sphere, two stress components are non-zero: circumferential/hoop stress (tangential stress) and longitudinal stress (axial stress). In the case of the cylindrical pressure vessel, the ends are closed with end caps called heads, which are commonly hemispherical in shape, as shown in Fig. 8.1. As the name suggests, the 'hoop stress' acts along the circumferential direction and is perpendicular to the long axis of the cylinder.

Fig. 8.1 Cylindrical pressure vessel with hemispherical end caps

A gas cylinder (LPG cylinder, Ref. Fig. 8.2) can be considered a cylindrical pressure vessel to store the cooking gas at a pressure range from 12 – 18 bar. Due to the pressure in the cylinder, both circumferential and longitudinal stresses are generated, which are tensile stresses in nature. It is found that the circumferential stress is more than the longitudinal stress and therefore is often the cause of the cylinder's failure. According to the Bureau of Indian Standards (BIS), carbon steel is used to make the LPG cylinders.

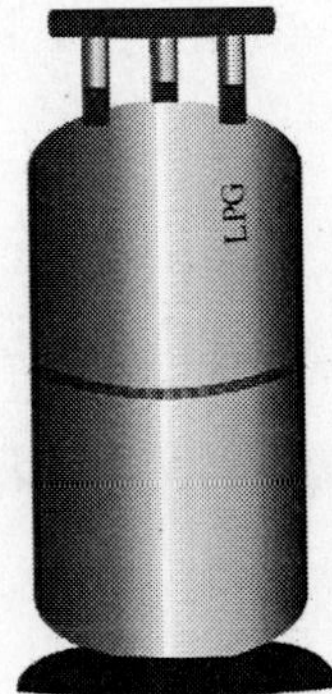

Fig. 8.2 Schematic of the household LPG cylinder

8.2 Thin-walled pressure vessels

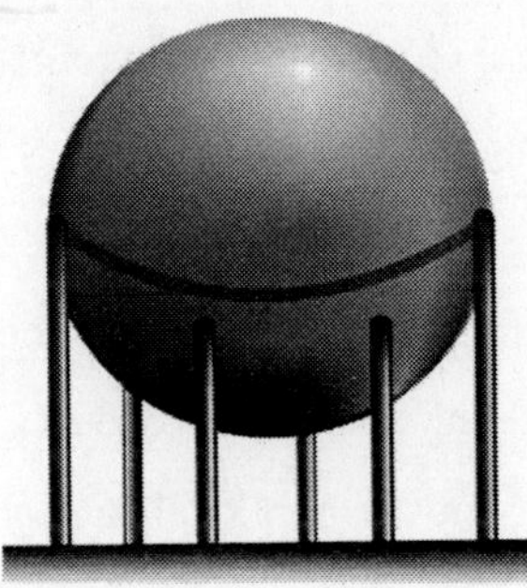

Fig. 8.3 A spherical pressure vessel

Components of aeronautical and marine vehicles, such as aircraft fuselage, rocket and balloon skins, submarine hulls, and soda cans, can be considered thin-walled pressure vessels.

A spherical pressure vessel (Fig.. 8.3) is the most structurally efficient form in shape. Three factors make a cylindrical vessel considerably less efficient: (1) the stresses in the wall change with direction, (2) a cylinder has a greater surface area per unit volume than a sphere, resulting in a higher heat transfer rate, and (3) at the ends, the corners are highly concentrated with stress. Nevertheless, cylindrical shapes are popular as they are easier to manufacture.

There are a few assumptions that need to be considered before the analysis of the thin-walled cylindrical and spherical pressure vessel.

a) Wall thickness: The wall is assumed to be thin compared to the other dimensions of the vessel. If r is the radius of the cylinder or sphere, and the t is the wall thickness, then the ratio of r to t should exceed 10, i.e. $\frac{r}{t} \gg 1$. This assumption implies that the circumferential and longitudinal stress components do not vary across the thickness of the wall.
b) Internal pressure: The operating pressure p inside the vessel is uniform everywhere. If the vessel is subjected to external pressure, then the pressure p is calculated by subtracting the external pressure from the absolute internal pressure; the gauge pressure is considered the operating (or the internal) pressure for the analysis. It should be noted that when the external pressure is more than the absolute internal pressure, as in the case of a submarine hull, the outcome of the present analysis may not be applicable as wall buckling can arise.
c) Material: The material of the pressure vessel is linearly elastic, isotropic, and homogenous. For anisotropic and non-homogenous materials, the present analysis is not applicable. Additionally, the wall thickness is constant.

Although the radial stress acts on the wall, they are significantly less compared to the other two stress components – circumferential stress and longitudinal stress. So, it is assumed to be zero in thin-walled pressure vessel analysis.

8.3 Thin-walled cylinders

Let us consider a pressurized thin-walled cylindrical pressure vessel of length L, inner radius R and thickness t, as shown in Fig. 8.4. It is subjected to an internal pressure of p.

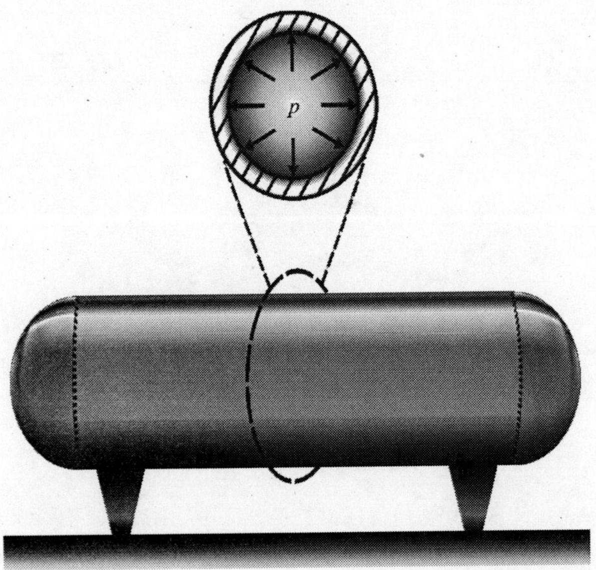

Fig. 8.4 Thin-walled cylindrical pressure vessel

Imagine a top half cross-section of the cylinder which is obtained by cutting the cylinder with $y - z$ planes whose normals are the longitudinal axis (x-axis), as shown in Fig. 8.5a and then slicing with a $x - y$ plane containing the longitudinal axis (Fig. 8.5b).

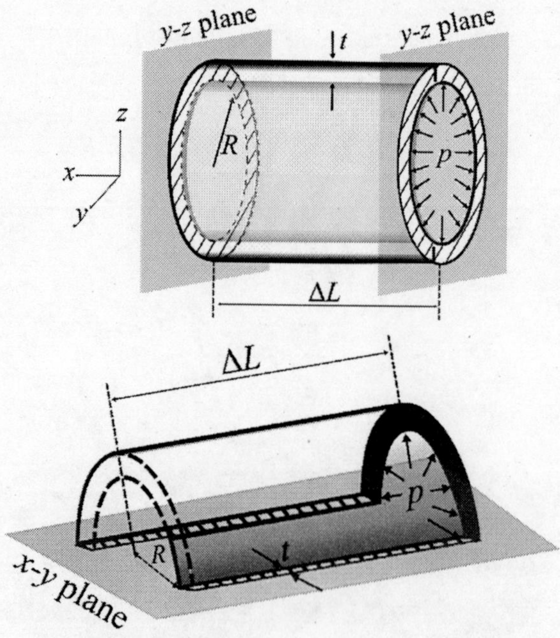

Fig. 8.5 Thin-walled cylinder: (a) cut by $y-z$ planes, and (b) cut by $x-y$ plane

Let F_T and F_R represent the component of the tangential forces and the radial forces, respectively, exerted by the other half, as shown in Fig. 8.6 a and Fig. 8.6 b.

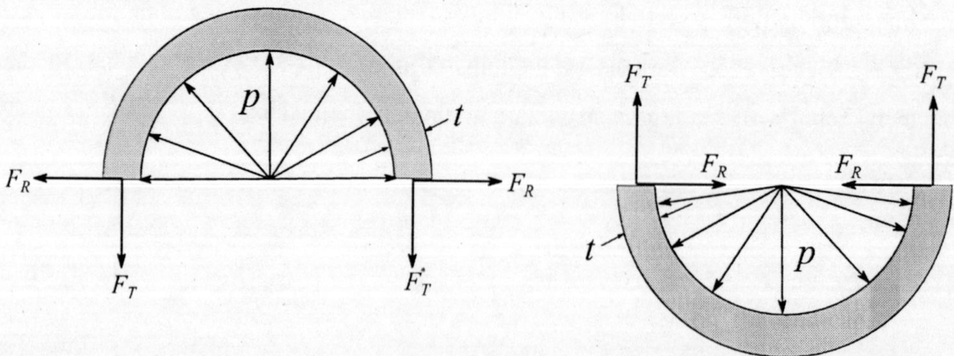

Fig. 8.6 Thin-walled cylinder: (a) top half cross-section, (b) bottom half cross-section (out-of-plane length = ΔL)

Because of symmetry in the load and geometry, the force component F_R should be zero. Now to find the tangential force F_T, consider an infinitesimal arc of length $R\Delta\theta$ as shown in Fig. 8.7.

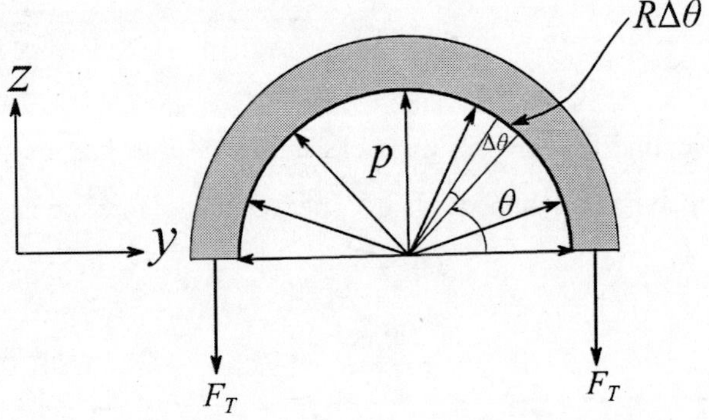

Fig. 8.7 Differential area element of the cylinder

The thin-walled cylinder is under static equilibrium. Therefore, the net force along the z-direction is zero. This is used to find the resultant tangential force – F_T acting on the top half cross-section due to the lower half. Let F_p be the force, due to the internal pressure, acting on the top half cross-section. Then,

$$\Delta F_p = p2R\Delta L \tag{8.1}$$

where ΔL is the length of the part that has been considered for the analysis. The force F_p is calculated taking into account the projected area of the surface of the top half cross-section on which the pressure is acting. The projected area is rectangular and is equal to $(2R)\Delta L$. More elaborately, the z-direction force component (ΔF_p^z) acting on a differential element can be considered and integrated to obtain the ΔF_p. The ΔF_p^z is given by

$$\Delta F_p^z = p\Delta L(R\Delta\theta)\sin\theta \tag{8.2}$$

Then, in the limit $\Delta\theta \rightarrow 0$, the F_p is obtained by

$$F_p = \int_0^{\pi} p\Delta LR\, sin\,\theta d\theta = p2R\Delta L \tag{8.3}$$

Since the pressure vessel is under static equilibrium, $\sum F_z = 0$. Therefore,

$$\begin{gathered} F_p - 2F_T = 0 \\ F_T = pRL \end{gathered} \tag{8.4}$$

If we unfold the cylindrical pressure vessel's top or bottom half cross-section, it would assume a thin rectangular-shaped plate. The resultant force component F_T can be visualized to act, as shown in Fig. 8.8a.

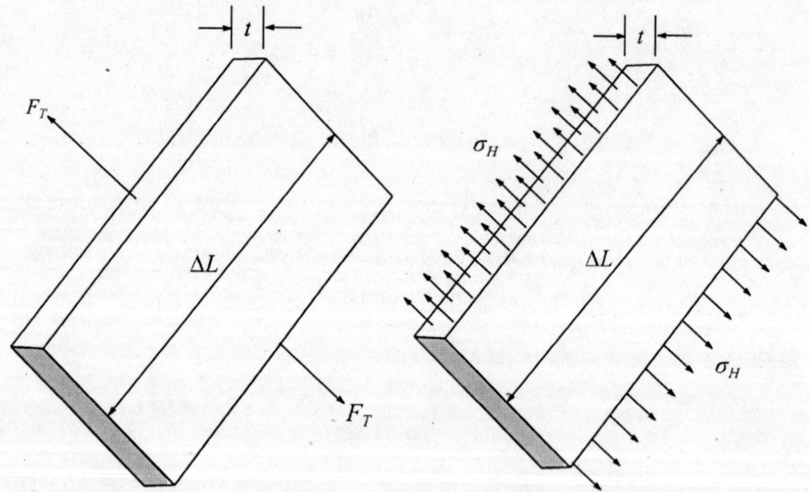

Fig. 8.8 Generation of hoop stress due to (a) the unfolded top half of the cylinder, (b) the hoop stress on the wall

The tangential force F_T is the resultant of the circumferential/hoop stress on the wall denoted by σ_H Fig. 8.8b. The F_T is given by

$$F_T = \sigma_H t \Delta L \tag{8.5}$$

Combining Eq. (8.4) and (8.5), we get

$$\sigma_H = \frac{pR}{t} \tag{8.6}$$

The Eq. (8.6) implies that the hoop stress, σ_H, is proportional to the internal pressure p and the internal radius R. As the internal radius increases, the net radial force experienced by the cylinder also increases, and therefore the hoop stress will increase accordingly.

In addition to the hoop stress, the cylinder walls are subjected to the longitudinal stress denoted by σ_L. It can be determined by considering the axial force acting on the walls of the cylinder. Since the cylinder is closed, the end-caps of the cylinder also experience a longitudinal or axial force due to the internal pressure (Ref. Fig. 8.9).

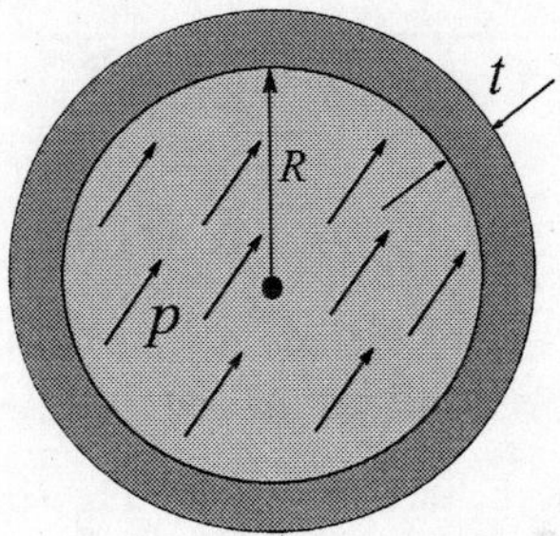

Fig. 8.9 End-cap of the cylindrical pressure vessel

The end cap of the cylinder can be hemispherical or flat. Irrespective of the shape, the longitudinal force experienced by the end cap will be $p\pi r^2$; the force exerted is simply the magnitude of pressure times the project area, which is circular in the present case.

Due to the internal pressure on the end-cap, the end-cap pulls the cylinder with a longitudinal force of magnitude $p\pi r^2$ in the axial direction. Therefore, the longitudinal stresses denoted by σ_L gets generated in the walls, as shown in Fig. 8.10.

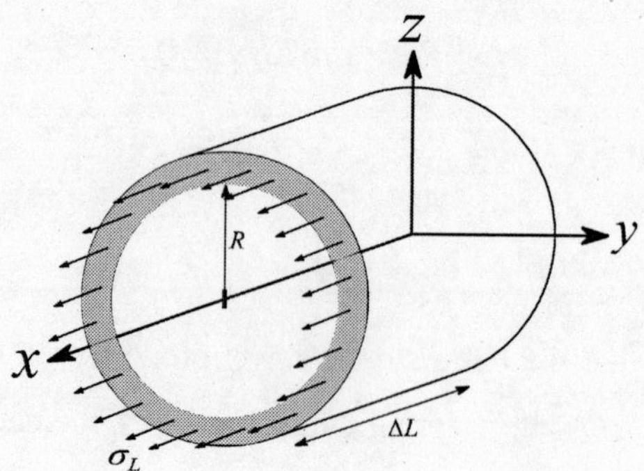

Fig. 8.10 Longitudinal stresses in the walls of the cylinder

If we consider the force equilibrium along the z-direction i.e. $\sum F_x = 0$, then

$$p\pi R^2 - \sigma_L(2\pi Rt) = 0$$
$$\sigma_L = \frac{pR}{2t} \tag{8.7}$$

The longitudinal stress (σ_L) is half of the hoop stress (σ_H). For this reason, the weld is along the circumferential direction in the LPG cylinder; therefore, any increase in the longitudinal stress can be accommodated.

In fact, σ_H and σ_L turns out to be the principal stresses in the case of the thin-walled cylindrical pressure vessel subjected to internal pressure p. The normal stress (radial stress) in the third direction was assumed to be zero. Therefore, thin-walled pressure vessels are the typical applications of plane stress. The maximum in-plane shear stress is given by

$$\tau_{max}^{in-plane} = \frac{\sigma_H - \sigma_L}{2} = \left[\frac{pR}{2t} - \frac{pR}{4t}\right] = \frac{pR}{4t} \tag{8.8}$$

Any general planar element on the wall will experience normal and shear stress, except those aligned in the principal direction, as shown in Fig. 8.11.

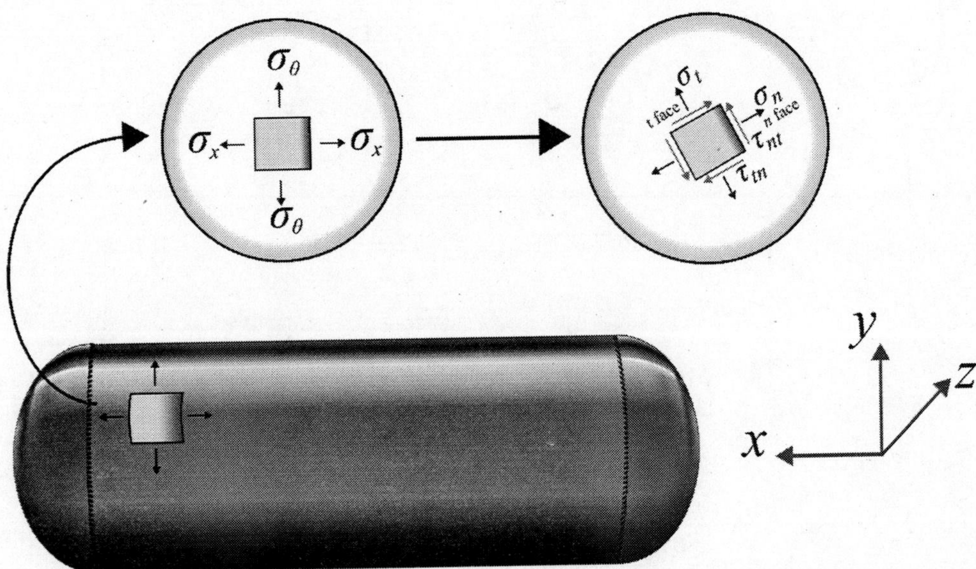

Fig. 8.11 Normal and shear stress on any general plane element on the wall

If Mohr's circle is drawn considering the hoop stress and the longitudinal stress, then the normal and shear stress components on the wall of the cylinder can be determined.

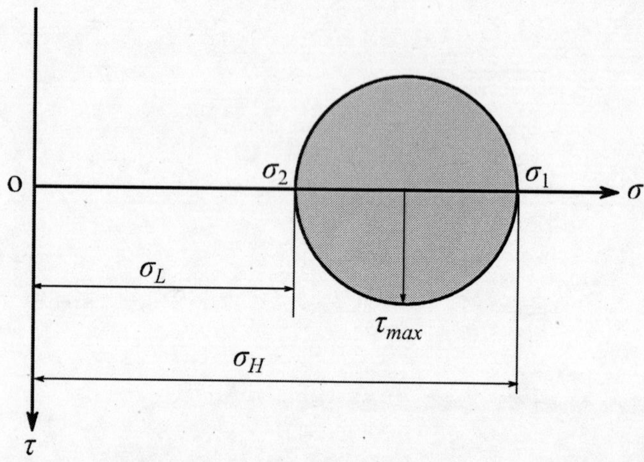

Fig. 8.12 Mohr's circle for determining the planar normal and shear stress stresses

Fig. 8.12 shows the Mohr's circle to determine the normal and shear stress components along a section that is oriented at an arbitrary angle to the circumferential direction (θ – direction).

Example 8.1: A thin cylinder of inner radius 500 mm and thickness 10 mm is subjected to an internal pressure of 5 MPa. What will be the hoop stress?

Solution: Given, $R = 500$ mm $= 0.5$ m, $t = 10$ mm $= 0.01$ m, $p = 5$ MPa

Using the Eq. (8.6), $\sigma_H = \frac{5\times0.5}{0.01} = 250$ MPa.

Example 8.2: A thin cylinder of inner radius 500 mm and thickness 10 mm is subjected to an internal pressure of 5 MPa. What is the maximum in-plane shear stress and the maximum shear stress?

Solution: From Example 8.1, the hoop stress $\sigma_H = 250$ MPa. The longitudinal stress σ_L can be obtained using the Eq. (8.7). It is given by

$$\sigma_L = \frac{pR}{2t} = \frac{5 \times 0.5}{2 \times 0.01} = 125 \text{ MPa}$$

Using the Eq. (8.8), the maximum in-plane stress can be obtained as

$$\tau_{max}^{in-plane} = \frac{pR}{4t} = \frac{5 \times 0.5}{4 \times 0.01} = 62.5 \text{ MPa}$$

It must be noted that the maximum shear stress (τ_{max}) will not be the same as the maximum in-plane stress. To find out the τ_{max}, the maximum principal stress (σ_1), which is the hoop stress – σ_H, and the minimum principal stress (σ_3), which is the zero radial stress components are considered.

$$\tau_{max} = \frac{\sigma_1 - \sigma_3}{2} = \frac{\sigma_H}{2} = \frac{pR}{2t} = 125 \text{ MPa}$$

Strains in the cylinder due to internal pressure

The circumferential and longitudinal (axial) strains can be calculated using

$$\begin{aligned} \epsilon_H &= \frac{1}{E}(\sigma_H - \nu\sigma_L) = \frac{pR(2-\nu)}{2Et} \\ \epsilon_L &= \frac{1}{E}(\sigma_L - \nu\sigma_H) = \frac{pR(1-2\nu)}{2Et} \end{aligned} \tag{8.9}$$

where ϵ_H and ϵ_L are circumferential and longitudinal strains, respectively. E and ν are the modulus of elasticity/Young's modulus and Poisson's ratio, respectively.

If ϵ_H or ϵ_L can be measured using strain gauges, then the internal pressure can be calculated by

$$p = \frac{2tE\epsilon_H}{R(2-\nu)} \tag{8.10}$$

$$p = \frac{2tE\epsilon_L}{R(1-2\nu)}$$

8.4 Thin-walled spherical pressure vessels

A similar method can be used to generate an expression for stresses experienced by the walls of a thin-walled spherical vessel under internal pressure, as shown in Fig. 8.13. A spherical pressure vessel is just a variant of a cylindrical pressure vessel. The sphere is cut into two hemispheres by $x-z$ plane. In fact, any cutting plane passing through the centre of the sphere yields two hemispheres.

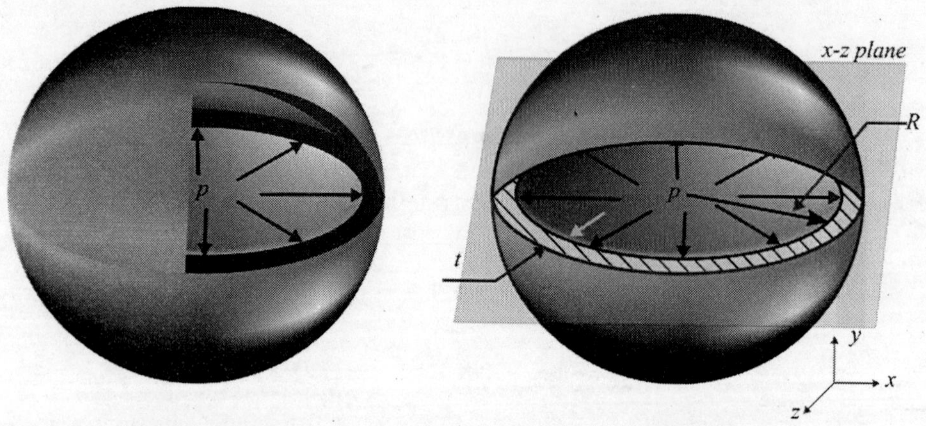

Fig. 8.13 (a) Internal pressure in the spherical pressure vessel, (b) Sphere cut by the $x-z$ plane

Since the sphere is in the static equilibrium under the action of external forces, here, due to the internal pressure p, the summation of the internal and external forces along the y-direction is zero. Therefore,

$$\sigma_t(2\pi Rt) = p\pi R^2 \tag{8.11}$$

$$\sigma = \sigma_t = \frac{pR}{2t}$$

where σ or σ_t is the tangential stress acting on the wall that resists the internal pressure (Fig. 8.14).

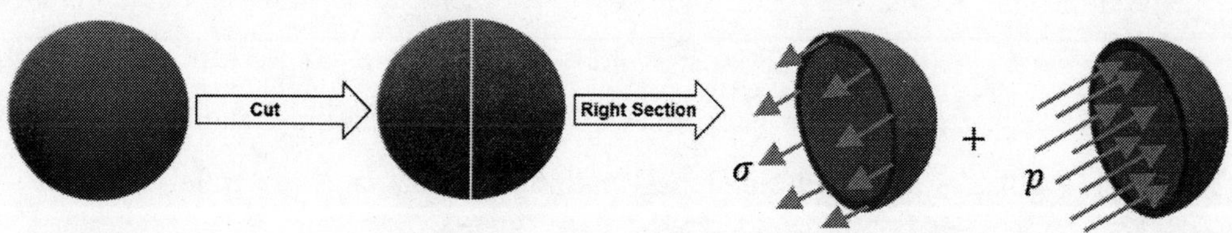

Fig. 8.14 Stress σ acting on the wall of the sphere

Unlike cylindrical pressure vessels, the magnitude of normal stress components acting on any planar wall element of the spherical vessel remains the same. Consequently, the shear stress on any section is zero, and Mohr's circle becomes a point located at a distance of $\frac{pr}{2t}$ from the origin of $\sigma - \tau$ plane (Ref: Fig. 8.15).

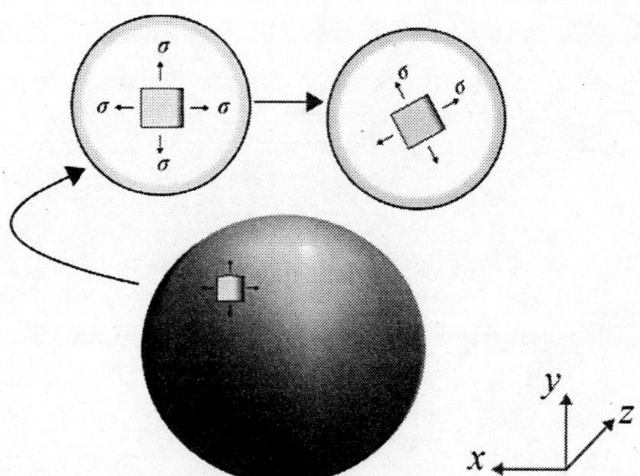

Fig. 8.15 Stress transformation in a thin-walled sphere

Strains in the sphere due to internal pressure

The thin-walled spherical pressure vessel expands when subjected to internal pressure. This results in the circumferential strain (or tangential strain) in two perpendicular in-plane directions ϵ_c and the radial strain ϵ_r. If we consider an internal circumferential fibre of radius r, within the wall, as shown in Fig. 8.16, the circumferential strain can be calculated by determining the ratio of the change in the circumferential length to the original length. For an infinitesimal arc length of $r\Delta\theta$, the circumferential strain can be written as

$$\epsilon_c = \frac{(r+u_r)\Delta\theta - r\Delta\theta}{r\Delta\theta} = \frac{u_r}{r} \tag{8.12}$$

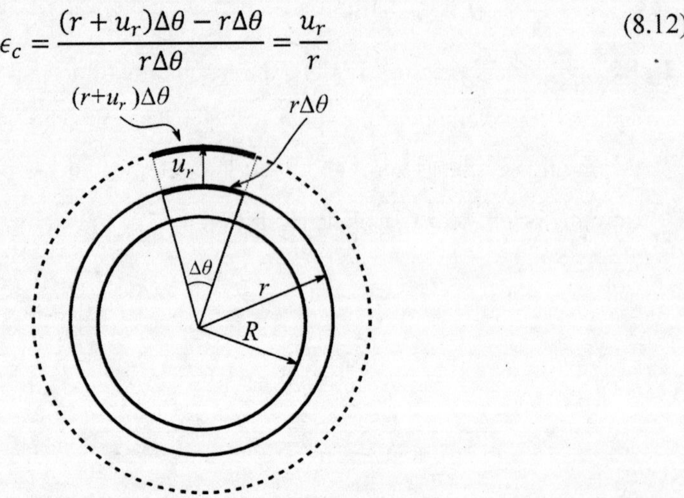

Fig. 8.16 Expansion of the sphere

The stress-strain relation using the Hooke's law can be written as

$$\begin{Bmatrix}\epsilon_c\\ \epsilon_c\\ \epsilon_r\end{Bmatrix} = \begin{bmatrix}\frac{1}{E} & -\frac{\nu}{E} & -\frac{\nu}{E}\\ -\frac{\nu}{E} & \frac{1}{E} & -\frac{\nu}{E}\\ -\frac{\nu}{E} & -\frac{\nu}{E} & \frac{1}{E}\end{bmatrix}\begin{Bmatrix}\sigma_t\\ \sigma_t\\ \sigma_r\end{Bmatrix} = \frac{pR}{2Et}\begin{Bmatrix}1-\nu\\ 1-\nu\\ -2\nu\end{Bmatrix} \tag{8.13}$$

Using Eqs. (8.12) and (8.13), we get

$$\epsilon_c = \frac{u_r}{r} = \frac{pr(1-\nu)}{2Et} \tag{8.14}$$

This is the circumferential strain for points located at a radial distance of r ($R < r < R + t$). Though this is applicable at the mid-radius, it can be taken as an approximate value at other internal locations.

Example 8.3: A thin spherical pressure of inner radius 200 mm is subjected to an internal pressure of 10 MPa. What will be the hoop stress? The wall thickness of the vessel is 15 mm.

Solution: Given $R = 200$ mm $= 0.2$ m, $p = 10$ MPa, and $t = 15$ mm $= 0.015$ m. For the spherical vessel, we know

$$\sigma_H = \sigma_L = \sigma = \frac{pR}{2t} = \frac{10 \times 0.2}{2 \times 0.015} = 66.67 \text{ MPa}$$

Example 8.4: A thin-walled spherical vessel of internal radius R is subjected to an internal pressure p. The wall-thickness of the vessel is t. What is the volumetric strain, i.e. the ratio of the change in the volume to the original volume due to p? Take E as the Young's modulus and ν as the Poissons's ratio?

Solution: Let V be the original volume and dV be the volume change, then

$$V = \frac{4}{3}\pi R^3$$

The change in the volume due to a change in the radii r would be

$$\mathrm{d}V = 4\pi r^2 \mathrm{d}R$$

Using Eq. (8.14) and dividing the above equation with V, and, we get

$$\frac{dV}{V} = 3\frac{dR}{R} = \frac{3pR(1-\nu)}{2Et}$$

8.5 Thick-walled cylindrical pressure vessels

Thick-wall cylinders find their applications in gun barrels, tubes, pressure vessels, etc. In many situations, the cylinder is subjected to a uniform internal pressure p_1 and a uniform external pressure p_2; the wall-thickness generally remains constant. Under such scenarios, the problem becomes axisymmetric, i.e., the deformations are independent of θ – the azimuthal angle: the angle from the x-axis in the $x-y$ plane, or quite simply, the deformations are symmetrical with respect to the longitudinal axis of the cylinder.

We are interested in determining the stresses in the walls. Also, the determination of the radial component of the displacement at any material point is equally important. If the cylinder is closed at the ends due to end-caps, under the action of external forces, it will undergo limited radial displacements at the ends, as the end-caps restrict the displacements. However, the locations far away from the end caps are not influenced. Therefore, the stresses, strains, and displacements expression that we will obtain as part of the thick-walled cylinder analysis are valid in the proximity of the end caps.

The usage of cylindrical coordinates will facilitate the easy determination of stresses and displacements. Using the standard vertical coordinate z, the cylindrical coordinate system extends polar coordinates into three-dimensional space. This yields coordinates (r, θ, z) that consists:

	Coordinate	Range	Remarks
1	r (radius)	$0 \leq r < \infty$	Distance from the $z-$axis
2	θ (azimuth)	$-\pi < \theta \leq \pi$	Angle from the $x-$axis in the $x-y$ plane
3	z (height)	$-\infty < z < \infty$	Length along the z - axis

The axis of revolution or the longitudinal axis is taken as z – axis. The displacement and stress field variables for a thick cylinder subjected to pressure are symmetrical about the z – axis. The governing partial differential equations of equilibrium are obtained considering an infinitesimal cylindrical element, as shown in Fig. 8.17.

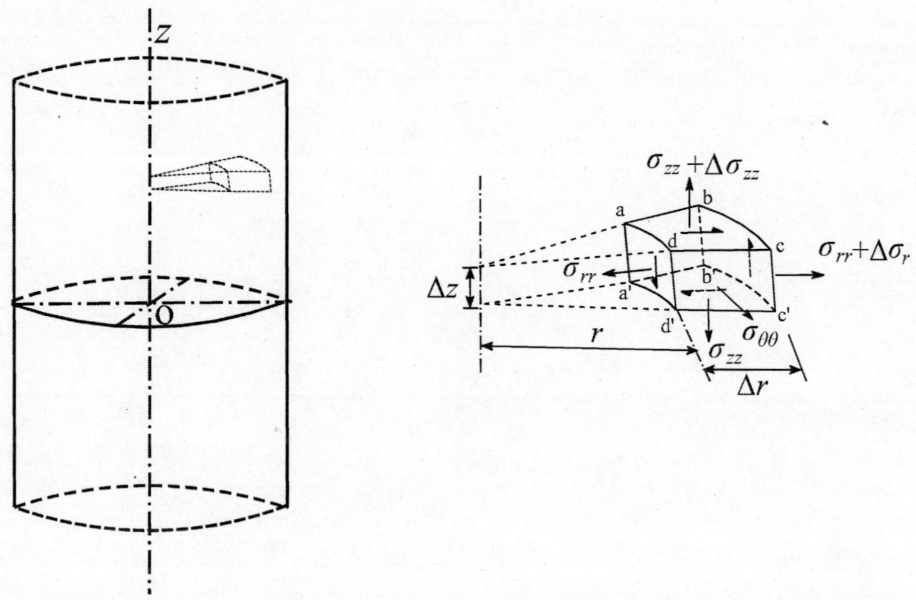

Fig. 8.17 Infinitesimal cylindrical element showing the normal stress components

On face aa'd'd,

Normal stress component: σ_{rr}

Tangential stress components: $\tau_{rz}\ and \tau_{r\theta}$

On face bb'c'c,

Normal stress: $(\sigma_{rr} + \frac{\partial \sigma_r r}{\partial r} \Delta r)$

Tangential stress components: $\tau_{rz} + \frac{\partial \tau_{rz}}{\partial r}\Delta r$ and $\tau_{r\theta} + \frac{\partial \tau_{r\theta}}{\partial r}\Delta r$

On face dcc'd',

Normal stress: $\sigma_{\theta\theta}$

Tangential stress components: $\tau_{r\theta}$ and $\tau_{\theta z}$

On face abb'a,

Normal stress: $\sigma_{\theta\theta} + \frac{\partial \sigma_{\theta\theta}}{\partial \theta}\Delta\theta$

Tangential stress components: $\tau_{r\theta} + \frac{\partial \tau_{r\theta}}{\partial \theta}\Delta\theta$ and $\tau_{\theta z} + \frac{\partial \tau_{\theta z}}{\partial \theta}\Delta\theta$

On face a'b'c'd'

Normal stress: σ_{zz}

Tangential stress: τ_{rz} and $\tau_{\theta z}$

On face abcd

Normal stress: $\sigma_{zz} + \frac{\partial \sigma_{zz}}{\partial z}\Delta z$

Tangential stress: $\tau_{rz} + \frac{\partial \tau_{rz}}{\partial z}\Delta z$ and $\tau_{\theta z} + \frac{\partial \tau_{\theta z}}{\partial z}\Delta z$

Area of face aa'd'd is $r\Delta\theta\Delta z$

Area of face bb'c'c is $(r + \Delta r)\Delta\theta\Delta z$

Area of faces abcd and a'b'c'd' is $(r + \Delta r/2)\Delta\theta\Delta r$

Area of faces dcc'd' and abb'e' is $\Delta r\Delta z$

Let ρ_r, ρ_θ and ρ_z be the body force components per unit volume.

Since the element is in equilibrium, the sum of all the forces acting along the three directions namely r, θ and z is zero. The force balance ($\sum F_r = 0$) along the r is given by

$$\begin{aligned}(\sigma_{rr} + \frac{\partial \sigma_{rr}}{\partial r}\Delta r)(r + \Delta r)\Delta\theta\Delta z - \sigma_{rr} r\Delta\theta\Delta z + (\tau_{rz} + \frac{\partial \tau_{rz}}{\partial z}\Delta z)(r \\ + \Delta r/2)\Delta\theta\Delta r - \tau_{rz}(r + \Delta r/2)\Delta\theta\Delta r \\ - \left(\sigma_{\theta\theta} + \frac{\partial \sigma_{\theta\theta}}{\partial \theta}\Delta\theta\right)\sin\left(\frac{\Delta\theta}{2}\right)\Delta r\Delta z - \sigma_{\theta\theta}\sin\left(\frac{\Delta\theta}{2}\right)\Delta r\Delta z \\ + \left(\tau_{r\theta} + \frac{\partial \tau_{r\theta}}{\partial \theta}\Delta\theta\right)\cos\left(\frac{\Delta\theta}{2}\right)\Delta r\Delta z - \tau_{r\theta}\cos\left(\frac{\Delta\theta}{2}\right)\Delta r\Delta z \\ + \rho_r\left(r + \frac{\Delta r}{2}\right)\Delta r\Delta\theta\Delta z = 0\end{aligned} \quad (8.15)$$

As $\Delta r, \Delta\theta$ and Δz tend to zero, this gives

$$r\frac{\partial \sigma_{rr}}{\partial r} + r\frac{\partial \tau_{rz}}{\partial z} + \frac{\partial \tau_{\theta}}{\partial \theta} + \sigma_{rr} - \sigma_{\theta\theta} + r\rho_r = 0$$

$$\boxed{\frac{\partial \sigma_{rr}}{\partial r} + \frac{\partial \tau_{rz}}{\partial z} + \frac{1}{r}\frac{\partial \tau_{r\theta}}{\partial \theta} + \frac{\sigma_{rr} - \sigma_{\theta\theta}}{r} + \rho_r = 0} \quad (8.16)$$

Likewise, along the tangential direction, $\sum F_\theta = 0$

$$\begin{aligned}\left(-\sigma_{\theta\theta}\cos\left(\frac{\Delta\theta}{2}\right) + \left(\sigma_{\theta\theta} + \frac{\partial \sigma_{\theta}}{\partial \theta}\Delta\theta\right)\cos\left(\frac{\Delta\theta}{2}\right)\right)\Delta r\Delta z + \tau_{r\theta}\Delta\theta\Delta z \\ + \left(\tau_{r\theta} + \frac{\partial \tau_{r\theta}}{\partial r}\Delta r\right)(r + \Delta r)\Delta\theta\Delta z - \tau_{\theta z}\left(r + \frac{\Delta r}{2}\right)\Delta\theta\Delta r \\ + \left(\tau_{\theta z} + \frac{\partial \tau_{\theta z}}{\partial z}\Delta z\right)\left(r + \frac{\Delta r}{2}\right)\Delta\theta\Delta r + \rho_\theta\left(r + \frac{\Delta r}{2}\right)\Delta r\Delta\theta\Delta z \\ = 0\end{aligned} \quad (8.17)$$

Simplification of Eq. (8.17) gives

$$\boxed{\frac{1}{r}\frac{\partial \sigma_{\theta\theta}}{\partial \theta} + \frac{\partial \tau_{r\theta}}{\partial r} + \frac{\partial \tau_{\theta z}}{\partial z} + \frac{2\tau_{r\theta}}{r} + \rho_\theta = 0} \quad (8.18)$$

Along the axial direction (z – axis), $\sum F_z = 0$. This gives

$$\left(\sigma_{zz} + \frac{\partial \sigma_z}{\partial z}\Delta z\right)\left(r + \frac{\Delta r}{2}\right)\Delta\theta\Delta r + \left(\tau_{rz} + \frac{\partial \tau_{rz}}{\partial r}\Delta r\right)(r + \Delta r)\Delta\theta\Delta z - \tau_{rz} r\Delta\theta\Delta z - \sigma_{zz}\left(r + \frac{\Delta r}{2}\right)\Delta\theta\Delta r + \rho_z\left(r + \frac{\Delta r}{2}\right)\Delta r\Delta\theta\Delta z = 0 \tag{8.19}$$

Simplification of Eq. (8.17) gives

$$\frac{\partial \sigma_{zz}}{\partial z} + \frac{\partial \tau_{rz}}{\partial r} + \frac{\tau_{rz}}{r} + \rho_z = 0 \tag{8.20}$$

Due to the axisymmetric nature of the problems, the solutions are independent of θ, and the equilibrium equation along the circumferential direction is automatically satisfied. The radial component of displacement remains uniform under the action of uniform pressure. This results in $\tau_{rz} = 0$, and accordingly, the equilibrium equation along the z – direction under zero body force component becomes

$$\frac{\partial \sigma_{zz}}{\partial z} = 0 \tag{8.21}$$

Equation. (8.21) can imply two conditions: (a) $\sigma_{zz} = 0$, or (b) σ_{zz} is constant along the axis of the cylinder. The former occurs in the case of an open cylinder (cylinder without end-caps)/plane stress condition. The latter condition applies when the cylinder is closed (with end-caps) or plane strain condition.

Therefore, to solve for the stresses: circumferential, radial, and longitudinal components and the radial displacements resulting due to internal p_1 and external pressure p_2, we consider the equilibrium equation along the radial direction, neglecting the body forces.

$$r\frac{\mathrm{d}\sigma_{rr}}{\mathrm{d}r} = \sigma_{\theta\theta} - \sigma_{rr} \tag{8.22}$$

In the Eq. (8.22), the partial derivative symbol ∂ is replaced with ordinal derivative symbol $'\mathrm{d}'$ because the field variables – stresses and displacements are only functions of r.

After the deformation, a particle at a radial location r would displace by the amount u_r in the radial direction. Likewise, another particle at a location $(r + \Delta r)$ will displace by $u_r + \frac{\mathrm{d}u_r}{\mathrm{d}r}\Delta r$. These particles, initially separated by length Δr, have undergone a change in length due to deformation by $\frac{\mathrm{d}u_r}{\mathrm{d}r}\Delta r$. Now, to determine the circumferential strain, let's consider the initial circumference as $2\pi r$. After the deformation, since the radius becomes $(r + u_r)$, the change in the circumference is $2\pi(r + u_r) - 2\pi r = 2\pi u_r$.

Accordingly, the strain–displacement relations for a thick-walled cylinder is

$$\begin{aligned} \varepsilon_{rr} &= \frac{\mathrm{d}u_r}{\mathrm{d}r} \\ \varepsilon_{\theta\theta} &= \frac{u_r}{r} \\ \varepsilon_{zz} &= \frac{\mathrm{d}u_z}{\mathrm{d}z} \end{aligned} \tag{8.23}$$

where u_r and u_z are radial and axial components of the displacement vector. If we combine the first two equations of the Eq. (8.23), we obtain the strain-compatibility equation as

$$\frac{\mathrm{d}}{\mathrm{d}r}(r\varepsilon_{\theta\theta}) = \varepsilon_{rr} \tag{8.24}$$

The constitutive relations considering the material to linear-elastic are

$$\begin{aligned} \varepsilon_{rr} &= \frac{1}{E}[\sigma_{rr} - v(\sigma_{\theta\theta} + \sigma_{zz})] \\ \varepsilon_{\theta\theta} &= \frac{1}{E}[\sigma_{\theta\theta} - v(\sigma_{rr} + \sigma_{zz})] \end{aligned} \tag{8.25}$$

If we substitute the expressions of Eq. (8.25) in Eq. (8.24), we get

$$\frac{\mathrm{d}}{\mathrm{d}r}(\sigma_{rr} + \sigma_{\theta\theta}) = 0, \text{ or} \tag{8.26}$$

$$\sigma_{rr} + \sigma_{\theta\theta} = C_1$$

where C_1 is the integration constant. The constative relation for ε_{zz} can be considered later depending on the nature of the problem: open-ended or closed-ended cylinder.

If we eliminate $\sigma_{\theta\theta}$ from the second expression of Eq. (8.26) and Eq. (8.22), we obtain

$$\frac{\mathrm{d}}{dr}(r^2\sigma_{rr}) = C_1 r \tag{8.27}$$

Integration of Eq. (8.27) gives

$$\sigma_{rr} = \frac{C_1}{2}\left(1 - \frac{a^2}{r^2}\right) + \frac{C_2}{r^2} \tag{8.28}$$

where C_2 is the second integration constant. The integration constants C_1 and C_2 can be found from the surface traction boundary conditions: (a) at $r = a, \sigma_{rr} = -p_1$ and (b) at $r = b, \sigma_{rr} = -p_2$.

$$C_1 = \frac{2}{b^2 - a^2}(p_1 a^2 - p_2 b^2) \tag{8.29}$$

$$C_2 = -p_1 a^2$$

Substituting expressions for C_1 and C_2 in Eq. (8.27), σ_{rr} can be expressed as

$$\sigma_{rr} = \frac{p_1 a^2 - p_2 b^2}{b^2 - a^2} - \frac{a^2 b^2}{r^2}\left(\frac{p_1 - p_2}{b^2 - a^2}\right) \tag{8.30}$$

Substituting the expression for σ_{rr} in the Eq. (8.26), we get the expression for $\sigma_{\theta\theta}$ as

$$\sigma_{\theta\theta} = \frac{p_1 a^2 - p_2 b^2}{b^2 - a^2} + \frac{a^2 b^2}{r^2}\left(\frac{p_1 - p_2}{b^2 - a^2}\right) \tag{8.31}$$

Equations (8.30) and (8.31) are Lame's equations. Though the stress components σ_{rr} and $\sigma_{\theta\theta}$ are functions of r, the sum of σ_{rr} and $\sigma_{\theta\theta}$ is a constant.

$$\sigma_{rr} + \sigma_{\theta\theta} = 2\left(\frac{p_1 a^2 - p_2 b^2}{b^2 - a^2}\right) \tag{8.32}$$

The variation of $\sigma_{\theta\theta}$ and σ_{rr} with radial distance r in a thick-walled cylinder subjected to internal pressure p_1 and external pressure p_2 is shown in Fig. 8.18a and Fig. 8.18b respectively.

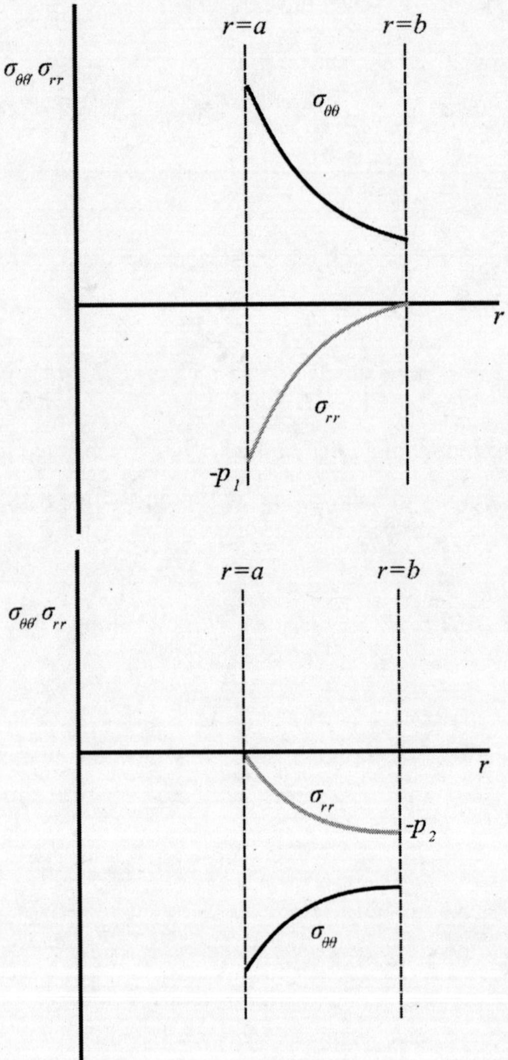

Fig. 8.18 $\sigma_{\theta\theta}$ and σ_{rr} variation with r in thick-walled cylinder subjected to (a) internal pressure p_1 only, (b) external pressure p_2 only

8.5.1 Open-ended cylinder/plane stress case

The ϵ_{zz} can be obtained from the constitutive relation that relates ϵ_{zz} with stress compoenents. It is given by

$$\varepsilon_{zz} = \frac{1}{E}[\sigma_{zz} - \nu(\sigma_{rr} + \sigma_{\theta\theta})] \tag{8.33}$$

In the case of an open-ended cylinder, the longitudinal stress $\sigma_{zz} = 0$. Therefore, ε_{zz} is

$$\varepsilon_{zz} = \frac{-2\nu}{E}\left(\frac{p_1 a^2 - p_2 b^2}{b^2 - a^2}\right) \tag{8.34}$$

The radial displacement u_r can be obtained by substituting the mathematical expression of σ_{rr}, $\sigma_{\theta\theta}$ and σ_{zz} into the first expression of Eq. (8.25), and making use of the first expression of Eq. (8.23).

$$u_r = \frac{1-\nu}{E}\left(\frac{p_1 a^2 - p_2 b^2}{b^2 - a^2}\right) r + \frac{1+\nu}{E}\left(\frac{p_1 - p_2}{b^2 - a^2}\right)\frac{a^2 b^2}{r} \tag{8.35}$$

8.5.2 Closed-ended cylinder

Since the cylinder is closed at either end with end-caps, because of internal pressure p_1 and external pressure p_2, the force equilibrium along the longitudinal direction gives

$$\begin{gathered}\int_a^b \sigma_{zz} 2\pi r\, dr = \pi(p_1 a^2 - p_2 b^2) \\ \sigma_{zz} = \frac{p_1 a^2 - p_2 b^2}{b^2 - a^2}\end{gathered} \tag{8.36}$$

Using Eq. (8.33), the ε_{zz} can be written as

$$\varepsilon_{zz} = \frac{1-2\nu}{E}\left(\frac{p_1 a^2 - p_2 b^2}{b^2 - a^2}\right) \tag{8.37}$$

Again, the radial displacement u_r can be obtained by substituting the mathematical expression of σ_{rr}, $\sigma_{\theta\theta}$ and σ_{zz} into the first expression of Eq. (8.25), and making use of the first expression of Eq. (8.23).

$$u_r = \frac{1-2v}{E}\left(\frac{p_1a^2 - p_2b^2}{b^2 - a^2}\right)r + \frac{1+v}{E}\left(\frac{p_1 - p_2}{b^2 - a^2}\right)\frac{a^2b^2}{r} \tag{8.38}$$

8.5.3 Plane strain case

In the case of plane strain case, which is applicable when the cylinder is long, $\varepsilon_{zz} = 0$, therefore, making use of Eq. (8.33) σ_{zz} is

$$\sigma_{zz} = v(\sigma_{rr} + \sigma_{\theta\theta}) = 2v\left(\frac{p_1a^2 - p_2b^2}{b^2 - a^2}\right) \tag{8.39}$$

By employing the same procedure for finding the radial displacements in the previous two scenarios for open-ended cylinder/plane-stress and closed-end cylinder, we obtain

$$u_r = \frac{(1+v)}{E}\left[(1-2v)\left(\frac{p_1a^2 - p_2b^2}{b^2 - a^2}\right)r + \left(\frac{p_1 - p_2}{b^2 - a^2}\right)\frac{a^2b^2}{r}\right] \tag{8.40}$$

Example 8.5: A thick-walled cylinder has an inside diameter of 50 mm and an outside diameter of 100 mm. If the cylinder is subjected to an internal pressure of 300 MPa, find the stress components σ_{rr} and $\sigma_{\theta\theta}$ at $r = 25$ mm i.e. at $r = a$, $r = 40$ mm and $r = 50$ mm i.e. at $r = b$. Take $E = 300$ GPa and $v = 0.29$.

Solution: The internal pressure $p_1 = 300$ MPa, and the external pressure $p_2 = 0$. Eqs. (8.30) and (8.31) gives

$$\sigma_{rr} = \frac{p_1a^2}{b^2 - a^2} - \frac{a^2b^2}{r^2} = \frac{p_1a^2}{r^2}\left(\frac{r^2 - b^2}{b^2 - a^2}\right)$$

$$\sigma_{\theta\theta} = \frac{p_1 a^2}{b^2 - a^2} + \frac{a^2 b^2}{r^2}\left(\frac{p_1}{b^2 - a^2}\right) = \frac{p_1 a^2}{r^2}\left(\frac{r^2 + b^2}{b^2 - a^2}\right)$$

This gives, (i) at $r = 25$ mm, $\sigma_{rr} = -300$ MPa and $\sigma_{\theta\theta} = 500$ MPa

(ii) at $r = 40$ mm, $\sigma_{rr} = -56.25$ MPa and $\sigma_{\theta\theta} = 256.25$ MPa

(ii) at $r = 50$ mm, $\sigma_{rr} = 0$ MPa and $\sigma_{\theta\theta} = 200$ MPa

Example 8.6: A thick-walled closed cylinder has an inside diameter of 400 mm and an outside diameter of 800 mm. The cylinder is subjected to an internal pressure of 150 MPa. Find the maximum shear stress and the radial displacement at $r = a = 400$ mm. Take $E = 69.9$ GPa and $\nu = 0.33$.

Solution: The maximum shear stress can be obtained if we know the principal stresses. $\sigma_{\theta\theta}, \sigma_{rr}$ and σ_{zz} are the principal stresses. For $p_2 = 0$ and $r = a$, we have

$$\sigma_{rr} = \frac{p_1 a^2}{b^2 - a^2} - \frac{a^2 b^2}{r^2} = p_1\left(\frac{a^2 - b^2}{b^2 - a^2}\right) = -p_1 = -150 \text{ MPa}$$

$$\sigma_{\theta\theta} = \frac{p_1 a^2}{b^2 - a^2} + \frac{a^2 b^2}{r^2}\left(\frac{p_1}{b^2 - a^2}\right) = p_1\left(\frac{a^2 + b^2}{b^2 - a^2}\right) = 150\frac{(200^2 + 400^2)}{(400^2 - 200^2)} = 250 \text{ MPa}$$

From the second expression for Eq. (8.36), we can write

$$\sigma_{zz} = \frac{p_1 a^2 - p_2 b^2}{b^2 - a^2} = \frac{p_1 a^2}{b^2 - a^2} = 150\frac{200^2}{400 - 200^2} = 50 \text{ MPa}$$

The maximum shear stress is given by

$$\tau_{max} = \frac{\sigma_{max} - \sigma_{min}}{2} = \frac{250 - (-150)}{2} = 200 \text{ MPa}$$

The radial displacement for a closed-end thick cylinder can be found using Eq. (8.38). At $r = a$, it is given by

$$u_{r=a} = \frac{1-2v}{E}\left(\frac{p_1 a^2}{b^2-a^2}\right)a + \frac{1+v}{E}\left(\frac{p_1}{b^2-a^2}\right)\frac{a^2 b^2}{a}$$

$$= \left[\frac{(1-0.66)(150)(200^3)}{69900(400^2-200^2)} + \frac{(1+0.33)(150\times 200)(400^2)}{69900(400^2-200^2)}\right]$$

$$= 0.8097 \text{ mm}$$

8.6 Thick-walled spherical vessels

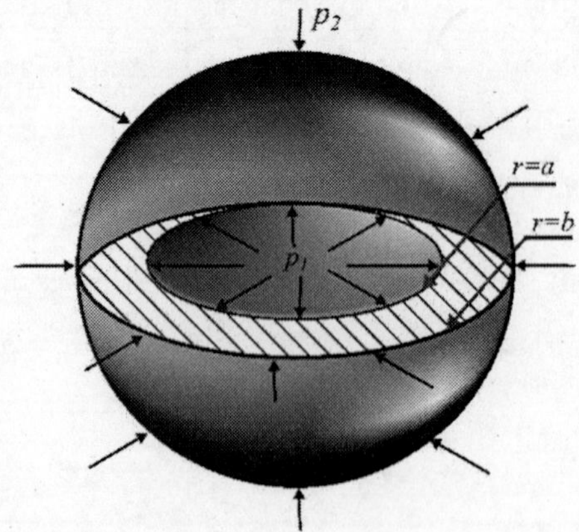

Fig. 8.19 Thick-walled spherical vessel

In the last section of this unit, the thick-walled spherical vessel is analysed to determine the stresses and displacements when subjected to internal pressure p_1 and external pressure p_2 (Ref: Fig. 8.19). In this regard, the usage of the spherical coordinate system is convenient.

Spherical coordinates, also known as spherical polar coordinates, are a system of curvilinear coordinates that describe points on a sphere or spheroid naturally. θ is defined as the azimuthal angle in the xy - plane from the x-axis and its values in the range of $-\pi < \theta \leq \pi$. ϕ is defined as the polar angle measured from the positive z – axis with $0 < \phi \leq \pi$, and r is the distance (radius) from a point to the origin.

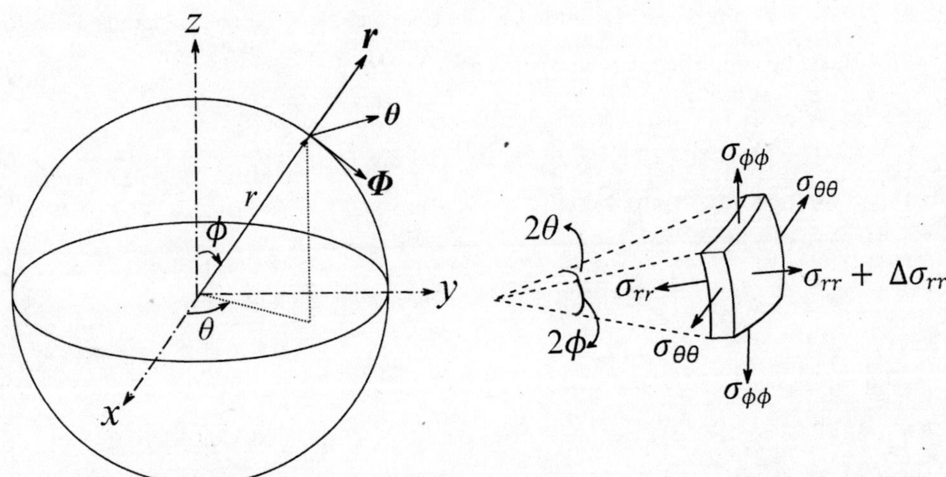

Fig. 8.20 Infinitesimal spherical element showing the normal stress components

Fig. 8.20 shows the normal stress components on an infinitesimal element. Due to the spherical symmetry, the circumferential stress $\sigma_{\theta\theta} = \sigma_{\phi\phi}$. The governing differential equilibrium equations along the circumferential directions are not relevant here. Considering the force balance along the radial direction ($\sum F_r = 0$), we get

$$\begin{aligned}&(\sigma_{rr} + \Delta\sigma_{rr})(r + \Delta r)2\varphi(r + \Delta r)2\theta - \sigma_{rr}(2\varphi r)(2\theta r)\\ &\quad - 2\left(r + \frac{\Delta r}{2}\right)2\varphi\Delta r\sigma_{\varphi\varphi}\sin\varphi - 2\left(r + \frac{\Delta r}{2}\right)2\theta\Delta r\sigma_{\phi\phi}\sin\theta\\ &\quad + \rho_r 4\theta^2 r^2\Delta r = 0\end{aligned} \tag{8.41}$$

Neglecting the radial body force component ρ_r and $\sigma_{\theta\theta} = \sigma_{\phi\phi}$ and $\Delta\sigma_r = \frac{d\sigma_r}{dr}\Delta r$ in the Eq. (8.41), we obtain

$$r^2\frac{\Delta\sigma_{rr}}{\Delta r}(4\varphi\theta) + 2r\sigma_r(4\varphi\theta) - 4r(\varphi^2\sigma_{\varphi\varphi} + \theta^2\sigma_{\theta\theta}) = 0 \tag{8.42}$$

Since σ_r depends on only the radial coordinate r, $\Delta\sigma_r = \frac{d\sigma_r}{dr}\Delta r$, and making use of the spherical symmetry, $\sigma_{\theta\theta} = \sigma_{\phi\phi}$. The spherical symmetry also implies that the variation of field variables along the azimuthal and polar angles will be the same. Therefore, Eq. (8.42) can be simplified can be written as

$$\frac{\mathrm{d}\sigma_{rr}}{\mathrm{dr}} r^2 + 2r\sigma_r - 2r\sigma_{\theta\theta} = 0 \tag{8.43}$$

Eq. (8.43) can be further simplified to

$$\frac{1}{r^2}\frac{\mathrm{d}(r^2\sigma_{rr})}{\mathrm{d}r} = \frac{2}{r}\sigma_{\theta\theta} \tag{8.44}$$

The strain-displacement relation of the cylindrical coordinates can be extended to the sphere. In this case, the circumferential strain is calculated considering the initial circumference of any great circle passing through the point of interest (located at radial distance r) in the sphere. The initial circumference of the great circle is $2\pi r$. After the deformation, the circumference becomes $2\pi(r + u_r)$. Therefore, the circumferential strain would remain the same as that of the thick-walled cylinder. The strain components in the case of the sphere will be

$$\begin{aligned} \epsilon_{rr} &= \frac{\mathrm{d}u_r}{\mathrm{d}r} \\ \epsilon_{\theta\theta} = \epsilon_{\phi\phi} &= \frac{u_r}{r} \end{aligned} \tag{8.45}$$

The constitutive relations are

$$\begin{aligned} \varepsilon_{rr} &= \frac{1}{E}\left[\sigma_{rr} - v\left(\sigma_{\theta\theta} + \sigma_{\phi\phi}\right)\right] \\ \varepsilon_{\theta\theta} &= \frac{1}{E}\left[\sigma_{\theta\theta} - v\left(\sigma_{rr} + \sigma_{\phi\phi}\right)\right] \end{aligned} \tag{8.46}$$

The first expression of Eqs. (8.45) and (8.46) is combined to eliminate $\sigma_{\theta\theta}$ from Eq. (8.44), which can be written as

$$(1-\nu)\frac{\mathrm{d}^2(r^2\sigma_{rr})}{\mathrm{d}r^2}+\frac{2\nu}{r}\frac{\mathrm{d}(r^2\sigma_{rr})}{\mathrm{d}r}-2\nu\frac{\mathrm{d}(r\sigma_{rr})}{\mathrm{d}r}-2\sigma_{rr}=0 \tag{8.47}$$

Substituting the relation $\frac{\mathrm{d}(r\sigma_{rr})}{\mathrm{d}r}=\frac{1}{r}\frac{\mathrm{d}(r^2\sigma_{rr})}{\mathrm{d}r}-\frac{r^2\sigma_{rr}}{r^2}$ in Eq. (8.47), we get

$$\frac{\mathrm{d}^2(r^2\sigma_{rr})}{\mathrm{d}r^2}-2\frac{r^2\sigma_{rr}}{r^2}=0 \tag{8.48}$$

Eq. (8.48) is a linear homogenous ordinary differential equation with a solution

$$\sigma_{rr}=C_1+\frac{C_2}{r^3} \tag{8.49}$$

From the Eq. (8.44), we can write

$$\sigma_{\theta\theta}=\frac{1}{2r}\frac{\mathrm{d}}{\mathrm{d}r}\left(C_1r^2+\frac{C_2}{r}\right)=C_1-\frac{C_2}{2r^3} \tag{8.50}$$

The constants C_1 and C_2 can be found from the boundary conditions of the thick-walled sphere subjected to internal pressure p_1 and external pressure p_2 i.e., $r=a, \sigma_{rr}=-p_1$ and $r=b, \sigma_{rr}=-p_2$.

$$\begin{aligned}-p_1&=C_1+\frac{C_2}{a^3}\\-p_2&=C_1+\frac{C_2}{b^3}\end{aligned} \tag{8.51}$$

The radial and circumferential stresses can be finally expressed as

$$\begin{aligned}\sigma_{rr}&=\frac{p_1a^3-p_2b^3}{b^3-a^3}+\frac{a^3b^3}{r^3}\left(\frac{p_2-p_1}{b^3-a^3}\right)\\\sigma_{\phi\phi}=\sigma_{\theta\theta}&=\frac{p_1a^3-p_2b^3}{b^3-a^3}-\frac{a^3b^3}{2r^3}\left(\frac{p_2-p_1}{b^3-a^3}\right)\end{aligned} \tag{8.52}$$

Making use of $\epsilon_{\theta\theta}=\frac{u_r}{r}$, the radial displacement u_r can be obtained by substituting Eq. (8.52) in the second expression of the Eq. (8.46) as

$$u_r = \frac{1-\nu}{E}\left(\frac{p_1 a^3 - p_2 b^3}{b^3 - a^3}\right) r - \frac{1+\nu}{E}\left(\frac{a^3 b^3}{2r^2}\right)\left(\frac{p_2 - p_1}{b^3 - a^3}\right) \tag{8.53}$$

Example 8.7: A thick-walled sphere of internal radius 5 cm is subjected to an internal pressure p. The allowable stress is 800 MPa. If the thickness of the sphere is 2 cm, determine the maximum value of p.

Solution: The maximum tensile stress corresponds to the circumferential stress at $r = a$, when subjected to internal pressure, as one can observe from the Eq. (8.52). Therefore, given $a = 5$ cm and $b = 7$ cm, at $r = a$

$$\sigma_{\theta\theta} = \frac{p_1 a^3}{b^3 - a^3} - \frac{a^3 b^3}{2a^3}\left(\frac{-p_1}{b^3 - a^3}\right) = \frac{p_1}{2}\left(\frac{2a^3 + b^3}{b^3 - a^3}\right) = 1.36p_1$$

The maximum value of $\sigma_{\theta\theta}$ is 800 MPa.

$$1.36p_1 = 800 \text{ MPa}$$

So, the maximum internal pressure would be 588.19 MPa.

Know More

Exercises

Multiple Choice Questions

8. 1. A thin pipe of 750 mm diameter is used to carry water under a pressure head of 30 m. What is the wall thickness of the pipe if the allowable normal stress is 20 MPa?

(a) 11.036 mm
(b) 5.518 mm
(c) 12.025 mm
(d) 14.5 mm

8.2. The ratio of the hoop stress to the longitudinal stress in thin-walled cylinders is
(a) 1
(b) ½
(c) 2
(d) ¼

8.3. What is the ratio of maximum stress created in a thin cylindrical and thin spherical pressure vessel if both the vessels have the same internal diameter, wall thickness, and material, and are subjected to the same internal pressure?
(a) 1
(b) ½
(c) ¼
(d) 2

8.4. The ratio of volumetric strain to diametrical strain in a thin spherical shell subjected to internal pressure is
(a) 3:1
(b) 1:1
(c) 4:1
(d) 1:3

8.5. For a thin cylinder of $\nu = 0.3$, the ratio of circumferential strain to longitudinal strain is

(a) 4.25
(b) 2.25
(c) 2.5
(d) 5

8.6. The sum of radial stress and circumferential stress components in the case of a thick cylinder subjected to internal pressure is

(a) independent of the pressure
(b) depends on the radius
(c) constant
(d) depends on the material

8.7. For a thick cylinder subjected to internal pressure, the hoop stress is maximum at

(a) the outer radius
(b) the inner radius
(c) the centre of the wall
(d) both at the inner and outer radii

8.8. Which of the following is correct for a thick cylinder (closed at the ends) subjected to internal pressure?

(a) Both the hoop stress and radial stress are tensile
(b) Both the hoop stress and radial stress are compressive
(c) The longitudinal stress is compressive
(d) Both the hoop stress and longitudinal stress are tensile

8.9. A thick cylinder subjected to internal pressure p has an internal diameter of d and an external diameter of $3d$? The maximum hoop stress is

(a) $2p$
(b) $\frac{5}{4}p$
(c) $\frac{5}{3}p$
(d) $2.5p$

8.10. A thick hollow sphere of a relatively large outer radius compared to an inner radius is subjected to internal pressure p. The circumferential stress will be approximately

(a) p
(b) $p/2$
(c) $2p$
(d) $3p$

Answer for Multiple Choice Questions

8.1 (b), 8.2 (c), 8.3 (d), 8.4 (a), 8.5 (a), 8.6 (c), 8.7 (b), 8.8 (d), 8.9 (b), 8.10 (b).

Numerical Problems

8.1. A thin gas cylinder is subjected to an internal pressure of 10 MPa. If the highest allowable working stress is set to 100 MPa, what is the minimum wall thickness of a cylinder? The internal radius is 100 mm. (**Ans.** t = 10 mm)

8.2. A cylindrical tank with closed ends is pressurized with 500 kPa of compressed air. The tank's inner radius is 2 metres, and its wall thickness is 10 millimetres. What is the maximum in-plane shear stress? (**Ans.** τ_{max} = 25 MPa)

8.3. A spherical shell (thin wall) is subjected to an internal pressure of constant magnitude. If the shell's radius increases by 1% and the wall thickness decreases by 1%, what will be the percentage change in hoop stress? (**Ans.** ≈ 2%)

8.4. The internal pressure of a thin spherical pressure vessel is 15 MPa, and the ratio of wall thickness to radius is 0.1. What is the value of the longitudinal and hoop stresses? (**Ans.** σ = 75 MPa)

8.5 A pressure tank is fabricated by wrapping the plates spirally. They are welded at the seams, as shown in Fig. P1, where β = 60°. The tank is subjected to a gauge pressure of 1 MPa, and has an inner diameter of 500 mm and wall thickness of 8 mm. Find the (a) normal stress perpendicular to the weld, and (b) the shear stress parallel to the weld. (**Ans.** 85.94 MPa, 13.53 MPa)

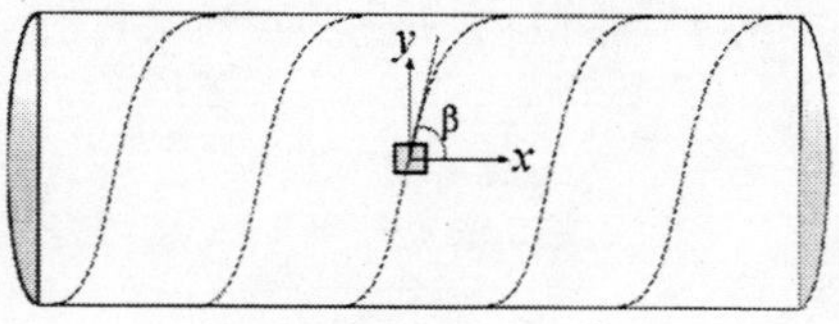

Fig. P8.1

8.6. For the problem given in 5, determine the maximum gage pressure in the tank if the allowable normal stress perpendicular to the weld and the allowable shear stress parallel to the weld is 100 MPa and 25 MPa, respectively. **(Ans.** 1.16 MPa)

8.7. Show that the volumetric strain in the case of a thin-walled cylinder of radius R and wall-thickness t, subjected to gage pressure p is $\frac{pR}{2Et}(5-4\nu)$. Take E as the Young's modulus and ν as the Poisson's ratio.

8.8. A thick-walled cylinder has an inside diameter of 50 mm. The outer diameter is twice the inner diameter. If the cylinder is subjected to an internal pressure of 300 MPa and an external pressure of 50 MPa, find the stress components σ_{rr} and $\sigma_{\theta\theta}$ at $r = 25$ mm i.e. at $r = a$, $r = 40$ mm and $r = 50$ mm i.e. at $r = b$. Take $E = 300$ GPa and $\nu = 0.29$. (**Ans.** 1. $\sigma_{rr@r=25} = -300$ MPa, $\sigma_{\theta\theta@r=25} = 366.67$ MPa, 2. $\sigma_{rr@r=40} = -96.875$ MPa, $\sigma_{\theta\theta@r=40} = 163.54$ MPa and 3. 1. $\sigma_{rr@r=50} = -50$ MPa, $\sigma_{\theta\theta@r=50} = 116.67$ MPa)

8.9. A thick-walled closed cylinder has an inside diameter of 400 mm. The outer diameter is twice the inner diameter. The cylinder is subjected to an internal pressure of 150 MPa and external pressure of 50 MPa. Find the principal stresses, maximum shear stress, and the radial displacement at $r = a = 400$ mm. Take $E = 69.9$ GPa and $\nu = 0.33$. (**Ans.** $\sigma_1 = \sigma_{\theta\theta} = 116.67$ MPa, $\sigma_2 = \sigma_{zz} = -16.67$ MPa, $\sigma_3 = \sigma_{rr} = -150$ MPa, $\tau_{max} = 133.33$ MPa and $u_r = 0.491$ mm)

8.10. A large elastic medium with a spherical cavity is subjected to an internal pressure p_1. Show that $\sigma_{rr} = -p_1\left(\frac{a}{r}\right)^3$ and $\sigma_{\theta\theta} = \frac{p_2}{2}\left(\frac{a}{r}\right)^3$.

REFERENCES FOR FURTHER LEARNING

1. E. P. Popov, Engineering Mechanics of Solids, 2nd edition, Pearson Education India, 2015.
2. F. P. Beer, E. R. Johnston (Jr.), J.T. DeWolf, D.F. Mazurek and S. Sanghi, Mechanics of Materials, 7th edition, McGraw Hill Education (India) Private Limited, 2017.
3. S. Timoshenko, Strength of Materials, Vol. 1: Elementary Theory and Problems, CBS; 3rd Edition, 2004.
4. S. Timoshenko and D.H. Young, "Elements of Strength of Materials", 5th edition, East West, 2003.
5. J. M. Gere, B. J. Goodno, Mechanics of Materials, SI Edition, 8th edition,Nelson .Engineering; International edition, 2012
6. J.M. Gere and S. Timoshenko, Mechanics of Materials (5th Ed.) Brooks/Cole, 2001.
7. A. Mubeen, Mechanics of Solids, 2nd edition, Pearson India, 2011
8. Parnes, R., Solid Mechnaics in Engineering, John Wiley & Sons, Baffins Lane, Chichester, England, 2001.
9. S. H. Crandall, N. C. Dahl, and T. J. Lardner, An Introduction to The Mechanics Of Solids, 2nd Ed., Tata McGraw Hill, 2008.
10. H. Shames and J. M. Pitarresi, Introduction to Solid Mechanics, Prentice Hall of India, 2003.
11. R.C. Hibbeler, Mechanics of Materials (10th Edition), Pearson, 2016.
12. L.S. Srinath, Advanced Mechanics of Solids, 3rd edition, McGraw Hill Education, 2017: added as suggested by Dr. Nelson.

CO AND PO ATTAINMENT TABLE

Course outcomes (COs) for this course can be mapped with the programme outcomes (POs) after the completion of the course and a correlation can be made for the attainment of POs to analyze the gap. After proper analysis of the gap in the attainment of POs necessary measures can be taken to overcome the gaps.

Table for CO and PO attainment

Course Outcomes	**Expected Mapping with Programme Outcomes: CE** *(1- Weak Correlation; 2- Medium correlation; 3- Strong Correlation)*											
	PO-1	PO-2	PO-3	PO-4	PO-5	PO-6	PO-7	PO-8	PO-9	PO-10	PO-11	PO-12
CO-1												
CO-2												
CO-3												
CO-4												

Course Outcomes	**Expected Mapping with Programme Outcomes: ME** *(1- Weak Correlation; 2- Medium correlation; 3- Strong Correlation)*											
	PO-1	PO-2	PO-3	PO-4	PO-5	PO-6	PO-7	PO-8	PO-9	PO-10	PO-11	PO-12
CO-1												
CO-2												

The data filled in the above table can be used for gap analysis.

INDEX